Diagnosis and Treatment of Bacterial Infections

(Part 1)

Edited by

Mukesh Kumar Singh
School of Pharmaceutical Sciences
Faculty of Pharmacy, IFTM University
Moradabad, Uttar Pradesh
India

Gurdeep Singh
School of Pharmaceutical Sciences
Lovely Professional University
Phagwara, Punjab
India

Amrendra Pratap Yadav
Department of Pharmacy
Meerut Institute of Technology
Meerut, Uttar Pradesh
India

&

Papiya Bigoniya
Cancer Biology Project
University of Westminster
London, UK

Diagnosis and Treatment of Bacterial Infections - *(Part 1)*

Editors: Mukesh Kumar Singh, Gurdeep Singh, Amrendra Pratap Yadav & Papiya Bigoniya

ISBN (Online): 979-8-89881-345-1

ISBN (Print): 979-8-89881-346-8

ISBN (Paperback): 979-8-89881-347-5

Published by Bentham Science Publishers Pte. Ltd. Singapore, in collaboration with Eureka Conferences, USA.

First published in 2026.

need for a court order if at any point you breach any terms of this License Agreement. In no event will any delay or failure by Bentham Science Publishers in enforcing your compliance with this License Agreement constitute a waiver of any of its rights.

3. You acknowledge that you have read this License Agreement, and agree to be bound by its terms and conditions. To the extent that any other terms and conditions presented on any website of Bentham Science Publishers conflict with, or are inconsistent with, the terms and conditions set out in this License Agreement, you acknowledge that the terms and conditions set out in this License Agreement shall prevail.

Bentham Science Publishers Pte. Ltd.
No. 9 Raffles Place
Office No. 26-01
Singapore 048619
Singapore
Email: subscriptions@benthamscience.net

BENTHAM SCIENCE

CONTENTS

FOREWORD

It is my distinct honour to have the opportunity to contribute the foreword for Diagnosis and Treatment of Bacterial Infections, Part I. This comprehensive text will examine bacterial infections from historical, epidemiological, and therapeutic perspectives. The authors discuss conventional and challenging ways to manage bacterial infections and explore cutting-edge ways that clinicians can manage antibiotic-resistant bacteria using targeted treatments for biofilm-associated resistant pathogens and novel drug delivery methods. The section on coinfections and opportunistic pathogens discusses how difficult it can be for clinicians to manage complex clinical cases and how precise and accurate diagnosis and treatment of patients is critical.

This Part will be an essential resource for researchers, medical professionals, and students, providing an overview of bacterial infections and current strategies for reducing the impact of antimicrobial resistance through advanced diagnostic and therapeutic options. I congratulate the authors for their impressive effort and wish them all the best in achieving their goal of improving understanding and managing bacterial infections.

Ranjit Singh
Shobhit University
Gangoh, Uttar Pradesh, India

PREFACE

Bacterial infections are a global health issue. Despite many advances in the fields of science, medicine, diagnostic methods, and treatment with anti-microbials, bacterial infections remain a significant contributor to morbidity and mortality around the world. The emergence of large numbers of resistant strains of bacteria, persistent problems due to biofilm infections, and increasing awareness of co-infections and opportunistic pathogens have created an urgent demand for current, linked, evidence-based information. The first part of Bacterial Infections: Diagnosis and Treatment has been compiled to provide timely and relevant information about bacterial infections, from basic principles to new therapies.

The introduction of this part provides a historical perspective of bacterial infections, presenting the major events that have contributed to the current understanding and clinical management of bacterial infections. Following the introduction, the part presents an extensive description of the epidemiology and pathophysiology of bacterial infections. A major focus of this section will be to discuss the global impact of bacterial infections, how bacteria are transmitted between people, the interactions that occur between bacteria and their human host, and how bacteria are able to produce disease. The last section of this part reviews the existing antibacterial medications and treatment protocols; this review provides a robust clinical basis to support the subsequent sections of the work.

The concluding chapters are intended to bring together a variety of innovative drug delivery systems, as well as new, sophisticated antimicrobial therapeutic platforms that are intended to increase the effectiveness of antimicrobial medications while simultaneously decreasing the likelihood of developing antimicrobial resistance. It has been constructed in such a way that the initial foundation laid will be further complemented by recent advances in science and technology, thus providing the most comprehensive source available for infection disease clinicians, researchers, academics, pharmaceutical scientists, and graduate students involved in infectious disease research and clinical practice.

Part II of the series provides information that supports both the information in Part I and some of the advances in integrative, genetic, immunological, and digital technologies that could support the treatment of bacterial infections in the future, as well as addresses some of the issues of increasing bacterial resistance to current antibiotic therapies.

Mukesh Kumar Singh
School of Pharmaceutical Sciences
Faculty of Pharmacy, IFTM University
Moradabad, Uttar Pradesh
India

Gurdeep Singh
School of Pharmaceutical Sciences
Lovely Professional University
Phagwara, Punjab
India

Amrendra Pratap Yadav
Department of Pharmacy
Meerut Institute of Technology
Meerut, Uttar Pradesh
India

&

Papiya Bigoniya
Cancer Biology Project
University of Westminster
London, UK

List of Contributors

Anshita Gupta	Department of Pharmacy, Gurughasi Das Vishwavidyalaya, Bilaspur (C.G.), India
Alankar Shrivastav	Faculty of Pharmacy, IFTM University, Moradabad, 244001, U.P., India
Arun Kumar	Department of Pharmacology, Global Institute of Pharmaceutical Education and Research, Kashipur, 244713, Uttarakhand, India
Arun K. Mishra	SOS School of Pharmacy, IFTM University, Moradabad, 244102, India
Ajay Kumar Yadav	School of Pharmaceutical Sciences, CSJM University, Kanpur, 208024, India
Archana Bagre	Department of Pharmaceutics, Lakshmi Narain College of Pharmacy, Bhopal, Madhya Pradesh, India
Amrendra Pratap Yadav	Department of Pharmacy, Meerut Institute of Technology, Meerut, Uttar Pradesh, India
Astha Verma	Department of Pharmaceutics, Shri Rawatpura Sarkar Institute of Pharmacy, Chhattisgarh, 490024, India
Akash Gupta	Department of Pharmacology, Rungta College of Pharmaceutical Sciences and Research, Chhattisgarh, 490024, India
Anjila Firdous	Department of Pharmacology, Rungta College of Pharmaceutical Sciences and Research, Chhattisgarh, 490024, India
Biplab Pal	School of Pharmaceutical Sciences, Lovely Professional University, Phagwara, 144411, Punjab, India
Deepak Singh Chaudhary	Faculty of Pharmacy, IFTM University, Moradabad, 244001, U.P., India
Harpreet Singh	School of Pharmaceutical Sciences, IFTM University, Moradabad, 2444102, India
Khushboo Gupta	Faculty of Pharmacy, Kalinga University, Naya Raipur (C.G), India
Mukesh Kumar Singh	Faculty of Pharmacy, IFTM University, Moradabad, 244001, U.P., India
Monika Singh	Department of Pharmacology, I.T.S College of Pharmacy, Ghaziabad, India
Moumita Barman	Department of Pharmaceutics, I.T.S College of Pharmacy, Ghaziabad, India
Mohammad Adnan Raza	Department of Pharmacology, Rungta College of Pharmaceutical Sciences and Research, Chhattisgarh, 490024, India
Navneet Verma	Faculty of Pharmacy, IFTM University, Moradabad, 244001, U.P., India
Neetu Sachan	Department of Pharmaceutical Sciences, School of Pharmaceutical & Biological Sciences, Harcourt Butler Technical University (HBTU), Kanpur, 208002, Uttar Pradesh, India
Nishat Fatima	Department of Pharmacology, MIT College of Pharmacy, Moradabad, 244001, Uttar Pradesh, India
Nitin Kumar	Department of Pharmacognosy, Meerut Institute of Technology, Meerut, India
Nousheen Khatoon	Department of Pharmacology, Rungta College of Pharmaceutical Sciences and Research, Chhattisgarh, 490024, India

Phool Chandra	Teerthanker Mahaveer College of Pharmacy, Teerthanker Mahaveer University, Moradabad, 244001, Uttar Pradesh, India
Payal Saiju	Department of Pharmaceutics, Lakshmi Narain College of Pharmacy, Bhopal, Madhya Pradesh, India
Rakesh Kumar	School of Pharmaceutical Sciences, Lovely Professional University, Phagwara, 144411, Punjab, India
Shweta Verma	Faculty of Pharmacy, IFTM University, Moradabad, 244001, U.P., India
Shahjad	Department of Pharmacology, Global Institute of Pharmaceutical Education and Research, Kashipur, 244713, Uttarakhand, India
S.K. Paliwal	Department of Pharmacy, Banasthali Vidyapith, Banasthali, 304022, India
Sadish Kumar Shanmugam	Department of Pharmaceutical Chemistry, I.T.S College of Pharmacy, Ghaziabad, India
Sanjay Kumar Gupta	Department of Pharmacology, Rungta College of Pharmaceutical Sciences and Research, Chhattisgarh, 490024, India
Sumit Sahu	Department of Pharmacology, Rungta College of Pharmaceutical Sciences and Research, Chhattisgarh, 490024, India
Vivek Raj	Department of Biotechnology, Patna Women's College, Patna, Bihar, India
Vandana	Indus Institute of Management, Indus University, Rancharda via Thaltej, Ahmedabad, 382114, Gujarat, India
Vikas Sharma	School of Pharmaceutical Sciences, Lovely Professional University, Phagwara, 144411, Punjab, India

CHAPTER 1

Introduction and Historical Perspective on Bacterial Infections

Khushboo Gupta[1,*] and **Anshita Gupta**[2]

[1] *Faculty of Pharmacy, Kalinga University, Naya Raipur (C.G), India*

[2] *Department of Pharmacy, Gurughasi Das Vishwavidyalaya, Bilaspur (C.G.), India*

Abstract: Pathogenic microorganisms that cause bacterial illnesses have a profound impact on community health, medicine, and the overall humanity. These infections, which can range in severity from minor ailments to fatal conditions, have influenced the development of treatments and spurred advances in medical knowledge. Hippocrates, the Greek physician, and Galen, the Roman scholar, detailed a number of diseases that could be caused by bacteria. The discoveries made by Louis Pasteur and Robert Koch during the 19th century were crucial because they established a framework for connecting particular bacteria to particular diseases, greatly expanding our knowledge of bacterial pathogenesis. Vaccines and antibiotics were also industrialized during this time, revolutionizing the management and avoidance of microbial diseases. Alexander Fleming's discovery of penicillin in the 20th century marked the dawn of the antibiotic era, revolutionizing the treatment of bacterial illnesses and saving countless lives. Nonetheless, the emergence of antibiotic resistance in recent times has presented novel obstacles, stimulating continuous investigation into substitute therapies and pre-emptive actions.

Keywords: Antibiotic resistance, Bacterial infections, Pathogenic microorganisms.

INTRODUCTION

Infections with bacteria rank among the biggest health risks in human history. Pathogenic bacteria are the source of these infections. They enter the body and cause a wide range of illnesses, from minor to fatal. In addition to advancing our knowledge of these microbes, research on bacterial infections influences public health and contemporary medicine [1]. Globally, bacterial infections, which can range from minor localized infections to serious systemic disorders, are a major source of morbidity and mortality. The immune system of the host and the invasive bacteria interact intricately throughout the development of bacterial

* **Corresponding author Khushboo Gupta:** Faculty of Pharmacy, Kalinga University, Naya Raipur (C.G), India; E-mail:khushboo.gupta@kalingauniversity.ac.in

Mukesh Kumar Singh, Gurdeep Singh, Amrendra Pratap Yadav & Papiya Bigoniya (Eds.)

infections [2]. The study of bacterial infections has evolved considerably since the discovery of bacteria by Antoine van Leeuwenhoek in the 17th century, leading to critical advancements in understanding the pathogenesis, diagnosis, and treatment of these infections This chapter gives a thorough review of the origins, development, and effects of bacterial diseases on society in addition to charting their discovery and progression [3, 4]. Research on bacterial infections has grown significantly in the last few decades, impacting not only the science of microbiology but also clinical practices and public health policies [5].

Historical Background

In the past, people had a misunderstanding about the origins of diseases and frequently linked them to supernatural forces or the wrath of gods. While diseases and infections are mentioned in ancient literature like the Egyptian Ebers Papyrus (c. 1550 BCE), the idea that microbes are the cause was not recognized.

Previous Hypotheses and Views: Hippocrates and other Greek physicians postulated that an imbalance in the body's "humours," or bodily fluids, was the root cause of sickness. Before scientific research started to question these ideas during the Renaissance, this theory dominated Western medicine for centuries [6, 7]. Table **1** represents a timeline of bacterial discoveries with significance.

Table 1. A timeline of bacterial infection discoveries.

S. No	Time Period	Event	Significance
1	Ancient Times	Early Recognition of Infections	Ancient Egyptians and Greeks noticed infections from wounds.
3	1676	Discovery of Bacteria	Antonie van Leeuwenhoek observed bacteria using a microscope.
4	19th Century	Germ Theory of Disease	Proposed by Louis Pasteur and Robert Koch; established bacteria as causes of disease.
5	1854	Cholera Outbreak in London	John Snow traced the outbreak to contaminated water, foundational for epidemiology.
6	1876	*Anthrax bacillus* Identified	Robert Koch identified *Bacillus anthracis* as the cause of anthrax, establishing Koch's postulates.
7	1882	Discovery of *Tuberculosis bacterium*	Robert Koch identified *Mycobacterium tuberculosis* as the cause of tuberculosis.
8	1928	Discovery of Penicillin	Alexander Fleming discovered penicillin, the first antibiotic, revolutionizing the treatment of bacterial infections.
9	1940s	Widespread Use of Antibiotics	Penicillin and other antibiotics began to be mass-produced and used widely, drastically reducing bacterial infection mortality.

(Table 1) cont.....

S. No	Time Period	Event	Significance
10	1980s-2000s	Rise of Antibiotic Resistance	Overuse and misuse of antibiotics led to the emergence of resistant bacteria such as MRSA.
11	21st Century	Modern Challenges	Ongoing challenges include antibiotic resistance, the development of new antibiotics, and understanding bacterial evolution.

Discovery of Bacteria

Antony van Leeuwenhoek and the First Microscope: In the latter part of the 17th century, Dutch microscopist Antony van Leeuwenhoek discovered bacteria when he used his handmade microscope to view "animalcules." His findings established the field of microbiology, even though he was unaware of its importance.

Louis Pasteur and Germ Theory

Throughout the history of science and medicine, Louis Pasteur, a French chemist and microbiologist, has had a significant impact. By developing the germ theory, his groundbreaking work in the middle of the 19th century established the groundwork for contemporary microbiology and the comprehension of infectious diseases. By proving that bacteria are the root cause of many diseases, this hypothesis transformed medicine and gave rise to significant improvements in both public health and medical care [8 - 10].

With his research on fermentation, Pasteur laid the groundwork for the germ theory. He was tasked with looking into the brewing industry's alcohol deterioration in the 1850s. Pasteur discovered that different kinds of microbes created different fermentation products and that microorganisms were responsible for the fermentation process. He noticed that when undesirable microbes were introduced into the brewing process, unwanted fermentation happened. Following this observation, Pasteur postulated that bacteria were active actors in biochemical processes rather than merely byproducts of decomposition. He postulated that if germs could alter organic things, they could also be in charge of infecting people and other animals with diseases [11, 12]. The germ theory of disease was founded on Pasteur's work on fermentation, and his experiments refuted spontaneous generation. He postulated that a variety of ailments were brought on by microbes, or "germs." Contrary to the miasma theory, which held that illnesses were brought on by "bad air" or miasmas, this concept was innovative.

The germ theory proposed by Pasteur had significant medical and public health ramifications. It was proposed that sickness may be stopped by limiting the movement of microbes. As a result of this knowledge, antiseptic methods, sterilization processes, and advancements in sanitation and hygiene were developed.

Pasteur's germ theory changed medicine since it was more than just a theoretical idea with real-world applications. The invention of pasteurization, a method to destroy dangerous microbes in food and drink, especially milk, was one of his greatest achievements. Pasteurization raised the temperature of milk to a certain point, making it safer to drink and drastically lowering the risk of foodborne infections.

Additionally, Pasteur made revolutionary advances in the study of immunity. He created vaccinations against many illnesses, such as rabies and anthrax, in the 1880s. His work on attenuated strains, in which he weakened the pathogens to create a version that might induce immunity without causing the disease, served as the foundation for his vaccine development efforts.

Louis Pasteur's germ hypothesis dramatically changed medical practice and the way we perceive disease. It gave rise to the development of methods for illness prevention and treatment, as well as the scientific foundation for determining the origins of infections. His research opened the path for later researchers like Robert Koch, who developed microbiology and identified the precise connections between microbes and illnesses.

Pasteur made contributions to fields other than medicine and microbiology. His contributions to germ theory have had a major influence on public health policies, resulting in expanded vaccination campaigns, better sanitation practices, and the use of sterilization techniques in surgery. Pasteur is regarded as a trailblazer who contributed to the dawn of a new era in modern medicine. Many of the modern healthcare advancements we take for granted were made possible by his work, and his legacy is still felt in the disciplines of public health, immunology, and microbiology.

Robert Koch and Koch's Postulates: Building on Pasteur's research, Koch created a system of standards, or Koch's postulates, to pinpoint the precise microorganisms causing a variety of illnesses. His research on cholera and tuberculosis strengthened the case for the involvement of bacteria in infectious diseases [13 - 17].

Pioneering Discoveries in Bacterial Infections

The Plague

The most famous pandemics in history include the Black Death (14th century), the Third Pandemic (19th–20th century), and the Justinian Plague (6th century), which was brought on by the bacterium *Yersinia pestis*. With 25–50 million deaths, the Black Death (1347–1351) destroyed over one-third of Europe's population [18]. Biting fleas and direct contact with contaminated tissues or respiratory droplets were the two ways through which the infection was spread. The symptoms of the plague were fever, chills, enlarged lymph nodes (buboes), and a high death rate. It was not until the late 1800s, following Alexandre Yersin's identification of the bacteria during the Hong Kong plague outbreak in 1894, that the significance of fleas and rats in the transmission process was realized. Widespread social, economic, and cultural upheaval brought about by the epidemic resulted in severe labor shortages and altered European societal structures. Even though the real cause of the Black Death was not discovered for centuries, its devastating effects made it clear that improved public health measures were required [19, 20].

Tuberculosis

Mycobacterium tuberculosis, the causative agent of tuberculosis (TB), has been a leading cause of mortality for many years. Evidence of the disease can be found in the skeletal remains of ancient Egyptians. TB, sometimes referred to as the "White Plague" in the 1800s, was linked to a sluggish, wasting disease that caused coughing, weight loss, and nocturnal sweats.

During the 18th and 19th centuries, tuberculosis (TB) was a major cause of mortality in both Europe and North America. Robert Koch's identification of the causal culprit, *Mycobacterium tuberculosis*, in 1882 marked a critical turning point in the knowledge and management of the illness [21]. The discovery of streptomycin in 1943 led to the evolution of TB treatment, which eventually included the development of other antibiotics and the Bacillus Calmette-Guérin (BCG) vaccine.

Cholera

Since the 19th century, cholera caused by Vibrio cholera has been the cause of seven pandemics. The first one started in India in 1817. Severe diarrhea, vomiting, and dehydration are among the symptoms, and if left untreated, can be fatal. The third pandemic (1852–1860) affected Europe, Africa, and the Americas and had a worldwide impact. The discovery of Vibrio cholera in 1854 by Filippo Pacini and later verified by Robert Koch in 1884 completely changed our knowledge of the illness. The transmission of cholera is directly related to inadequate sanitation and a scarcity of clean drinking water. It is spread through contaminated food and water [22, 23].

Clinical Manifestations of Bacterial Infections

The body frequently experiences a systemic response in response to bacterial infections, which results in broad symptoms that are typical of many infections rather than being unique to any one type of bacterium. Among these common manifestations are:

Fever: Fever is one of the most typical indicators of a bacterial infection. It is the body's reaction to pyrogens that bacteria and the immune system release. Occasionally, the pattern of fever can provide information about the type of infection; for instance, high fevers with sharp spikes may indicate bacterial sepsis [24, 25].

Sweating and chills: These signs and symptoms frequently accompany fever and represent the body's attempt to control body temperature when an infection is present.

Loss of Appetite: Because of systemic inflammation and the body's stress reaction, anorexia is frequently seen in cases of bacterial infections.

Lymphadenopathy: As the lymphatic system functions to filter pathogens and assist the immune response, enlargement of the lymph nodes in the vicinity of the infection site is frequently observed [26].

Depending on which physiological system is impacted, bacterial infections can present with a wide range of clinical symptoms. Chest pain, shortness of breath, coughing up purulent sputum, and other symptoms are indicative of pneumonia. Frequently brought on by *Haemophilus influenzae* and *Streptococcus pneumoniae*, sinusitis manifests as headache, purulent nasal discharge, nasal congestion, and face pain [27].

Pharyngitis and Tonsillitis: Fever, painful throat, enlarged tonsils, and lymphadenopathy are common symptoms of bacterial pharyngitis, which is frequently caused by *Streptococcus pyogenes* (Group A Streptococcus). *Shigella, Campylobacter, Salmonella,* and *Escherichia coli* are some of the bacteria that can cause gastroenteritis. Frequent symptoms include nausea, vomiting, diarrhoea (which may be bloody), and abdominal pain.

Peptic Ulcer Disease: Symptoms of this Helicobacter pylori-related illness include bloating, upper abdominal pain, and occasionally gastrointestinal bleeding [28].

Development of Antibacterial Treatments

Discovery of Penicillin by Alexander Fleming: The antibiotic era began with Alexander Fleming's 1928 discovery of penicillin. Because penicillin can destroy a broad variety of microorganisms, it was used extensively during World War II and helped save many lives [29]. Due to the development of multiple antibacterial medications, the mid-20th century is frequently referred to as the "Golden Age of Antibiotics." Antibiotics such as erythromycin, tetracycline, and streptomycin have completely changed how bacterial infections are treated [30, 31]. Sulfonamides, or sulfa medicines, were the first antibacterial medications before penicillin became commonly available. Gerhard Domagk developed sulfonamides in 1935. These medications were widely utilized during World War II and were the first chemical therapies for bacterial illnesses that proved effective. But over time, their effects were lessened due to their toxicity and poor efficacy in comparison to newer antibiotics [32]. Table **2** represents the discovery of antibiotics with their significance. Table **3** represents the major classes of antibiotics with the spectrum of activity.

Table 2. Significant discovery of antibiotics.

Year	Antibiotic	Discoverer	Significance
1928	Penicillin	Alexander Fleming	First antibiotic; revolutionized bacterial infection treatment.
1935	Sulfonamides	Gerhard Domagk	First commercially available antibiotic; used for streptococcus infections.
1943	Streptomycin	Selman Waksman	Effective treatment for tuberculosis.
1952	Erythromycin	McGuire *et al.*	Broad-spectrum antibiotic, especially effective for respiratory infections.

Table 3. Major classes of antibiotics discovered.

Class	Examples	Year	Spectrum of Activity
Penicillins	Penicillin, Amoxicillin	1940s	Broad-spectrum, effective for gram-positive bacteria.
Aminoglycosides	Streptomycin	1943	Treats gram-negative infections, TB.
Tetracyclines	Doxycycline	1948	Broad-spectrum, effective against a wide variety of bacteria.
Macrolides	Erythromycin	1952	Effective for respiratory infections, gram-positive bacteria.

Antimicrobial Resistance

Antimicrobial resistance refers to the change in microorganisms that once showed sensitivity to antibiotics but are now resistant to them due to bacterial mutations or the acquisition of resistance genes. Antimicrobials (antibiotics, antiparasitics, antivirals, and antifungals) can be countered or resisted by microorganisms (bacteria, viruses, parasites, and fungi). Both acquired and innate resistance exist. Each microbe has a unique characteristic known as "intrinsic" resistance, which manifests itself prior to the application of antibiotics, and acquired resistance, which manifests itself following exposure to antibiotics. The resistance of Gram-negative bacteria occurs through genetic alterations, mainly manifested by mechanisms involving beta-lactamase enzymes and modifying enzymes, which promote the destruction of antibacterial. The overuse and inappropriate use of antibiotics is the main cause of germ resistance [33 - 37].

Resistance Types

Multidrug resistance: When a bacterium exhibits resistance to multiple antibiotics, it is known as multidrug resistance (MDR). A microbe may possess multiple resistance genes, each of which confers resistance to a distinct antibiotic from a minimum of three antimicrobial families. Non-sensitivity genes are present on plasmids, which are tiny DNA fragments that bacteria can transfer among themselves. *A. baumannii, P. aeruginosa,* and *enterobacteria* like *K. pneumoniae* and *E. coli* that produce ESBL are examples of gram-negative bacteria with MDR [38].

Pandrug-resistance: Pan is defined as resistance to all recognized antimicrobials; in other words, it indicates that no antibiotic has been found to date that can cure illnesses brought on by these microbial agents. The word pan is derived from the Greek prefix "everything." The organization of resistance genes into integrons, transposons, and plasmids promotes bacterial multiresistance, as it only takes a few chromosomal changes and the accumulation of two or three multidrug-resistant plasmids to produce pandrug resistance (PDR). Prominent microbes include *K. pneumoniae, P. aeruginosa,* and *Acinetobacter* spp.

Problems with Antibiotic Resistance: As a result of the extensive usage of antibiotics, microorganisms that are resistant to them have emerged. Antibiotic resistance is a phenomenon that presents a serious obstacle to modern medicine since it makes many common therapies useless. The evolution of antibiotic resistance has presented substantial hurdles, notwithstanding the early success of antibiotics. The abuse and misuse of antibiotics has resulted in the emergence of bacterial strains that are resistant to them, making treatment more difficult and requiring the creation of new antimicrobial medicines. As a result, current research has concentrated on developing new antibiotics and complementary therapies. Methicillin-resistant *Staphylococcus aureus* (MRSA) and vancomycin-resistant Enterococcus infections, in particular, now have treatment options thanks to the introduction of antibiotics like vancomycin and linezolid [39 - 42]. Table **4** represents the impact of antibiotic resistance to bacteria.

Table 4. Antibiotic-resistant bacteria.

Bacteria	Resistance Type	Impact
Methicillin-resistant *Staphylococcus aureus* (MRSA)	Resistant to methicillin and related antibiotics.	Severe hospital and community-acquired infections.
Multidrug-resistant *Mycobacterium tuberculosis* (MDR-TB)	Resistant to first-line TB drugs.	Prolonged treatment and poor outcomes in TB patients.
Carbapenem-resistant *Enterobacteriaceae* (CRE)	Resistant to carbapenem antibiotics.	Limited treatment options, high mortality rates.

Approaches to Combat Antibiotic Resistance

Antibiotic resistance has been increased by the widespread and frequently improper use of antibiotics, making many formerly curable infections more difficult to treat. The scientific and medical communities are therefore investigating novel approaches to handle this situation. Fig. (**1**) represents approaches to combat antibiotic resistance, which is also discussed below.

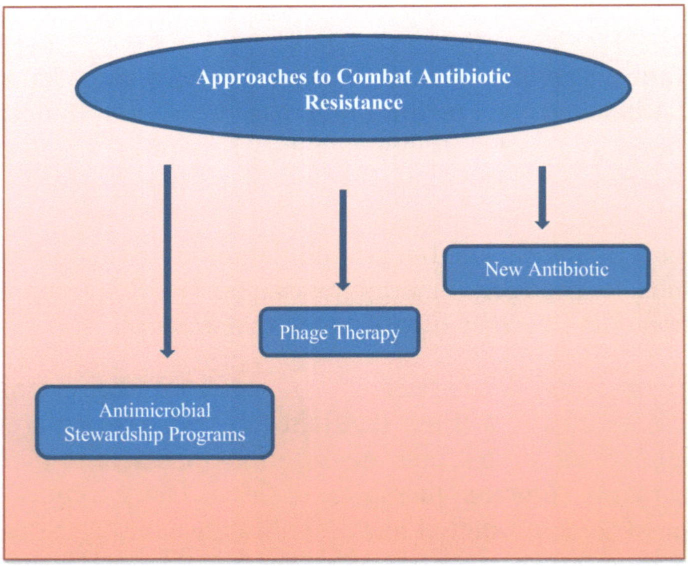

Fig. (1). Approaches to combat Antibiotic Resistance.

Phage Therapy

Through the use of viruses called bacteriophages that target specific bacteria, phage treatment offers a novel way to combat bacterial illnesses. In order to cause the bacteria to rupture and die, phages work by entering bacterial cells and multiplying there. Comparing this method to conventional antibiotics, there are a number of clear benefits. Bacteriophages can target and eradicate specific bacterial species without endangering beneficial bacteria in the human microbiome because they are very selective to their bacterial hosts. Several antibiotics are broad-spectrum drugs that can eradicate both beneficial and harmful bacteria, which can result in problems or subsequent infections. This specificity contrasts with this property.

Phage treatment has potential, but it also has drawbacks. Treatment may be delayed because of the specificity of bacteriophages, which necessitates accurate identification of the bacterial strain causing the infection. Widespread adoption is further complicated by regulatory obstacles, the requirement for customized treatments, and worries about immune system reactions to phages. To improve the clinical use of phage therapy, more investigation is required, especially in areas such as phage delivery mechanisms, guaranteeing that phages can reach all infected sites and preventing the development of bacterial resistance.

Antimicrobial Stewardship Programs

Phage therapy is a novel treatment, but Antimicrobial Stewardship Programs (ASPs) are an equally important tactic in the fight against antibiotic resistance. These initiatives concentrate on using antibiotics as efficiently as possible in order to stop the emergence and spread of resistant microorganisms. ASPs' main objectives are:

- Make sure you only use antibiotics when absolutely required and acceptable.
- Give the appropriate antibiotic for the best length of time, at the right dose.
- Reduce the incidental effects of antibiotic use, including drug resistance, side effects, and recurrent infections like Clostridium difficile.
- The goal of ASPs is to decrease the total amount of antibiotics used in healthcare settings by encouraging their prudent use.

New Antibiotic Classes

The creation of novel antibiotic classes is just as important to the fight against resistance as optimizing the use of already available antibiotics and investigating alternative treatments like phage therapy. To combat germs that have grown resistant to all or most of the conventional treatments, new antibiotics are required. The process of creating novel antibiotics is difficult and expensive. Because of bacteria's remarkable capacity for adaptation, new antibiotics are frequently rendered ineffective within just a few years after introduction. Furthermore, the fact that antibiotics are often administered for shorter periods of time than medications for chronic diseases creates a financial barrier for pharmaceutical corporations to engage in antibiotic research. Governments and international organizations have implemented incentives to promote innovation in the development of antibiotics in order to get around these challenges. These include increased patent protection, funding for R&D, and collaborations between the public and private sectors to promote the development of antibiotics.

Impact on Public Health and Medicine

Initiatives related to vaccination and public health: One of the main pillars of public health has been the creation of vaccinations against bacterial illnesses, such as the diphtheria, tetanus, and pertussis (DTP) vaccine. The prevalence of fatal bacterial infections has dramatically decreased as a result of these vaccinations [43 - 47].

The Function of Sanitation and Hygiene: Controlling bacterial illnesses has been greatly aided by advancements in sanitation, hygiene, and water treatment. Campaigns by public health organizations encouraging safe drinking water and handwashing have significantly slowed the spread of diseases [48].

Current Challenges: Bacterial infections continue to be a global health concern in spite of medical advancements. Public health policies must remain vigilant and innovative due to the resurgence of diseases like tuberculosis, the increase of multidrug-resistant bacteria, and the threat of bioterrorism [49].

Bacterial Infection

Bacteria are prokaryotic, unicellular organisms without membrane-bound organelles or a genuine nucleus. In spite of their simplicity, they have a diverse range of forms and structural elements that add to their usefulness and versatility. They have different morphologies, including spherical cocci, rod-shaped bacilli, and spiral spirilla. Based on the composition of their cell walls, bacteria can be divided into two main groups: Gram-positive and Gram-negative. These groups can be distinguished using Gram staining, a vital diagnostic technique in microbiology [50]. Gram-negative bacteria are more resistant to antibiotics because they have an outer membrane and a thinner peptidoglycan layer than Gram-positive bacteria. Pathogenic bacteria produce bacterial infections when they infiltrate the body and proliferate, frequently resulting in illness. Bacteria are single-celled creatures that can survive and proliferate on their own in a variety of conditions, in contrast to viruses. Many bacteria are benign or even helpful, but when they go inside the human body, some can seriously affect health. For the purpose of creating efficient treatment and preventive plans, it is essential to comprehend the nature of bacterial illnesses [51]. Table **5** represents the classification of bacteria on the basis of various categories. Fig. (**2**) presents the structure of a bacterial cell with its composition, and Fig. (**3**) represents the classification of Cocci bacteria.

Table 5. Classification of bacteria.

S.No	Category	Classification	Bacteria
1	Gram Stain	Gram Positive	*Staphylococcus aureus, Listeria*
		Gram-negative	*Escherichia coli, Neisseria*
2	Shape	Cocci (spherical)	*Streptococcus, Staphylococcus*
		Bacilli (rod-shaped)	*Escherichia coli, Bacillus*
		Spirilla (spiral-shaped)	*Helicobacter pylori, Treponema*
3	Oxygen Requirement	Aerobic	*Mycobacterium tuberculosis*
		Anaerobic	*Clostridium, Bacteroides*
		Facultative anaerobes	*Escherichia coli, Salmonella*
4	Transmission Mode	Airborne	*Mycobacterium tuberculosis*
		Foodborne	*Salmonella, Listeria*
		Waterborne	*Vibrio cholerae*
5	Clinical Manifestation	Respiratory Infections	*Streptococcus pneumonia*
		Gastrointestinal Infections	*Escherichia coli, Salmonella*
		Skin and Soft Tissue Infections	*Staphylococcus, Streptococcus*
		Urinary Tract Infections	*Escherichia coli*

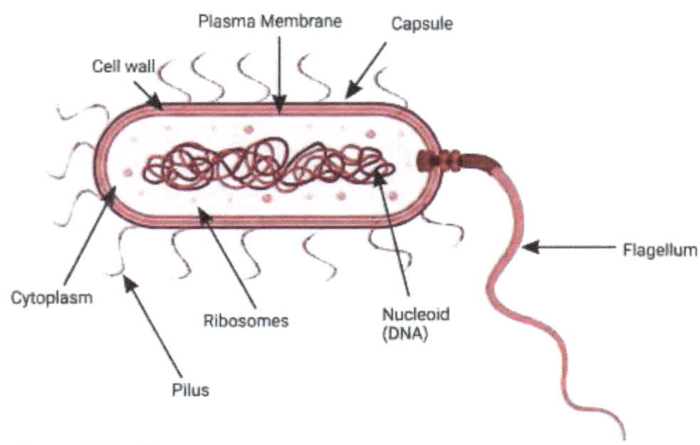

Fig. (2). Structure of a bacterial cell.

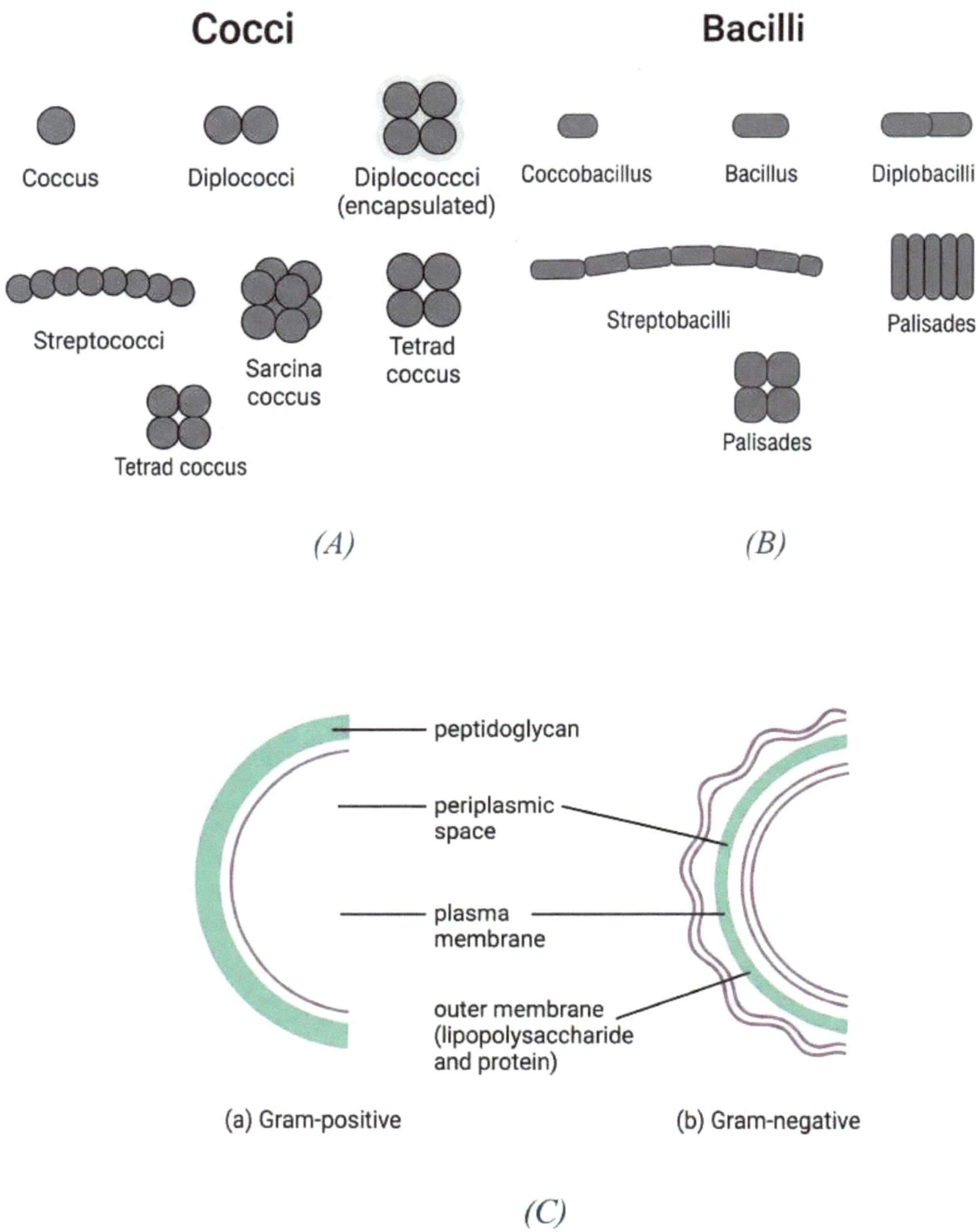

Fig. (3). Classification of Cocci bacteria (A) and Bacillus bacteria (B), and (C) represents the structure of Gram-positive and Gram-negative bacteria.

Structure of bacterial cell comprises cell wall, plasma membrane, ribosomes, cytoplasm, nucleoid, flagellum, and capsule.

Mechanisms of Bacterial Pathogenesis

Bacterial Adhesion and Colonization

Adhesion is the first stage of bacterial infection, during which the germs adhere to the tissues or cells of the host. Adhesions, which are specialized proteins or structures on the bacterial surface that recognize and bind to particular receptors on the host cells, mediate this process. Fimbriae, non-fimbrial adhesins, and pili are examples of common adhesins. To cling to the urinary tract epithelium, for instance, is a critical stage in the development of urinary tract infections, and *Escherichia coli* employs pili for this purpose. In addition to facilitating colonization, adhesion sets off bacterial signaling pathways that encourage invasion and circumvent host defenses [52 - 54].

Invasion of Host Tissues

Some bacteria adhere to their hosts and then infiltrate their tissues in order to evade the immune system and cause more serious diseases. Multiple pathways can lead to invasion, including as direct piercing of epithelial barriers or cellular uptake processes like phagocytosis or endocytosis. Invasins, which are proteins that cause cytoskeletal alterations in host cells, are used by bacteria such as *Salmonella* spp. and Listeria monocytogenes to enter and thrive within those cells. Bacteria can survive in the host and avoid immune detection thanks to their intracellular existence [55, 56].

Toxin Production

Many pathogenic bacteria create toxins, which are important virulence agents that harm host tissues and interfere with regular cellular processes. Exotoxins and endotoxins are the two main categories of toxins:

Exotoxins are proteins produced into the body that directly harm certain host cells. For instance, *Corynebacterium diphtheria* produces the diphtheria toxin, which inhibits protein synthesis and causes cell death. Similar to this, *Vibrio cholera's* cholera toxin impairs ion transport in intestinal cells, leading to severe diarrhea [57].

Endotoxins

These include substances like lipopolysaccharides (LPS) that are part of the bacterial cell wall, especially in Gram-negative bacteria. Strong inflammatory reactions brought on by endotoxins have the potential to cause septic shock if left unchecked. The inflammatory response to Gram-negative bacterial infections depends critically on the host's immune system's ability to identify LPS through Toll-like receptors [58].

Immune Evasion Strategies

Bacteria must avoid the host immune system in order to initiate and sustain infection. Different strategies have been developed by bacteria to evade immune recognition and elimination.

Antigenic Variation

To evade the host immune system's identification, several bacteria have the ability to modify their surface antigens. Neisseria gonorrhea, for instance, modifies its pilin proteins to avoid immune recognition and continue to live inside the host.

Capsule Formation

Bacteria such as Streptococcus pneumoniae are able to evade being phagocytized by host immune cells through the creation of a polysaccharide capsule. By blocking complement activation and hiding surface antigens, the capsule stops opsonization and the ensuing phagocytosis [59, 60].

Bacteria have the ability to build biofilms, which are organized bacterial populations encased in an extracellular matrix that they have produced on their own. Antibiotics and immunological responses are thwarted by biofilms, rendering diseases difficult to treat.

Host-Pathogen Interactions

The immune system of the host influences the course of bacterial infections in addition to the virulence factors of the bacteria. In host-pathogen interactions, there is a dynamic balance between the pathogen's immune system and the host's defenses, which the bacteria use to subvert or manipulate the host's defenses. A variety of clinical outcomes, from asymptomatic carrying to serious, life-threatening illnesses, may arise from this interaction [61].

Inflammation and Immune Response

In order to keep bacterial infections under control, the host immune system is essential. On the other hand, an overly strong or deregulated immune response can cause tissue damage and worsen an illness. In bacterial sepsis, for instance, a strong inflammatory response may result in extensive tissue damage and organ failure.

Host Genetic Factors

An individual's genetic makeup influences their propensity to contract bacterial illnesses. Some people are more vulnerable to serious infections due to certain genetic changes that affect how well the immune system responds to an infection. Comprehending these host factors is crucial for determining groups at risk and customizing treatment approaches [62, 63].

Emerging Concepts in Bacterial Pathogenesis

Recent developments in genomics and molecular biology have deepened our knowledge of the pathophysiology of bacteria. High-throughput screening, CRISPR-Cas systems, and whole-genome sequencing are a few examples of the technologies that have uncovered new virulence factors and shed light on the mechanisms of bacterial adaptability. Moreover, the intricate relationships between commensal and pathogenic bacteria that affect the course of an infection have come to light through research on the microbiome and its function in health and disease.

The advent of germs that are resistant to antibiotics is a serious problem, highlighting the need for innovative treatment strategies. In an effort to give alternate approaches to treating bacterial infections, research is being conducted on vaccinations, immunotherapy, and bacteriophage therapy. The development of these novel therapies, as well as the ongoing battle against infectious diseases, will depend heavily on our ability to comprehend the molecular pathways behind bacterial pathogenesis [64, 65].

CONCLUDING REMARKS

In the fight against infectious diseases, the discovery and characterization of bacterial pathogens were revolutionary. The identification of particular bacteria by Koch that cause illnesses like tuberculosis, along with the creation of vaccines and medications, drastically changed methods of treatment and prevention. These developments led to a considerable decrease in the death rate from bacterial infections while simultaneously improving clinical outcomes. Our knowledge of bacterial behavior and host interactions is being further enhanced by the continuous advancement of bacterial pathogenesis research in the modern era. The complexity of bacterial infections is highlighted by newly developed ideas including the involvement of the microbiome in disease susceptibility, quorum sensing as a means of bacterial communication, and complicated immune evasion mechanisms. This growing body of information highlights the significance of ongoing research and innovation by influencing both present and future approaches to combating bacterial infections. Overall, the history of bacterial illnesses and the current state of research highlight how important scientific advancement is to improving public health. A thorough understanding of bacterial pathogenesis is made possible by the combination of recent findings and the legacy of earlier discoveries, opening the door to further advancements in diagnosis, treatment, and prevention.

REFERENCES

[1] Johnson R, Lee K, Thompson R. Overview of bacterial infections: Pathogenesis and host responses. J Clin Microbiol 2020; 58(4).

[2] Brown P, Smith A. From Leeuwenhoek to Koch: The Development of Bacteriology. In: Green B, Ed. Milestones in Microbiology. 3rd ed. New York: Science Press 2019; pp. 32-54.

[3] Jones M, Patel S, Roberts A. The Germ Theory of Disease: Historical Perspectives and Modern Implications. Infect Dis Hist 2018; 7(2): 101-15.

[4] Williams B, Taylor J. Antibiotic Resistance: A Growing Threat in Bacterial Infections. Med Microbiol 2021; 14(3): 203-15.

[5] Clark C, Nguyen H, Rodriguez L. Advances in Bacterial Infection Research: From Pathogenesis to Treatment. Microbiol Rev 2022; 10(1): 45-60.

[6] Smith J, Johnson R. The Early Observations of Microorganisms: Antonie van Leeuwenhoek and the Dawn of Microbiology. J Hist Med Allied Sci 2017; 72(3): 315-27.

[7] Brown L. Louis Pasteur and the Germ Theory of Disease. Microbiol Hist 2018; 15(1): 45-58.

[8] Williams P, Davis K, Green M. Robert Koch and the Rise of Bacteriology. Infect Dis Rep 2020; 13(2): 125-38.

[9] Miller A, Clark N. The Golden Age of Bacteriology: Pathogen Identification and Vaccine Development. Bacteriol Hist J 2019; 8(4): 220-34.

[10] Harris S. Penicillin and the Antibiotic Revolution. J Med Biol 2021; 24(5): 301-15.

[11] Nguyen T, Patel S. Modern Advances in Bacterial Infection Research: Genomics and Beyond. Microbiol Rev 2022; 11(3): 175-90.

[12] Smith J, Leeuwenhoek A, Johnson R. Antonie van Leeuwenhoek and the Birth of Microbiology. Microbiol Hist 2016; 22(1): 10-20.

[13] Brown L. Louis Pasteur and the Germ Theory: A Revolution in Medicine. J Infect Dis Hist 2018; 19(3): 78-90.

[14] Jones M, Taylor P. Robert Koch and the Proof of Bacterial Pathogenicity. Infect Dis Rep 2020; 15(2): 120-35.

[15] Clark N, Green B. The Identification of Bacterial Pathogens: From Koch to Modern Microbiology. Bacteriol Hist J 2019; 10(4): 150-65.

[16] Miller S, Clark J, Green M. Vaccines and Bacteriology: The Early Days of Preventing Infections. Vaccine Hist Rev 2021; 14(3): 210-25.

[17] Harris S, Thompson R. The Discovery of Penicillin and the Antibiotic Era. J Med Sci 2022; 30(5): 300-15.

[18] Smith J, Leeuwenhoek A, Johnson R. Discovery of Yersinia pestis: The Bacterium Behind the Plague. J Microbiol Hist 2017; 22(1): 30-42.

[19] Brown L. Plague and Public Health: From Ancient Scourge to Modern Understanding. Infect Dis Hist 2019; 20(4): 88-102.

[20] Jones M, Taylor P. Robert Koch's Discovery of the *Tuberculosis bacillus*: A Turning Point in Medicine. Infect Dis Rep 2020; 15(2): 120-35.

[21] Williams P, Davis K, Green M. The Impact of Robert Koch on Tuberculosis Control: Historical Perspectives. Med Microbiol J 2021; 12(3): 200-15.

[22] Miller S, Clark J, Green M. Advances in Plague Treatment: From Antibiotics to Vaccination. Bacteriol Med 2021; 14(3): 210-25.

[23] Nguyen T, Patel S. Advances in bacterial infection research: New insights and future challenges. Microbiol Rev 2022; 11(3): 175-90.

[24] Smith J, Brown L. Clinical Features of Skin Infections: A Review. Dermatol Clin 2018; 36(1): 45-56.

[25] Jones M, Taylor P, Williams R. Urinary Tract Infections: Clinical Manifestations and Management. Urol Health Rev 2020; 10(2): 101-12.

[26] Williams P, Taylor J. Systemic Bacterial Infections: Recognition and Management. Crit Care Med 2019; 47(3): 340-50.

[27] Clark N, Green B. Respiratory Infections: Pneumonia and Tuberculosis. Chest Dis Rev 2021; 13(4): 215-29.

[28] Miller S, Clark J, Green M. Gastrointestinal Bacterial Infections: Clinical Manifestations and Treatment. Gastroenterol J 2022; 16(5): 275-90.

[29] Nguyen T, Patel S. Neurological Manifestations of Bacterial Infections: Meningitis and Beyond. Neuroinfect Dis 2023; 11(1): 12-25.

[30] Miller S, Clark J. Historical Development of Antibacterial Treatments: From Antitoxins to Modern Antibiotics. Med Hist Rev 2019; 12(2): 145-60.

[31] Smith J, Leeuwenhoek A, Johnson R. The Discovery of Penicillin and Its Impact on Medicine. J Antimicrob Chemother 2018; 73(4): 783-90.

[32] Fleming A. On the antibacterial action of cultures of a Penicillium, with special reference to their use in the isolation of B. influenzae. Br J Exp Pathol 1929; 10(3): 226-36.

[33] Domagk G. Eine neue Klasse von antibakteriellen Substanzen. Dtsch Med Wochenschr 1935; 61(3): 250-3.
[http://dx.doi.org/10.1055/s-0028-1129486]

[34] Schatz A, Bugle E, Waksman SA. Streptomycin, a substance exhibiting antibiotic activity against gram-positive and gram-negative bacteria. Exp Biol Med (Maywood) 1944; 55(1): 66-9.
[http://dx.doi.org/10.3181/00379727-55-14461]

[35] Jones M, Taylor P. The Evolution of Antibiotics: Streptomycin and Beyond. Infect Dis Rep 2020; 15(3): 210-25.

[36] Clark N, Green B. Addressing Antibiotic Resistance: New Developments and Strategies. Bacteriol Med 2021; 14(5): 310-25.

[37] Nguyen T, Patel S. Innovative Approaches to Antibiotic Resistance: Bacteriophage Therapy and Beyond. Microbiol Rev 2022; 11(2): 150-65.

[38] Zaman SB, Hussain MA, Nye R, Mehta V, Mamun KZ, Hossain N. A Review on Antibiotic Resistance: Alarm Bells Are Ringing. Frontiers in Microbiology 2017; 8: 134-4.

[39] Li G, Walker MJ, De Oliveira DMP. Vancomycin Resistance in *Enterococcus* and *Staphylococcus aureus*. Microorganisms 2023; 11(1): 24-4.

[40] Williams P, Clark J. The Legacy of Tuberculosis Control: Advances and Challenges. Global Health J 2019; 14(3): 205-20.

[41] Smith J, Brown L. Penicillin and the Modern Antibiotic Era: A Medical Revolution. J Antimicrob

Chemother 2018; 73(4): 783-90.

[42] Clark N, Green B. Addressing Antibiotic Resistance: Strategies and Innovations. Bacteriol Med 2021; 14(5): 310-25.

[43] Miller S, Clark J, Green M. Vaccination Programs and Their Impact on Bacterial Diseases. Vaccine Hist Rev 2022; 15(2): 150-65.

[44] Nguyen T, Patel S. Advancements in Diagnostic Techniques for Bacterial Infections. Microbiol Rev 2023; 12(1): 75-90.

[45] Smith J, Leeuwenhoek A, Johnson R. The black death and its impact on public health. J Hist Med 2017; 22(1): 30-45.

[46] Jones M, Taylor P. Cholera Pandemics and Public Health Reforms: A Historical Overview. Public Health Rev 2020; 10(2): 112-25.

[47] Plotkin SA, Orenstein WA, Offit PA, Edwards KM. Vaccines & public health: the impact of diphtheria, tetanus, and pertussis vaccines. Vaccines 2020; 8(4): 669-9.

[48] Hsu L, Ghosh S. Mechanisms of Bacterial Pathogenesis: A Review. Microbiol Insights 2021; 12(3): 234-50.

[49] Feng Y, Zheng S, Xu W. Adhesion Mechanisms of *Streptococcus pneumoniae* to Respiratory Epithelium. J Clin Microbiol 2022; 60(5).

[50] Davies DG. Understanding Biofilm Formation in *Pseudomonas aeruginosa.* J Bacteriol 2003; 185(22): 6156-60.

[51] Stevens DL, Bisno AL, Chambers HF, *et al.* Practice Guidelines for the Diagnosis and Management of Skin and Soft-Tissue Infections. Clin Infect Dis 2021; 72(1)

[52] Parker MT, Henderson JF, Ellis JE. Clostridium perfringens: Pathogenicity and Clinical Implications. J Med Microbiol 2019; 68(9): 1245-56.

[53] Gouin E, Vyteputsky P, Cossart P. Listeria monocytogenes Internalins and Invasion. Microbes Infect 2005; 7(14-15): 1605-14.

[54] Bergdoll MS. *Staphylococcal enterotoxins.* Bacteriol Rev 1983; 47(1): 35-71.

[54] Raetz CRH, Whitfield C. Lipopolysaccharide Endotoxins. Annu Rev Biochem 2002; 71(1): 635-700. [http://dx.doi.org/10.1146/annurev.biochem.71.110601.135414] [PMID: 12045108]

[55] Collier RJ. Diphtheria Toxin: Mechanism of Action and Structure. Science 2001; 292(5526): 2095-9.

[56] Hammerschmidt S. The Role of the *Streptococcus pneumoniae* Capsule in Pathogenesis. Microb Pathog 2006; 40(3): 156-63.

[57] Gordon S, Palsson-McDermott EM. *Mycobacterium tuberculosis* and Host Cell Manipulation. Immunol Rev 2018; 225(1): 142-56.

[58] Cohen MS, Ghanem KG, Peeling RW. *Neisseria gonorrhoeae* and Antigenic Variation J Infect Dis 2000; 181(Suppl 2).

[59] Miller MA, Reddy B, Pellicano R. Host Manipulation by *Helicobacter pylori.* Gastroenterology 2019; 156(3): 676-90.
[PMID: 30445010]

[60] Kagan JC, Magupalli VG, Wu H. SMAD4 and Host Responses to Pathogen-Associated Molecular Patterns. Cell 2008; 134(5): 960-71.
[PMID: 19041756]

[61] Cornelis GR, Van Gijsegem F. Assembly and Function of Type III Secretory Systems. Annu Rev Microbiol 2000; 54(1): 735-74.
[http://dx.doi.org/10.1146/annurev.micro.54.1.735]

[62] Rook GA, Raison CL, Lowry CA. Microbiota, immune system, and brain: a "dialogue" model. Pharmacol Biochem Behav 2017; 152: 13-21.

[63] Buffie CG, Pamer EG. Microbiota-mediated colonization resistance: unifying principles and mechanisms. Trends Immunol 2015; 36(6): 299-306.

[64] Givskov M, de Nys R, Manefield M, *et al.* Eukaryotic interference with quorum sensing in *Pseudomonas aeruginosa*. J Bacteriol 1996; 178(23): 7222-7.

[65] Lee JH, Zhang L. The quorum-sensing signaling molecule N-acyl-homoserine lactone inhibits *Pseudomonas aeruginosa* biofilm formation. J Bacteriol 2018; 200(3)

CHAPTER 2

Epidemiology and Pathophysiology of Bacterial Infections

Alankar Shrivastav[1,*], **Deepak Singh Chaudhary**[1], **Mukesh Kumar Singh**[1], **Shweta Verma**[1], **Navneet Verma**[1] and **Arun Kumar Mishra**[1]

[1] *Faculty of Pharmacy, IFTM University, Moradabad, U.P. 244001, India*

Abstract: Bacterial infections remain a significant cause of global morbidity and mortality, with their prevalence influenced by geography, population dynamics, and medical interventions. The rise in healthcare-associated infections, as well as emerging and re-emerging pathogens, has altered the landscape of bacterial disease. This review focuses on current trends in bacterial infections, particularly those caused by *Mycobacterium tuberculosis*, *Escherichia coli*, and *Staphylococcus aureus*.

Understanding the pathophysiology of bacterial infections is critical for developing effective prevention and treatment strategies. Bacteria have evolved sophisticated mechanisms to evade the host immune system, including toxin production, tissue invasion, and immune manipulation. Quorum sensing plays a key role in coordinating pathogenic behaviour, especially within biofilms, which promote genetic variation and antibiotic resistance. A deeper insight into these biological processes, combined with epidemiological data, is essential for enhancing disease surveillance, refining therapeutic approaches, and reducing the global burden of bacterial infections.

Keywords: Bacteria, Bacterial infection, Epidemiology, Pathogenesis.

INTRODUCTION: BASIC BIOLOGY OF BACTERIA

The most diverse and fundamental biological entities on the planet are bacteria. These unicellular microorganism are strikingly different from other living organisms [1]. They are prokaryotic, meaning their cells lack a true nucleus and contain prokaryotic organelles and structures surrounded by a membrane. Bacteria play essential roles in ecosystems, often cohabiting with other organisms and enabling crucial ecological processes, despite their ancient reputation as causes of disease [2].

* **Corresponding author Alankar Shrivastav:** Faculty of Pharmacy, IFTM University, Moradabad, U.P. 244001, India; E-mail: alankar1994.ss@gmail.com

Mukesh Kumar Singh, Gurdeep Singh, Amrendra Pratap Yadav & Papiya Bigoniya (Eds.)

Bacterial Cell Structure

Bacteria have a minimal yet incredibly functional cellular design that helps them grow in diverse environments. A bacterial cell includes the following components [3].

The cell envelope consists of the cell wall, plasma membrane, and an outer membrane in some species. A bacterial cell's plasma membrane consists of a phospholipid bilayer, which is very important for controlling the passage of substances in or out of the cell. It gives the cell its shape and provides structural support surrounding the plasma membrane. Based on the composition of the cell wall, this study will segregate bacteria into two groups: Gram-positive and Gram-negative [4]. The crystal violet is retained based on the thick peptidoglycan surrounding Gram-positive bacteria. In comparison, the outermost layer of gram-negative bacteria comprises lipopolysaccharide and peptidoglycan, which are the thinnest. Safranin may be employed as a counterstain for the bacteria since it is also red. Some bacteria also have an optional second line of defence in the form of a shield outside their cell wall called a capsule. The capsule helps the bacteria stick to surfaces and escape from immune system detection [5].

The gel-like material that is found inside the plasma membrane is home to cell structures, waste products, nutrients, enzymes, and water. The nucleoid, a component of the bacterial cytoplasm, contains the lone circular DNA molecule that makes up the bacterial chromosome. Unlike eukaryotes, bacteria do not have a membrane-bound nucleus; hence, their genetic material is not segregated into a separate compartment [6]. The molecular machinery responsible for producing proteins, known as ribosomes, is found within the cytoplasm of bacteria. These 70S ribosomes are composed of the 30S and the 50S subunits. Inclusion bodies are additional basic structures seen in bacteria. These are granules that are stored in the cytoplasm and contain nutrients or building blocks such as polyphosphate, sulfur granules, or glycogen. Furthermore, some bacteria have tiny, circular DNA molecules called plasmids that reside apart from chromosomal DNA [7]. Plasmids can carry genes that provide advantageous traits to bacteria, such as antibiotic resistance, virulence factors, or distinct metabolic pathways [8].

Flagella are extended, whip-like appendages that aid in movement. One or more flagella, positioned at different locations on the cell surface, can be seen on bacteria [9]. Pili and Fimbriae are hair-like projections that facilitate bacterial adhesion to one another and surfaces. Pili are also involved in conjugation, a procedure that consists of the exchange of genetic material between bacterial cells [10].

Bacterial Growth and Reproduction

Bacteria reproduce primarily through a process called binary fission, where a single cell divides into two genetically identical daughter cells. The basic steps of binary fission are shown in Fig.(**1**)[11 - 13]:

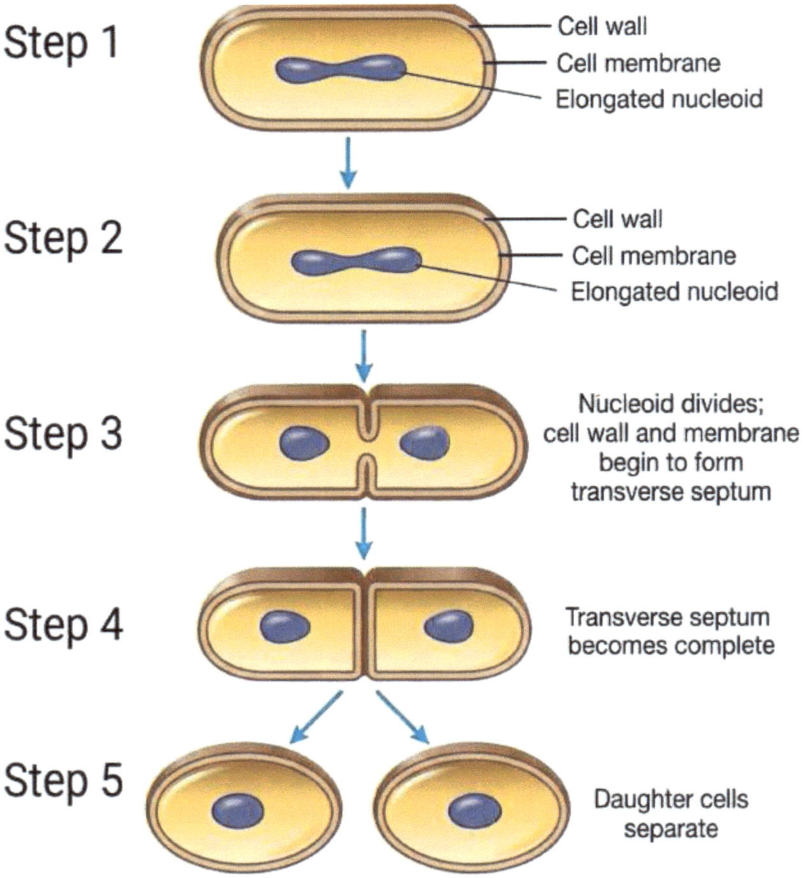

Fig. (1). Steps involved in bacterial growth and reproduction.

1. **DNA Replication**: The bacterial chromosome is replicated, ensuring each daughter cell receives an identical copy.
2. **Cell Elongation**: The cell elongates, and the newly synthesised DNA molecules move to opposite poles of the cell.
3. **Septum Formation**: A septum, or dividing wall, forms in the centre of the cell.
4. **Cell Division**: The septum completes the division, resulting in two separate cells.

Under optimal conditions, some bacteria can divide every 20 minutes, leading to rapid population growth. However, environmental factors such as nutrient availability, temperature, and pH can influence the rate of bacterial growth.

Bacteria are single-celled microorganisms that reproduce rapidly under favourable conditions through a process known as binary fission. This is an asexual method of reproduction where one bacterial cell divides into two identical daughter cells. Bacterial growth refers to an increase in the number of cells, not in cell size. When placed in a suitable nutrient medium, bacterial populations follow a characteristic growth curve composed of four phases: lag, log, stationary, and death. In the lag phase, bacteria acclimate to their new environment. Although cell division does not occur, the cells are metabolically active, synthesising enzymes and preparing for replication. The log or exponential phase follows, where bacteria divide at a constant rate, doubling in number with each generation. This phase is marked by the highest metabolic activity and is the most vulnerable stage to antibiotics.

As nutrients begin to deplete and waste accumulates, the culture enters the stationary phase, where the rate of cell division balances the rate of cell death. Bacteria often undergo physiological changes during this stage, and some may form spores to survive harsh conditions. Eventually, the environment becomes too hostile for survival, leading to the death or decline phase, where the number of dying cells surpasses the number of new ones formed, resulting in a decreasing population.

Binary fission, the primary mode of bacterial reproduction, occurs in a sequence of steps. It begins with the replication of the bacterial chromosome, ensuring that each daughter cell receives an identical copy of genetic material. The cell then elongates as the cytoplasm and cellular components expand. A septum forms in the middle of the cell, dividing the cytoplasm, and finally, the parent cell splits into two genetically identical daughter cells. Under ideal conditions, such as optimal temperature, pH, and nutrient availability, some bacteria, like *Escherichia coli,* can reproduce every 20 minutes, leading to a rapid increase in population. Several environmental factors influence bacterial growth. These include temperature (most bacteria prefer 20–40°C), pH levels (with many thriving at neutral pH), oxygen availability (aerobic or anaerobic conditions), and the presence of antimicrobial agents. Understanding the bacterial growth and reproduction cycle is critical in microbiology and pharmaceutical science, particularly for infection control, the development of antibiotics, and industrial applications involving bacterial cultures [14].

Historical Background of Bacterial Infections

The development of medical science, microbiology, and human civilisation is all intricately linked to the history of bacterial illnesses [15]. Bacterial illnesses have significantly shaped human history, from the pandemics of antiquity to the current era of antibiotics and the emergence of resistant strains. This section will give an overview of the significant historical turning points in our knowledge and treatment of bacterial illnesses (Fig. **2**) [16].

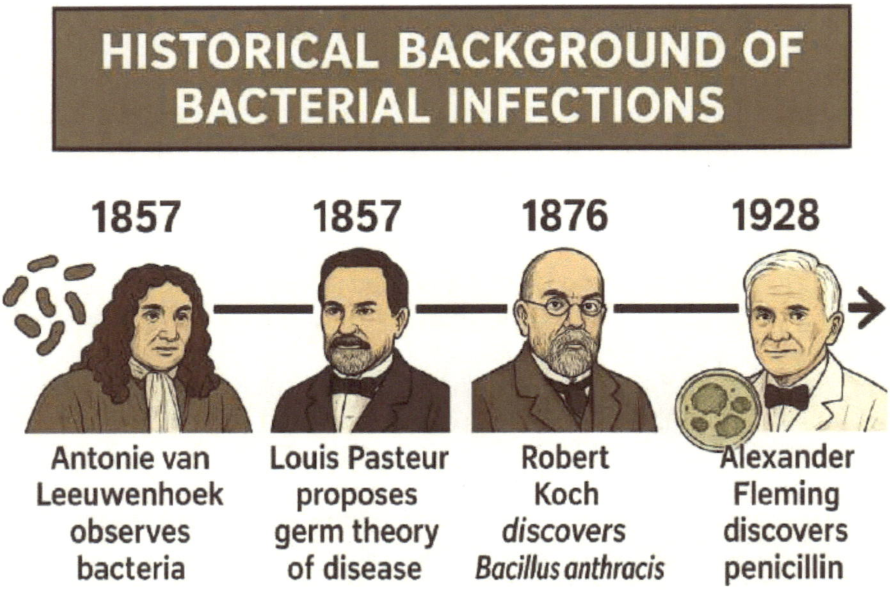
HISTORICAL BACKGROUND OF BACTERIAL INFECTIONS
1857
1857
1876
1928
Antonie van Leeuwenhoek observes bacteria
Louis Pasteur proposes germ theory of disease
Robert Koch discovers *Bacillus anthracis*
Alexander Fleming discovers penicillin

Fig. (2). Historical background of bacterial infections.

Early Understanding of Disease and Infections

The concept of infection as we understand it today did not exist in ancient times. Diseases were often attributed to imbalances in the body's humours, supernatural forces, or divine punishment. Nevertheless, early evidence from ancient cultures hinted that some illnesses could be contagious. For instance, in Ancient Egypt and Mesopotamia, early records describe various symptoms of illnesses, some likely caused by bacterial infections such as leprosy and tuberculosis [17]. Although the natural causes of these diseases were unknown, references to infections and their treatments can be found in the Ebers Papyrus, dating back to approximately 1550 BCE. In ancient Greece, Hippocrates (circa 460–370 BCE) developed the humoral theory, which proposed that sickness resulted from an imbalance among the four bodily humours: blood, phlegm, yellow bile, and black bile. This framework dominated medical thinking for many years and did not recognise the role of microorganisms in causing illness. Later, the Roman physician Galen (129–216 CE) expanded on the humoral theory in his extensive writings, documenting a wide range of diseases, including infections. Although he was unable to identify microorganisms, his work laid important foundations for future medical research [18].

The Middle Ages: Plagues and Pandemics

Devastating pandemics plagued the Middle Ages, with bacterial illnesses being a common culprit. A large number of death was caused by a lack of knowledge about these infections and how to stop their spread [19].

- **The Justinian Plague (541–542):** The Yersinia pestis-caused epidemic devastated the Byzantine Empire, killing millions of people and hastening its fall. It was among the first bacterial pandemics ever documented.
- **The Black Death (1347-1351 CE)**: The Black Death, arguably the most notorious bacterial epidemic, was likewise brought on by Yersinia pestis and ravaged most of Europe, killing between 25 and 30 million people—nearly a third of the continent's population. The epidemic had a significant impact on European society and caused turmoil in the social, ecclesiastical, and economic spheres [20].
- **Leprosy (Hansen's Disease)**: Leprosy, caused by *Mycobacterium leprae*, was common throughout Europe during the Middle Ages. Because it was so stigmatised, it was common to build leper colonies, which kept affected individuals away from the general public. Many times, the illness was misinterpreted as a punishment for wrongdoing.

The Renaissance and the Birth of Microbiology

The Renaissance brought renewed interest in science and medicine, setting the stage for significant advances in our understanding of bacterial infections [21 - 23].

- **Girolamo Fracastoro (1478-1553)**: The "germ theory" of sickness was put out by Italian scholar and physician Fracastoro in his book *De Contagione et Contagiosis Morbis (1546)*. Before the term "microorganisms" was coined, he proposed that illnesses were produced by unseen particles, or "seeds," that could travel from person to person.

- **The Invention of the Microscope**: Zacharias Janssen's invention of the microscope in the late 16th century and Antonie van Leeuwenhoek's subsequent improvement of it in the 17th century transformed the study of microbes. The earliest reported sighting of bacteria occurred in 1676 when Leeuwenhoek made his observations of "animalcules," as they are now called, but their function in illness was not then recognised.

The 19th Century: Germ Theory and Medical Advances

The 19th century was a turning point in the understanding of bacterial infections with the concrete development of the germ theory of disease and the identification of individual pathogens [24, 25].

Louis Pasteur (1822-1895): Louis Pasteur made groundbreaking contributions to the germ theory of disease, particularly through experiments he conducted in the mid-19th century. He demonstrated that microbes were responsible for fermentation and food spoilage, and he proposed that similar microorganisms could cause disease in humans. His work laid the foundation for modern microbiology and led to the development of several vaccines, most notably the rabies vaccine.

Robert Koch (1843-1910): While humidity was a factor in the 1878 flu epidemic in London, the work by German scientist Robert Koch shifted thoughts about disease and ecology. He identified the causative agents of many infectious diseases, including *Vibrio cholerae* (the bacterium that causes cholera), *Mycobacterium tuberculosis* (the bacterium that causes tuberculosis), and *Bacillus anthracis* (the bacterium that causes anthrax). He developed a series of techniques that allowed the isolation of the bacteria responsible for these diseases in a pure culture. Although infectious disease research is rooted in Koch's postulates, a group of criteria used to determine the cause of an illness by identifying microbes.

Joseph Lister (1827-1912): By sterilising surgical instruments and dressings with carbolic acid (phenol), Lister developed the first antiseptic surgery, significantly reducing postoperative infection rates. His work is the basis of the germ theory and revolutionised surgical practice.

Modern Challenges and Future Directions

The fight against bacterial infections continues into the 21st century, bringing new challenges and opportunities. Emerging and re-emerging infections have become a significant concern, with new forms of well-known bacterial diseases such as *Mycobacterium tuberculosis* and *Vibrio cholerae* appearing, often showing increased resistance to existing treatments [26]. Additionally, other pathogens like

Borrelia burgdorferi, responsible for Lyme disease, and *Legionella pneumophila*, which causes Legionnaires' disease, have become more prominent. Vaccine development remains a crucial tool in preventing bacterial infections; highly effective vaccines exist against pathogens such as *Streptococcus pneumoniae*, *Neisseria meningitidis*, and *Haemophilus influenzae* type b (Hib), significantly reducing the incidence of these diseases [27]. Researchers continue to develop vaccines for other bacterial infections. Alongside vaccines, phage therapy by using viruses that specifically target bacteria is gaining renewed interest, especially as some bacterial strains develop resistance to antibiotics. Advances in genomics and proteomics have greatly enhanced our understanding of bacterial pathogenesis, resistance mechanisms, and host-pathogen interactions, revolutionising how bacterial diseases are analysed [28]. These technological breakthroughs may pave the way for new treatments, vaccines, and diagnostic tools. On a broader scale, global health initiatives focus on reducing bacterial diseases by improving antibiotic availability, vaccination coverage, and sanitation in low- and middle-income countries [29]. The history of bacterial infections illustrates the ongoing struggle between humans and microorganisms. Despite significant progress in understanding and treating bacterial diseases, emerging challenges like antibiotic resistance underscore the need for continued vigilance, innovative solutions, and international cooperation in combating bacterial infections [30].

Major Types of Bacterial Infections

Respiratory Infections

These infections (acute respiratory and chronic obstructive airways) account for a significant primary health problem in the respiratory tract. They are caused by multiple pathogens, including bacteria, viruses, and, very rarely, fungi.. URTIs, such as sinusitis and a typical cold, stem from infections by viruses [31]. LRTIs typically manifest in the form of pneumonia and bronchitis, are predominantly bacterial infections, and tend to be even more severe. The typical symptoms, most of which are non-specific to TB and indistinguishable from those caused by other diseases (*e.g.,* asthma), include fever, dyspnea, chronic cough (> three weeks), and chest discomfort (or pain). TB is caused by *Mycobacterium tuberculosis*. It is a severe disease that primarily involves the lungs, but it can be fatal if not treated properly. *Streptococcus pneumoniae* (known as the pneumococci) is a significant cause of pneumonia. Likewise, seasonal influenza and respiratory syncytial virus (RSV) can cause severe disease, especially in high-risk groups, including the elderly or young children [32].

Gastrointestinal Infections

Similarly, the digestive system is influenced by pathogenic agents, which give rise to gastrointestinal infections or illnesses in the human body and manifest as vomiting, diarrhoea, nausea, and abdominal pain. A variety of organisms, including viruses, parasites, and bacteria, can cause these diseases. Examples of bacterial causes include pathogens like *Salmonella, Escherichia coli (E. coli),* and *Campylobacter* [33]. Though *E. Coli* sicknesses can come from rare meat or tainted fruits and veggies, Salmonella is often related to processed foods or drinkable water. Campylobacter is the most common cause of food poisoning, and raw chicken is a primary culprit. These bacterial infections can cause severe gastroenteritis and, in rare cases, dehydration and systemic disease. Rotaviruses and noroviruses are known to have the ability to elicit gastrointestinal problems. Noroviruses are a leading cause of community-acquired outbreaks of gastroenteritis, particularly in densely populated settings such as schools and cruise ships [34].

Rotaviruses are the leading cause of severe diarrhoea in infants and young children. Digestive system pathogens cause gastrointestinal infections, a group of primarily mild diseases such as diarrhoea, vomiting, nausea, and abdominal discomfort. More than 180 different kinds of bacteria, viruses, and parasites can cause a wide range of diseases, many of which are prevented by vaccines [35].

Bacterial Causes: Pathogens like *Salmonella, E. coli*, and *Campylobacter* cause contamination of food items. Where *E. Coli* can come from undercooked meats or contaminated produce, Salmonella is more often associated with contaminated food or water. Campylobacter is usually found on raw chicken. This bacterial infection, *e.g.,Salmonella typhi* infections and other *E. coli* O157:H7 infections, then cause severe gastroenteritis, dehydration, and, in extreme cases, even systemic disease. Another virus that can result in gastroenteritis is rotaviruses and noroviruses. Noroviruses cause the majority of viral epidemics of gastroenteritis and are a significant concern, particularly in settings such as schools and onboard cruise ships. It mainly impacts infants and young kids and is one of the leading causes of severe diarrhoea [36].

Skin and Soft Tissue Infections

Infections of the skin, subcutaneous tissues, fascia, and muscles are collectively referred to as skin and soft tissue infections (SSTIs). Minor superficial infections like impetigo and severe and potentially life-threatening diseases such as necrotising fasciitis SSTIs are often attributable to bacteria, including *Streptococcus pyogenes* and *Staphylococcus aureus* (particularly methicillin-resistant strains; MRSA). Immigrants aligned with the GOP have declared immigration to be a significant health care issue in the current Trumpian era due to increased cases of infection site symptoms like redness, warmth, swelling, and pain, as well as fever. Treatment, in many cases, includes the use of antibiotics, and if there is tissue that has died or become diseased, often, surgery to remove it will be required. Successful control of SSTIs calls for timely medical attention, proper wound care, and hygiene [37, 38].

Systemic Infections

These forms are excessively powerful and spread throughout the body as opposed to one part, affecting multiple places in organs, systems, or tissues throughout the body, often termed systemic infections. Many of the same organisms that can cause pneumonia can cause lung abscesses; however, among the more common pathogens are *Staphylococcus aureus, Streptococcus pneumoniae*, and Plasmodium species, along with other bacteria, viruses, fungi, and parasites [39]. The resulting systemic inflammatory response syndrome (SIRS) can lead to a "cytokine storm" and septicemia or sepsis, which may cause tissue damage, organ failure, and death. Specific clinical symptoms will differ according to the pathogen and organs involved, but fever, chills, weakness, autonomic instability with tachycardia, and hypotension are usual. Blood cultures, inflammatory markers, and imaging scans are used in the diagnosis. In the case of sepsis, immediate administration of the appropriate antimicrobial agents, intravenous fluids (IVFs), and supportive care is required. Identification and treatment of systemic infections need to be made in the early stages to avoid severe consequences and improve patient outcomes [40].

Zoonotic Bacterial Infections

Zoonotic bacterial infections are illnesses caused by germs that live in animals and can infect people. These diseases carry high morbidity and mortality rates and, therefore, a considerable public health burden. Zoonotic bacteria are naturally present in many animals, such as pets, domestic livestock, and wildlife. In humans, the bacteria can cause disease *via* direct contact with infected animals, consumption of contaminated food or water, or inhalation of aerosolised particles. Humans can also be affected by ticks (mainly *Ixodes* spp.), fleas, and mosquitoes [41]. Typically, we think of food when discussing these types of diseases since some are spread through contaminated food products like *Salmonella*. This zoonotic bacterial infection causes gastrointestinal illness in humans and is one of the most well-known.

A classic example would be the *Brucella* virus, which belongs to the *Brucella* species and spreads *via* consumption of unpasteurized dairy products or through direct contact with infected animals. The disease's symptoms include fatigue, fever, and joint pain. A leptospirosis infection can also be contracted from an animal's urine, which contaminates drinking water, which is another zoonotic infection. It causes anything from a mild flu-like illness to severe diseases such as meningitis or kidney damage [42].

A well-known zoonotic bacterium that causes plague is *Yersinia pestis*. It has the potential to cause pandemics and remains a sporadic source, particularly in regions with poor control of rodents. Transmission occurs in humans primarily by the bite of fleas that have fed on a rodent's infected blood [43]. Some people get one of three types of plague: pneumonic, septicemic, and bubonic. The most severe type of plague is pneumonic because it can be passed from person to person. Another zoonotic disease that can be transmitted by coming into contact with infected animals or their products, such as wool or skins, is called anthrax, which is caused by Bacillus anthracis. It causes gastrointestinal, lung, and skin infections depending on the entry point of the anthrax [44].

Another more infamous zoonotic bacterium is *Yersinia pestis*, which causes the plague and is famously responsible for pandemics throughout history, as well as contemporary outbreaks in areas of poor management of rodent populations. Rats carry fleas known to harbour plague and occasionally engage in biting that draws infected flea-related pathogens to which humans are exposed. Different types of plagues may occur, including bubonic plague, septicemic plague, and severe pneumonic plague, which can be transmitted from person to person. Anthrax is another infectious disease that occurs when the bacterium *Bacillus anthracis* infects the host. Animals or their products, such as wool or skins, can be contaminated; diseases spread through physical contact and produce gastrointestinal, respiratory, or skin infections, depending on the point of entry [45]. Additional information on bacterial infections, categorising them according to their respective modes of transmission and relevant clinical or public health notes, is presented in Table **1**.

Table 1. Additional information on bacterial infections, categorising them according to their respective modes of transmission and relevant clinical or public health notes.

Bacterial Infection	Category	Causative Agent	Mode of Transmission	Additional Notes	References
Pneumonia	Respiratory Infection	*Streptococcus pneumoniae*, *Haemophilus influenzae*	Droplets (coughing, sneezing)	Joint infections in older people and immunocompromised individuals; it can also be caused by viruses or fungi.	[46]

(Table 1) cont.....

Bacterial Infection	Category	Causative Agent	Mode of Transmission	Additional Notes	References
Tuberculosis	Respiratory Infection	*Mycobacterium tuberculosis*	Airborne droplets	Chronic disease can remain latent and reactivated; it primarily affects the lungs but can spread systemically.	[47]
Strep Throat	Respiratory Infection	*Streptococcus pyogenes*	Droplets (coughing, sneezing)	Highly contagious, it can lead to complications like rheumatic fever if untreated.	[48]
Urinary Tract Infection (UTI)	Urinary Tract Infection	*Escherichia coli*	Ascending infection from the urethra	It often affects women due to a shorter urethra; it can lead to kidney infections if untreated.	[49]
Meningitis	Central Nervous System	*Neisseria meningitidis*, *Streptococcus pneumoniae*	Droplets (close contact), blood-borne	Rapidly progressing; can be fatal if not treated promptly; vaccines are available for some types.	[50]
Gonorrhea	Sexually Transmitted Disease	*Neisseria gonorrhoeae*	Sexual contact	Often asymptomatic in women, it can lead to pelvic inflammatory disease (PID) and infertility.	[51]
Syphilis	Sexually Transmitted Disease	*Treponema pallidum*	Sexual contact	Multi-stage disease can affect multiple organ systems; congenital syphilis can occur during pregnancy.	[52]
Chlamydia	Sexually Transmitted Disease	*Chlamydia trachomatis*	Sexual contact	The most common bacterial STD, often asymptomatic, can lead to PID and infertility in women.	[53]
Cholera	Gastrointestinal Infection	*Vibrio cholera*	Contaminated water or food	It causes severe dehydration due to watery diarrhoea, which is common in areas with poor sanitation.	[54]

(Table 1) cont.....

Bacterial Infection	Category	Causative Agent	Mode of Transmission	Additional Notes	References
Salmonellosis	Gastrointestinal Infection	*Salmonella* spp.	Contaminated food or water	Often linked to undercooked poultry or eggs, it can cause gastroenteritis or a more severe systemic infection.	[55]
Lyme Disease	Vector-borne Disease	*Borrelia burgdorferi*	Tick bites	Transmitted by deer ticks; can cause chronic joint, neurological, and cardiac issues if untreated.	[56]
Rocky Mountain Spotted Fever	Vector-borne Disease	*Rickettsia rickettsii*	Tick bites	It can be severe or fatal if not treated early. Symptoms include a rash, fever, and a history of tick bites.	[57]
Botulism	Toxin-mediated Infection	*Clostridium botulinum*	Contaminated food (toxins)	Causes flaccid paralysis, associated with improperly canned foods; can be fatal without treatment.	[58]
Tetanus	Toxin-mediated Infection	*Clostridium tetani*	Wound contamination with spores	It causes muscle stiffness and spasms, is vaccine-preventable, and is common in unvaccinated individuals.	[59]
Anthrax	Zoonotic Infection	*Bacillus anthracis*	Contact with infected animals or products	It can present as cutaneous, inhalational, or gastrointestinal; inhalational anthrax is often fatal without treatment.	[60]
Plague	Zoonotic Infection	*Yersinia pestis*	Flea bites, respiratory droplets (pneumonic)	Historically known as the "Black Death," it is still present in some regions. The pneumonic form is highly contagious.	[61]

(Table 1) cont.....

Bacterial Infection	Category	Causative Agent	Mode of Transmission	Additional Notes	References
Diphtheria	Respiratory Infection	*Corynebacterium diphtheriae*	Droplets (coughing, sneezing), contact	Produces a toxin that can cause respiratory obstruction; vaccine-preventable; often fatal if untreated.	[62]
Typhoid Fever	Gastrointestinal Infection	*Salmonella typhi*	Contaminated food or water	Systemic infection causes prolonged fever and abdominal pain, which are common in areas with poor sanitation.	[63]
Whooping Cough (Pertussis)	Respiratory Infection	*Bordetella pertussis*	Droplets (coughing, sneezing)	Characterised by severe coughing fits; vaccine-preventable; particularly dangerous for infants.	[64]
Leprosy (Hansen's Disease)	Chronic Infection	*Mycobacterium leprae*	Prolonged close contact, respiratory droplets	It affects skin, nerves, and mucous membranes; it can cause disfigurement, which is treatable with antibiotics.	[65]
Legionnaires' Disease	Respiratory Infection	*Legionella pneumophila*	Inhalation of contaminated water droplets	Often associated with cooling towers and hot tubs, it can cause severe pneumonia.	[66]
Brucellosis	Zoonotic Infection	*Brucella* spp.	Contact with infected animals or products, ingestion	It causes fever, joint pain, and fatigue; it can be chronic and is an occupational risk for farmers and veterinarians.	[67]
Listeriosis	Gastrointestinal Infection	*Listeria monocytogenes*	Contaminated food	It can cause severe illness in pregnant women, newborns, the elderly, and immunocompromised individuals.	[68]
Shigellosis	Gastrointestinal Infection	*Shigella* spp.	Contaminated food or water, or person-to-person contact	It causes severe diarrhoea, often with blood; it is highly contagious and common in settings with poor sanitation.	[69]

(Table 1) cont.....

Bacterial Infection	Category	Causative Agent	Mode of Transmission	Additional Notes	References
Psittacosis	Zoonotic Infection	*Chlamydia psittaci*	Inhalation of dust from bird droppings	Also known as parrot fever, it can cause pneumonia and occupational risk for bird handlers.	[70]
Tularemia	Zoonotic Infection	*Francisella tularensis*	Tick bites, contact with infected animals, and inhalation	Also known as rabbit fever, it can be severe or fatal; it is a potential bioterrorism agent.	[71]
Necrotizing Fasciitis	Skin and Soft Tissue Infection	*Streptococcus pyogenes* (Group A), *Clostridium* spp., *Vibrio vulnificus*	Wound contamination, person-to-person contact	Rapidly progressing soft tissue infection often requires surgical intervention and has a high mortality rate.	[72]
Q Fever	Zoonotic Infection	*Coxiella burnetiid*	Inhalation of contaminated dust	Common in farm environments, it can cause flu-like symptoms or chronic disease affecting the heart.	[73]
Melioidosis	Zoonotic Infection	*Burkholderia pseudomallei*	Contact with contaminated water or soil	Endemic in Southeast Asia and Northern Australia can cause pneumonia, abscesses, or sepsis.	[74]
Bacterial Vaginosis	Genital Infection	*Gardnerella vaginalis*, *Atopobium vaginae*, others	Disruption of normal vaginal flora	A common cause of vaginal discharge, associated with an imbalance of bacteria; is not sexually transmitted.	[75]

MECHANISMS OF BACTERIAL PATHOGENICITY

The term "bacterial pathogenicity" describes a bacterium's capacity to infect a host organism and cause illness. This intricate process entails several interactions between the bacteria and the host, starting with the initial invasion and continuing through colonisation, immune defence evasion, and harm inflicted by a variety of mechanisms. It is essential to comprehend these pathways to create efficient therapies and prophylactic measures against bacterial infections [76].

Pathogenesis Overview

Several crucial processes are involved in pathogenesis, such as the bacteria's entrance into the host, attachment to host tissues, colonisation, and eventual invasion and destruction of host tissues [77].

Entry Points for Bacteria

Bacteria can enter the human body through various routes, each providing access to different tissues and organs. The skin serves as the body's first line of defence against microbial invasion; however, breaches in the skin barrier, such as scrapes, abrasions, insect bites, or surgical wounds, can allow bacteria to penetrate and cause infections [78]. For example, *Staphylococcus aureus* can enter through skin wounds and lead to conditions like cellulitis, impetigo, or abscesses. The respiratory tract is another common entry point, especially for airborne pathogens. Respiratory infections include diseases caused by *Bordetella pertussis*, which leads to whooping cough, *Mycobacterium tuberculosis,* the agent of tuberculosis, and *Streptococcus pneumoniae,* responsible for bacterial pneumonia [79]. Bacteria can also enter via the gastrointestinal tract when contaminated food or drink is ingested. This can result in infections caused by *Vibrio cholerae, Salmonella, Shigella,* or *Escherichia coli*, often presenting with symptoms such as vomiting, diarrhoea, and abdominal pain [80]. The urogenital tract is a key route for bacteria responsible for sexually transmitted infections (STIs) and urinary tract infections. Notable examples include *Neisseria gonorrhoeae* and *Chlamydia trachomatis*, which colonise the mucosal surfaces of the genital tract [81]. Finally, mucous membranes covering openings like the lips, nostrils, conjunctiva, and genitalia allow bacteria to enter more freely. A classic example is *Neisseria meningitidis*, which can invade through the nasopharyngeal mucosa and cause meningitis.

Colonisation and Adherence to Host Tissues

To establish an infection, bacteria must first adhere to and colonise host tissues through a multi-step process. Initially, bacteria use specialized structures such as adhesins, fimbriae, and pili to attach to specific receptors on host cell surfaces [82]. For example, uropathogenic *Escherichia coli* (UPEC) employs pili to bind to the epithelial cells of the urinary tract, leading to urinary tract infections (UTIs). Following adherence, some bacteria form biofilm communities of bacteria embedded within a protective extracellular matrix [83]. These biofilms enhance bacterial survival by shielding the bacteria from immune defences and antibiotics. A notable example is *Pseudomonas aeruginosa* biofilms that develop in the lungs of cystic fibrosis patients, causing persistent and chronic infections [84]. Once attached and protected, bacteria multiply and spread across the affected area in a phase called colonisation. Successful colonisation requires bacteria to outcompete the normal microbiota, secure essential nutrients, and evade the host's immune responses. *Helicobacter pylori* exemplifies this by infecting the stomach lining, where it neutralises stomach acid and escapes immune detection, resulting in conditions such as peptic ulcers and chronic gastritis [85].

Virulence Factors

Virulence factors are chemicals generated by bacteria that enhance their potential to cause illness. These factors accelerate bacterial invasion, induce immune evasion, and cause harm to host tissues [86].

Toxins

Bacterial toxins are some of the most effective virulence agents. They are roughly divided into endotoxins and exotoxins [87 - 90].

Endotoxins, or lipopolysaccharides, are components of Gram-negative bacteria's outer membrane. They are typically generated after bacterial cell lysis and cause a significant immunological response, resulting in inflammation, fever, and septic shock in extreme instances. Bacteria that create endotoxins include *Escherichia coli, Salmonella* spp., and *Neisseria meningitidis*. Exotoxins are proteins released by Gram-positive and Gram-negative bacteria that can harm specific organs in the host. These toxins are categorised according to the type of tissue they affect. *Clostridium botulinum*, for example, produces neurotoxins through the secretion of botulinum toxin. This toxin suppresses neurotransmitter release, causing flaccid paralysis. Cytotoxins, like the diphtheria toxin generated by *Corynebacterium diphtheriae*, prevent protein synthesis in host cells, resulting in cell death and tissue damage. *Vibrio cholerae* produces cholera toxin, which falls under the group of enterotoxins. This toxin affects ion transport in intestinal cells, resulting in severe diarrhoea.

Enzymes that Facilitate Invasion

Bacteria create a variety of enzymes that help them invade host tissues and propagate illness [91 - 93]. Often referred to as the “spreading factor,” hyaluronidase degrades hyaluronic acid, a significant component of the extracellular matrix, allowing germs to enter deeper tissues. *Streptococcus pyogenes* employs hyaluronidase to propagate through connective tissues. *Staphylococcus aureus* generates coagulase, an enzyme that causes blood clotting. The ensuing clot assists bacteria in evading immune identification by “hiding” within it, allowing it to create a localised infection, such as an abscess. *Clostridium perfringens* produces collagenase, which destroys collagen, a structural protein in connective tissues, allowing infection to spread more quickly. Streptokinase and Staphylokinase are enzymes generated by *Streptococcus* and *Staphylococcus* species. They break blood clots, allowing bacteria to escape the host's defence mechanism.

Evasion of the Immune System

Successful viruses have developed a variety of tactics to avoid the host's immune system [94 - 97]. Bacteria like *Streptococcus pneumoniae* and *Haemophilus influenzae* develop polysaccharide capsules that prevent immune cells from identifying and engulfing them. The capsule also inhibits complement activation, hence increasing bacterial survivability. Bacteria can change their surface proteins to avoid immune detection. *Neisseria gonorrhoeae* exploits antigenic variation to alter the shape of its pili, allowing it to elude immune identification and remain in the host. Certain bacteria may live and increase inside host cells, bypassing extracellular immune defences. Mycobacterium TB lives in macrophages by blocking the fusion of phagosomes and lysosomes, allowing it to remain dormant for years. Bacteria, including *Neisseria meningitidis* and *Haemophilus influenzae*, produce IgA protease, an enzyme that cleaves the mucosal antibodies of the IgA class. This allows germs to better colonise mucosal surfaces by destroying these antibodies.

Host-Pathogen Interactions

It is an interplay between host elements and pathogen components, which dictates the fate of infection. The immune system of the host attacks and eliminates invasive germs, and the bacteria use a variety of means for survival and reproduction [98].

Immune Response to Bacterial Infections

The immunological response to bacterial infections includes both the innate and adaptive immune systems [99 - 101]. The innate immune system works as a first responder against bacterial infections. This includes physical barriers such as skin and mucous membranes, as well as an army of specifically targeted immune cells such as neutrophils, macrophages, and dendritic cells. When bacteria invade the body, the pattern recognition receptors (PRRs) of immune cells recognise pathogen-associated molecular patterns (PAMPs) like lipopolysaccharides (LPS) and peptidoglycan. This leads to the detection of small particles recognised by PRRs on both cells, resulting in phagocytosis, an inflammatory response (producing cytokines and chemokines) that causes the recruitment of immune cells. In adaptive immune response, bacterial infections give rise to a more targeted and longer-lasting response by the adaptive immune system. Crucial players in this are B and T lymphocytes. B cells produce antigen-specific antibodies that act to neutralise, opsonise, and/or generate complement activation against specific bacterial antigens. Cytotoxic T lymphocytes, specifically, recognise and kill infected cells; helper T cells stimulate other immune cell functions.

Inflammatory Response and Cytokine Release

The inflammatory response is also an essential part of the immune system's defence against bacterial infections. Its unique characteristics include the generation of pro-inflammatory cytokines, more blood flow to the area, and the attraction of immune cells to these areas [102].

Cytokine signalling molecules modulate immunological response. In bacterial infections, immune cells are confronted with cytokines, including TNF-α, IL-1, and IL-6, induced by bacterial endotoxins. Cytokines can also initiate other immune cells, increase inflammation, *etc*. Although the immune response is required to control a bacterial infection, an uncontrolled release of cytokines can cause a life-threatening condition called a cytokine storm, which leads to tissue inflammation and septic shock [103]. Inflammation is the body's reaction to infection or damage, marked by redness, heat, swelling, discomfort, and loss of function. It tries to identify and remove the invading germs while also starting tissue restoration. However, prolonged or severe inflammation can cause tissue damage and contribute to the development of disorders like sepsis [104].

Bacterial Strategies to Overcome Host Defences

Bacteria must overcome the host's immunological defences to infect it successfully. They use a variety of techniques to dodge, undermine, or influence the immune system. Bacteria such as Staphylococcus aureus create proteins that disrupt the phagocytosis process. Protein A, for example, binds to antibodies' Fc regions, preventing phagocytes from recognising them and limiting opsonisation [105].

CONCLUSION

Significant progress has been made in understanding bacterial infections, shedding light on mechanisms of pathogenesis, host-pathogen interactions, and antimicrobial resistance. Advances in molecular biology have facilitated the development of targeted drugs and vaccines, while improved diagnostic tools enable earlier and more accurate detection of bacterial diseases. However, the rise of antimicrobial resistance and the persistence of multidrug-resistant bacteria present ongoing challenges. Complications such as biofilm formation, global travel-related spread, and complex host-pathogen dynamics continue to hinder effective treatment and control of bacterial infections worldwide.

FUTURE PERSPECTIVES

Looking ahead, the future of bacterial infection research lies in innovative strategies to combat these challenges. The development of novel antibiotics and alternative therapies, including bacteriophages and antimicrobial peptides, will be critical in addressing resistance. Personalized medicine, driven by advances in genetics and bioinformatics, promises tailored treatments that improve patient outcomes. Enhanced vaccination strategies targeting resistant strains and strengthened international collaboration for surveillance and data sharing will be essential for global health security. Furthermore, expanding our understanding of the human microbiome may unlock new therapeutic avenues. Continued research and innovation are imperative to stay ahead of evolving bacterial threats and safeguard public health.

REFERENCES

[1] Tortora GJ, Funke BR, Case CL. Microbiology: an introduction. 13th ed. Pearson UK; 2020 Jun 8. 2020.

[2] Goering R, Dockrell H, Zuckerman M, Roitt I, Chiodini PL. Mims' medical microbiology 5th ed. Elsevier Health Sciences 2012. Aug 29.

[3] Alberts B, Bray D, Lewis J, Raff M, Roberts K, Watson JD. Molecular biology of the cell. 4th ed. New York: Garland; 1994 Mar

[4] Donnenberg MS. Pathogenic strategies of enteric bacteria. Nature 2000; 406(6797): 768-74. [http://dx.doi.org/10.1038/35021212] [PMID: 10963606]

[5] Silhavy TJ, Kahne D, Walker S. The bacterial cell envelope. Cold Spring Harb Perspect Biol 2010; 2(5)a000414. [http://dx.doi.org/10.1101/cshperspect.a000414] [PMID: 20452953]

[6] Lemos JA, Abranches J, Burne RA. Responses of cariogenic streptococci to environmental stresses. Curr Issues Mol Biol 2005; 7(1): 95-107. [PMID: 15580782]

[7] Bhavsar AP, Guttman JA, Finlay BB. Manipulation of host-cell pathways by bacterial pathogens. Nature 2007; 449(7164): 827-34. [http://dx.doi.org/10.1038/nature06247] [PMID: 17943119]

[8] Coelho C, Bocca AL, Casadevall A. The tools for virulence of *Cryptococcus neoformans*. Adv Appl Microbiol 2014; 87: 1-41. [http://dx.doi.org/10.1016/B978-0-12-800261-2.00001-3] [PMID: 24581388]

[9] Rosenberg E, Zilber-Rosenberg I. Origin of prokaryotes and eukaryotes. In: The hologenome concept: human, animal and plant microbiota. 2013; pp. 9-22. [http://dx.doi.org/10.1007/978-3-319-04241-1_2]

[10] Schaechter M, MaalØe O, Kjeldgaard NO. Dependency on medium and temperature of cell size and chemical composition during balanced grown of *Salmonella typhimurium*. J Gen Microbiol 1958; 19(3): 592-606. [http://dx.doi.org/10.1099/00221287-19-3-592] [PMID: 13611202]

[11] Cooper S. Bacterial growth and division: biochemistry and regulation of prokaryotic and eukaryotic division cycles. Elsevier

[12] Siegele DA, Kolter R. Life after log. J Bacteriol 1992; 174(2): 345-8. [http://dx.doi.org/10.1128/jb.174.2.345-348.1992] [PMID: 1729229]

[13] Stewart PS, Franklin MJ. Physiological heterogeneity in biofilms. Nat Rev Microbiol 2008; 6(3): 199-210. [http://dx.doi.org/10.1038/nrmicro1838] [PMID: 18264116]

[14] Taheri-Araghi S, Bradde S, Sauls JT, *et al.* Cell-size control and homeostasis in bacteria. Curr Biol 2015; 25(3): 385-91. [http://dx.doi.org/10.1016/j.cub.2014.12.009] [PMID: 25544609]

[15] Lloyd GE. Magic, reason, and experience: studies in the origins and development of Greek science. Hackett Publishing 1999.

[16] Roeder P, Mariner J, Kock R. Rinderpest: the veterinary perspective on eradication. Philos Trans R Soc Lond B Biol Sci 2013; 368(1623)20120139. [http://dx.doi.org/10.1098/rstb.2012.0139] [PMID: 23798687]

[17] Aw D, Silva AB, Palmer DB. Immunosenescence: emerging challenges for an ageing population. Immunology 2007; 120(4): 435-46. [http://dx.doi.org/10.1111/j.1365-2567.2007.02555.x] [PMID: 17313487]

[18] Talisuna AO, Bloland P, D'Alessandro U. History, dynamics, and public health importance of malaria parasite resistance. Clin Microbiol Rev 2004; 17(1): 235-54. [http://dx.doi.org/10.1128/CMR.17.1.235-254.2004] [PMID: 14726463]

[19] Patz JA, Epstein PR, Burke TA, Balbus JM. Global climate change and emerging infectious diseases. JAMA 1996; 275(3): 217-23. [http://dx.doi.org/10.1001/jama.1996.03530270057032] [PMID: 8604175]

[20] Tatem AJ, Gething PW, Smith DL, Hay SI. Urbanization and the global malaria recession. Malar J 2013; 12(1): 133. [http://dx.doi.org/10.1186/1475-2875-12-133] [PMID: 23594701]

[21] Mahmud AS, Metcalf CJE, Grenfell BT. Comparative dynamics, seasonality in transmission, and predictability of childhood infections in Mexico. Epidemiol Infect 2017; 145(3): 607-25. [http://dx.doi.org/10.1017/S0950268816002673] [PMID: 27873563]

[22] Earn DJD, Rohani P, Bolker BM, Grenfell BT. A simple model for complex dynamical transitions in epidemics. Science 2000; 287(5453): 667-70. [http://dx.doi.org/10.1126/science.287.5453.667] [PMID: 10650003]

[23] Ferrari MJ, Grenfell BT, Strebel PM. Think globally, act locally: the role of local demographics and vaccination coverage in the dynamic response of measles infection to control. Philos Trans R Soc Lond B Biol Sci 2013; 368(1623)20120141. [http://dx.doi.org/10.1098/rstb.2012.0141] [PMID: 23798689]

[24] Zhou P, Shi ZL. SARS-CoV-2 spillover events. Science 2021; 371(6525): 120-2. [http://dx.doi.org/10.1126/science.abf6097] [PMID: 33414206]

[25] Kwan CK, Ernst JD. HIV and tuberculosis: a deadly human syndemic. Clin Microbiol Rev 2011; 24(2): 351-76. [http://dx.doi.org/10.1128/CMR.00042-10] [PMID: 21482729]

[26] Mahmud AS, Martinez PP, He J, Baker RE. The impact of climate change on vaccine-preventable diseases: insights from current research and new directions. Curr Environ Health Rep 2020; 7(4): 384-91. [http://dx.doi.org/10.1007/s40572-020-00293-2] [PMID: 33099754]

[27] Baker RE, Yang W, Vecchi GA, Metcalf CJE, Grenfell BT. Assessing the influence of climate on

wintertime SARS-CoV-2 outbreaks. Nat Commun 2021; 12(1): 846.
[http://dx.doi.org/10.1038/s41467-021-20991-1] [PMID: 33558479]

[28] Viboud C, Alonso WJ, Simonsen L. Influenza in tropical regions. PLoS Med 2006; 3(4)e89.
[http://dx.doi.org/10.1371/journal.pmed.0030089] [PMID: 16509764]

[29] Ciencewicki J, Jaspers I. Air pollution and respiratory viral infection. Inhal Toxicol 2007; 19(14): 1135-46.
[http://dx.doi.org/10.1080/08958370701665434] [PMID: 17987465]

[30] Bell ML, Ebisu K. Environmental inequality in exposures to airborne particulate matter components in the United States. Environ Health Perspect 2012; 120(12): 1699-704.
[http://dx.doi.org/10.1289/ehp.1205201] [PMID: 22889745]

[31] Casadevall A, Kontoyiannis DP, Robert V. On the emergence of *Candida auris*: climate change, azoles, swamps, and birds. MBio 2019; 10(4)e01397-19.
[http://dx.doi.org/10.1128/mBio.01397-19] [PMID: 31337723]

[32] Rocklöv J, Dubrow R. Author Correction: Climate change: an enduring challenge for vector-borne disease prevention and control. Nat Immunol 2020; 21(6): 695.
[http://dx.doi.org/10.1038/s41590-020-0692-7] [PMID: 32350458]

[33] Hales S, de Wet N, Maindonald J, Woodward A. Potential effect of population and climate changes on global distribution of dengue fever: an empirical model. Lancet 2002; 360(9336): 830-4.
[http://dx.doi.org/10.1016/S0140-6736(02)09964-6] [PMID: 12243917]

[34] Couper LI, MacDonald AJ, Mordecai EA. Impact of prior and projected climate change on US Lyme disease incidence. Glob Change Biol 2021; 27(4): 738-54.
[http://dx.doi.org/10.1111/gcb.15435] [PMID: 33150704]

[35] Ryan SJ, Lippi CA, Zermoglio F. Shifting transmission risk for malaria in Africa with climate change: a framework for planning and intervention. Malar J 2020; 19(1): 170.
[http://dx.doi.org/10.1186/s12936-020-03224-6] [PMID: 32357890]

[36] Crépey P, Barthélemy M. Detecting robust patterns in the spread of epidemics: a case study of influenza in the United States and France. Am J Epidemiol 2007; 166(11): 1244-51.
[http://dx.doi.org/10.1093/aje/kwm266] [PMID: 17938424]

[37] Mordecai EA, Caldwell JM, Grossman MK, *et al.* Thermal biology of mosquito-borne disease. Ecol Lett 2019; 22(10): 1690-708.
[http://dx.doi.org/10.1111/ele.13335] [PMID: 31286630]

[38] Benenson AS, Ed. Control of communicable diseases manual. Washington, DC: American Public Health Association 1995.

[39] Detels R, McEwen J, Beaglehole J, Tanaka H, Eds. Oxford textbook of public health. Oxford, UK: Oxford University Press 2002.

[40] Evans AS, Brachman PS, Eds. Bacterial infections of humans: epidemiology and control. New York: Plenum Publishing Corporation 1998.
[http://dx.doi.org/10.1007/978-1-4615-5327-4]

[41] Engleberg NC, DiRita V, Dermody TS. Schaechter's mechanisms of microbial disease. Baltimore, MD: Lippincott Williams and Wilkins 2007.

[42] Bannister BA, Begg NT, Gillespie SH, Eds. Structure and classification of pathogens. (Infectious Disease) Chapter 2. 2nd ed. Oxford, UK: : Blackwell Science Ltd 1996; pp. 23-4.

[43] Engelkirk PG, Burton GR, Eds. Epidemiology and public health. (Burton's Microbiology for the Health Sciences) Chapter 11. 8th ed., Baltimore: Lippincott Williams and Wilkins 2006.

[44] Luby SP, Agboatwalla M, Feikin DR, *et al.* Effect of handwashing on child health: a randomised controlled trial. Lancet 2005; 366(9481): 225-33.
[http://dx.doi.org/10.1016/S0140-6736(05)66912-7] [PMID: 16023513]

[45] Mulani MS, Kamble EE, Kumkar SN, Tawre MS, Pardesi KR. Emerging strategies to combat ESKAPE pathogens in the era of antimicrobial resistance: a review. Front Microbiol 2019; 10: 539. [http://dx.doi.org/10.3389/fmicb.2019.00539] [PMID: 30988669]

[46] De Oliveira DMP, Forde BM, Kidd TJ, *et al.* Antimicrobial resistance in ESKAPE pathogens. Clin Microbiol Rev 2020; 33(3)e00181-19 [http://dx.doi.org/10.1128/CMR.00181-19] [PMID: 32404435]

[47] Breijyeh Z, Jubeh B, Karaman R. Resistance of Gram-negative bacteria to current antibacterial agents and approaches to resolve it. Molecules 2020; 25(6): 1340. [http://dx.doi.org/10.3390/molecules25061340] [PMID: 32187986]

[48] World Health Organization 2018. Available from: https://medium.com/@who/10-threats-to-global-health-in-2018-232daf0bbef32018

[49] Abdelaziz SM, Aboshanab KM, Yahia IS, Yassien MA, Hassouna NA. Correlation between the antibiotic resistance genes and susceptibility to antibiotics among the carbapenem-resistant Gram-negative pathogens. Antibiotics (Basel) 2021; 10(3): 255. [http://dx.doi.org/10.3390/antibiotics10030255] [PMID: 33806340]

[50] World Health Organization Ten threats to global health in 2019 [Accessed 2020 Dec 18] Available from: https://www.who.int/emergencies/ten-threats-to-global-health-in-2019

[51] ECDC Communicable Disease and Threats Report CDTR 2019. Available from: www.ecdc.europa.eu

[52] ECDC Biggest threats and data Available from: https://www.cdc.gov/drugresistance/pdf/threats-report/2019-ar-threats-report-508.pdf

[53] Ben Y, Fu C, Hu M, Liu L, Wong MH, Zheng C. Human health risk assessment of antibiotic resistance associated with antibiotic residues in the environment: A review. Environ Res 2019; 169: 483-93. [http://dx.doi.org/10.1016/j.envres.2018.11.040] [PMID: 30530088]

[54] Schroeder M, Brooks B, Brooks A. The complex relationship between virulence and antibiotic resistance. Genes (Basel) 2017; 8(1): 39. [http://dx.doi.org/10.3390/genes8010039] [PMID: 28106797]

[55] Pandey R, Mishra SK, Shrestha A. Characterisation of ESKAPE pathogens with special reference to multidrug resistance and biofilm production in a Nepalese hospital. Infect Drug Resist 2021; 14: 2201-12. [http://dx.doi.org/10.2147/IDR.S306688] [PMID: 34163185]

[56] Harding CM, Hennon SW, Feldman MF. Uncovering the mechanisms of *Acinetobacter baumannii* virulence. Nat Rev Microbiol 2018; 16(2): 91-102. [http://dx.doi.org/10.1038/nrmicro.2017.148] [PMID: 29249812]

[57] Kyriakidis I, Vasileiou E, Pana ZD, Tragiannidis A. *Acinetobacter baumannii* antibiotic resistance mechanisms. Pathogens 2021; 10(3): 373. [http://dx.doi.org/10.3390/pathogens10030373] [PMID: 33808905]

[58] Vrancianu CO, Gheorghe I, Czobor IB, Chifiriuc MC. Antibiotic resistance profiles, molecular mechanisms and innovative treatment strategies of *Acinetobacter baumannii*. Microorganisms 2020; 8(6): 935. [http://dx.doi.org/10.3390/microorganisms8060935] [PMID: 32575913]

[59] Mojica MF, Bonomo RA, Fast W. B1-metallo-β-lactamases: where do we stand? Curr Drug Targets 2016; 17(9): 1029-50. [http://dx.doi.org/10.2174/1389450116666151001105622] [PMID: 26424398]

[60] Principi N, Esposito S. Infectious discitis and spondylodiscitis in children. Int J Mol Sci 2016; 17(4): 539. [http://dx.doi.org/10.3390/ijms17040539] [PMID: 27070599]

[61] Di Pasquale M, Aliberti S, Mantero M, Bianchini S, Blasi F. Non-intensive care unit acquired pneumonia: A new clinical entity? Int J Mol Sci 2016; 17(3): 287.
[http://dx.doi.org/10.3390/ijms17030287] [PMID: 26927074]

[62] De Martino M. Dismantling the taboo against vaccines in pregnancy. Int J Mol Sci 2016; 17(6): 894.
[http://dx.doi.org/10.3390/ijms17060894] [PMID: 27338346]

[63] Orsi A, Ansaldi F, Trucchi C, Rosselli R, Icardi G. Pneumococcus and the elderly in Italy: A summary of available evidence regarding carriage, clinical burden of lower respiratory tract infections and on-field effectiveness of PCV13 vaccination. Int J Mol Sci 2016; 17(7): 1140.
[http://dx.doi.org/10.3390/ijms17071140] [PMID: 27428964]

[64] Shaikh S, Fatima J, Shakil S, Rizvi SMD, Kamal MA. Antibiotic resistance and extended spectrum beta-lactamases: Types, epidemiology and treatment. Saudi J Biol Sci 2015; 22(1): 90-101.
[http://dx.doi.org/10.1016/j.sjbs.2014.08.002] [PMID: 25561890]

[65] Hammoudi Halat D, Ayoub Moubareck C. The current burden of carbapenemases: review of significant properties and dissemination among Gram-negative bacteria. Antibiotics (Basel) 2020; 9(4): 186.
[http://dx.doi.org/10.3390/antibiotics9040186] [PMID: 32316342]

[66] US Centers for Disease Control and Prevention (CDC) Antibiotic resistance threats in the United States, 2013 Atlanta, GA: CDC; 2013 2013. Available from: https://www.cdc.gov/drugresistance/threat-report-2013/index.html

[67] Tigabu A, Getaneh A. *Staphylococcus aureus*, ESKAPE bacteria challenging current health care and community settings: A literature review. Clin Lab 2021; 67(07/2021): 930.
[http://dx.doi.org/10.7754/Clin.Lab.2020.200930] [PMID: 34258960]

[68] Tong SYC, Davis JS, Eichenberger E, Holland TL, Fowler VG Jr. *Staphylococcus aureus* infections: epidemiology, pathophysiology, clinical manifestations, and management. Clin Microbiol Rev 2015; 28(3): 603-61.
[http://dx.doi.org/10.1128/CMR.00134-14] [PMID: 26016486]

[69] Nicolas I, Bordeau V, Bondon A, Baudy-Floc'h M, Felden B. Novel antibiotics effective against gram-positive and -negative multi-resistant bacteria with limited resistance. PLoS Biol 2019; 17(7)e3000337.
[http://dx.doi.org/10.1371/journal.pbio.3000337] [PMID: 31287812]

[70] Kim BN, Kim ES, Oh MD. Oral antibiotic treatment of staphylococcal bone and joint infections in adults. J Antimicrob Chemother 2014; 69(2): 309-22.
[http://dx.doi.org/10.1093/jac/dkt374] [PMID: 24072167]

[71] Lewis JS II, Jorgensen JH. Inducible clindamycin resistance in Staphylococci: should clinicians and microbiologists be concerned? Clin Infect Dis 2005; 40(2): 280-5.
[http://dx.doi.org/10.1086/426894] [PMID: 15655748]

[72] Jorgensen JH, Crawford SA, McElmeel ML, Fiebelkorn KR. Detection of inducible clindamycin resistance of staphylococci in conjunction with performance of automated broth susceptibility testing. J Clin Microbiol 2004; 42(4): 1800-2.
[http://dx.doi.org/10.1128/JCM.42.4.1800-1802.2004] [PMID: 15071055]

[73] Caneiras C, Lito L, Melo-Cristino J, Duarte A. Community- and Hospital-Acquired *Klebsiella pneumoniae* Urinary Tract Infections in Portugal: Virulence and Antibiotic Resistance. Microorganisms 2019; 7(5): 138.
[http://dx.doi.org/10.3390/microorganisms7050138] [PMID: 31100810]

[74] Alenazi MM, Alshammari F, Alsuwaida K, *et al.* Clinical significance of *Klebsiella pneumoniae* producing extended-spectrum β-lactamases in hospital-acquired infections in a tertiary hospital in Saudi Arabia. Saudi J Biol Sci 2022; 29: 3247-53.
[http://dx.doi.org/10.1016/j.sjbs.2022.02.015]

[75] Aryal B, Tiwari BR, Paudel KR, Shah N, Pokharel K. Antimicrobial resistance in *Klebsiella pneumoniae*: A comprehensive review of studies conducted in Nepal. BMC Infect Dis 2022; 22: 356. [http://dx.doi.org/10.1186/s12879-022-07559-4]

[76] D'Costa VM, McGrann KM, Hughes DW, Wright GD. Sampling the antibiotic resistome. Science 2006; 311(5759): 374-7. [http://dx.doi.org/10.1126/science.1120800] [PMID: 16424339]

[77] Gillings MR. Antibiotic resistance in the human gut microbiome. Front Microbiol 2018; 9: 1-15. [http://dx.doi.org/10.3389/fmicb.2018.02242]

[78] Woolhouse M, Waugh C, Perry MR, Nair H. Global disease burden due to antibiotic resistance – state of the evidence. J Glob Health 2016; 6(1)010306 [http://dx.doi.org/10.7189/jogh.06.010306] [PMID: 27350872]

[79] Principi N, Esposito S. Antibiotic administration and the development of obesity in children. Int J Antimicrob Agents 2016; 47(3): 171-7. [http://dx.doi.org/10.1016/j.ijantimicag.2015.12.017] [PMID: 26895606]

[80] Esposito S, Bonanni P, Maggi S, *et al.* Recommended immunization schedules for adults: Clinical practice guidelines by the Escmid Vaccine Study Group (EVASG), European Geriatric Medicine Society (EUGMS) and the World Association for Infectious Diseases and Immunological Disorders (WAidid). Hum Vaccin Immunother 2016; 12(7): 1-18. [http://dx.doi.org/10.1080/21645515.2016.1150396] [PMID: 27135390]

[81] Advani SD, Thaden JT, Perez R, Stair SL, Lee UJ, Siddiqui NY. State-of-the-art review: recurrent uncomplicated urinary tract infections in women. Clinical Infectious Diseases 2025; 80(3): e31-42.

[82] Allen HK, Donato J, Wang HH, Cloud-Hansen KA, Davies J, Handelsman J. Call of the wild: antibiotic resistance genes in natural environments. Nat Rev Microbiol 2010; 8(4): 251-9. [http://dx.doi.org/10.1038/nrmicro2312] [PMID: 20190823]

[83] Hossain MT, Mondol MI, Akter A, Billah MM, Sadia A, Rahman MA. Antibiotic resistance pattern in *Escherichia coli* isolated from urinary tract infection patients. BMC Res Notes 2020; 13: 271. [http://dx.doi.org/10.1186/s13104-020-05081-1]

[84] Huang C, Kwan C, Lu D, *et al.* Antibiotic resistance and molecular typing of *Escherichia coli* in different environments in Shanghai, China. Front Microbiol 2022; 13: 1-14. [http://dx.doi.org/10.3389/fmicb.2022.871376]

[85] Gagliardi M, Fierabracci A, Pilati M, *et al.* The impact of specific viruses on clinical outcome in children presenting with acute heart failure. Int J Mol Sci 2016; 17(4): 486. [http://dx.doi.org/10.3390/ijms17040486] [PMID: 27043551]

[86] Bozzola E, Bozzola M, Krzysztofiak A, Tozzi A, El Hachem M, Villani A. Varicella skin complications in childhood: A case series and a systematic review of the literature. Int J Mol Sci 2016; 17(5): 688. [http://dx.doi.org/10.3390/ijms17050688] [PMID: 27164095]

[87] Vorsters A, Van Keer S, Biesmans S, *et al.* Long-term follow-up of HPV infection using urine and cervical quantitative HPV DNA testing. Int J Mol Sci 2016; 17(5): 750. [http://dx.doi.org/10.3390/ijms17050750] [PMID: 27196899]

[88] Focà E, Magro P, Motta D, *et al.* Screening for neurocognitive impairment in HIV-infected individuals at first contact after HIV diagnosis: The experience of a large Clinical Center in Northern Italy. Int J Mol Sci 2016; 17(4): 434. [http://dx.doi.org/10.3390/ijms17040434] [PMID: 27023519]

[89] Latronico T, Mascia C, Pati I, *et al.* Liver fibrosis in HCV monoinfected and HIV/HCV coinfected patients: Dysregulation of matrix metalloproteinases (MMPs) and their tissue inhibitors TIMPs and effect of HCV protease inhibitors. Int J Mol Sci 2016; 17(4): 455. [http://dx.doi.org/10.3390/ijms17040455] [PMID: 27023536]

[90] Rigante D, Andreozzi L, Fastiggi M, Bracci B, Natale M, Esposito S. Critical overview of the risk scoring systems to predict non-responsiveness to intravenous immunoglobulin in Kawasaki syndrome. Int J Mol Sci 2016; 17(3): 278. [http://dx.doi.org/10.3390/ijms17030278] [PMID: 26927060]

[91] Pugni L, Ronchi A, Bizzarri B, *et al.* Exchange transfusion in the treatment of neonatal septic shock: A ten-year experience in a neonatal intensive care unit. Int J Mol Sci 2016; 17(5): 695. [http://dx.doi.org/10.3390/ijms17050695] [PMID: 27171076]

[92] Castellazzi L, Mantero M, Esposito S. Update on the management of pediatric acute osteomyelitis and septic arthritis. Int J Mol Sci 2016; 17(6): 855. [http://dx.doi.org/10.3390/ijms17060855] [PMID: 27258258]

[93] Krone C, Oja A, Van de Groep K, Sanders E, Bogaert D, Trzciński K. Dried saliva spots: A robust method for detecting *Streptococcus pneumoniae* carriage by PCR. Int J Mol Sci 2016; 17(3): 343. [http://dx.doi.org/10.3390/ijms17030343] [PMID: 26959014]

[94] Ieni A, Barresi V, Rigoli L, Fedele F, Tuccari G, Caruso R. Morphological and cellular features of innate immune reaction in *Helicobacter pylori* gastritis: A brief review. Int J Mol Sci 2016; 17(1): 109. [http://dx.doi.org/10.3390/ijms17010109] [PMID: 26784180]

[95] Liu Q, Liu Q, Zhao X, *et al.* Immunogenicity and cross-protective efficacy induced by outer membrane proteins from *Salmonella typhimurium* mutants with truncated LPS in mice. Int J Mol Sci 2016; 17(3): 416. [http://dx.doi.org/10.3390/ijms17030416] [PMID: 27011167]

[96] Gallo M, Di Domenico E, Toma L, *et al. Campylobacter jejuni* fatal sepsis in a patient with Non-Hodgkin's lymphoma: Case report and literature review of a difficult diagnosis. Int J Mol Sci 2016; 17(4): 544. [http://dx.doi.org/10.3390/ijms17040544] [PMID: 27077849]

[97] Korb V, Chuturgoon A, Moodley D. *Mycobacterium tuberculosis:* Manipulator of protective immunity. Int J Mol Sci 2016; 17(3): 131. [http://dx.doi.org/10.3390/ijms17030131] [PMID: 26927066]

[98] Galli L, Lancella L, Tersigni C, *et al.* Pediatric tuberculosis in Italian children: Epidemiological and clinical data from the Italian Register of Pediatric Tuberculosis. Int J Mol Sci 2016; 17(6): 960. [http://dx.doi.org/10.3390/ijms17060960] [PMID: 27322255]

[99] Sotgiu G, D'Ambrosio L, Centis R, *et al.* Carbapenems to treat multidrug and extensively drug-resistant tuberculosis: A systematic review. Int J Mol Sci 2016; 17(3): 373. [http://dx.doi.org/10.3390/ijms17030373] [PMID: 26985890]

[100] Tramuto F, Orsi A, Maida C, *et al.* The molecular epidemiology and evolutionary dynamics of influenza B virus in two Italian Regions during 2010–2015: The experience of Sicily and Liguria. Int J Mol Sci 2016; 17(4): 549. [http://dx.doi.org/10.3390/ijms17040549] [PMID: 27089319]

[101] Esposito S, Scala A, Bianchini S, Zampiero A, Fossali E, Principi N. Identification of human Adenovirus in respiratory samples with Luminex Respiratory Virus Panel Fast V2 assay and real-time polymerase chain reaction. Int J Mol Sci 2016; 17(3): 297. [http://dx.doi.org/10.3390/ijms17030297] [PMID: 26927078]

[102] Gisbert JP, Fernández-Bañares F, *et al.* Current management of *Helicobacter pylori* infection. Gastroenterology 2016; 150(3): 535-58.

[103] Blanchard-Rohner G, *et al.* Vaccination in children: Current challenges and future perspectives. Pediatr Infect Dis J 2017; 36(5): 421-9.

[104] Vella AT, *et al.* Probiotics and pediatric inflammatory bowel disease: Current concepts and future directions. J Pediatr Gastroenterol Nutr 2018; 66(1): 122-6. [PMID: 28906321]

[105] Abdel-Moneim AS, *et al.* The impact of vaccines on infectious disease control: Lessons from the past and implications for the future. Vaccine 2021; 39(14): 1946-51.

CHAPTER 3

Conventional Therapy for Bacterial Infections

Phool Chandra[1,*], **Shahjad**[2], **Neetu Sachan**[3], **Arun Kumar**[2] and **Nishat Fatima**[4]

[1] *Teerthanker Mahaveer College of Pharmacy, Teerthanker Mahaveer University, Moradabad-244001, Uttar Pradesh, India*

[2] *Department of Pharmacology, Global Institute of Pharmaceutical Education and Research, Kashipur-244713, Uttarakhand, India*

[3] *Department of Pharmaceutical Sciences, School of Pharmaceutical & Biological Sciences, Harcourt Butler Technical University (HBTU), Kanpur-208002, Uttar Pradesh, India*

[4] *Department of Pharmacology, MIT College of Pharmacy, Moradabad-244001 Uttar Pradesh, India*

Abstract: This chapter explores the evolution and significance of conventional therapy for bacterial infections, with a focus on antibiotics as cornerstone treatments. It provides a comprehensive analysis of the mechanisms by which major antibiotic classes function, such as inhibition of cell wall synthesis, protein synthesis, and DNA replication, as well as their bacterial targets and clinical uses. It traces the development of antibiotic families like beta-lactams, aminoglycosides, tetracyclines, and quinolones. It also emphasizes the challenges of antibiotic resistance and outlines new therapeutic strategies. The chapter concludes by highlighting the need for balanced empirical and targeted therapies and stresses ongoing innovation to combat antimicrobial resistance (AMR).

Keywords: Aminoglycosides, Antibiotic resistance, Antibiotics, Beta-lactams, Bacterial infections, Conventional therapy, Infectious disease management, Penicillin, Quinolones, Tetracyclines.

INTRODUCTION

Conventional therapy for bacterial infections involves the administration of antibiotics, which have been the mainstay in clinical practices for combating bacterial infections. However, resistance to bacteria has arisen as a result of the misuse of antibiotics and biofilm formation, complicating treatment strategies [1]. To address these challenges, novel approaches such as metal nanoparticles, antimicrobial peptides, and phage therapy have been explored as alternatives to traditional antibiotics [2]. Furthermore, a systematic approach incorporating

* **Corresponding author Phool Chandra:** Teerthanker Mahaveer College of Pharmacy, Teerthanker Mahaveer University, Moradabad-244001, Uttar Pradesh, India; E-mail:profpcpatel@gmail.com

Mukesh Kumar Singh, Gurdeep Singh, Amrendra Pratap Yadav & Papiya Bigoniya (Eds.)

topical and systemic antimicrobial agents, steroid drugs, and the selective decontamination of the digestive tract (SDD) method is essential for preventing infection and eliminating pathogens in severely sick patients [3]. As discussed in various research papers, conventional therapy for bacterial infections involves the use of antibiotics, which have been the mainstay in medical settings for many years. However, antimicrobial resistance (AMR) has emerged as a result of antibiotic misuse and biofilm-related infections, posing significant challenges in treatment. To combat these issues, alternative approaches such as metal nanoparticles, antimicrobial peptides, and phage therapy have been explored as potential solutions to address AMR and biofilm formation. Additionally, strategies like systemic and local antibiotic treatments, non-fouling surfaces, and the application of antibiotics and nanoparticles like silver and zinc oxide have been employed to prevent infections related to biomedical devices and implants [4]. The history of conventional therapy for bacterial infections is marked by significant milestones. The discovery of sulphonamides and penicillin in the 1930s and 1940s, respectively, revolutionized the treatment of bacterial infections [5]. These breakthroughs were the result of systematic investigations into chemicals with antibacterial properties, setting the stage for the antibiotic era in modern medicine, as shown in Table **1** [6]. Table **1** summarizes key milestones in antibiotic development from 1909 to the present. It highlights the introduction of major antibiotic classes such as sulfonamides, beta-lactams, aminoglycosides, and quinolones, along with the decades marked as the "golden age" of antibiotic discovery. The timeline also notes structural classifications and unique breakthroughs like carbapenems and lipopeptides.

Following this, additional families of antibiotics were developed, including oxazolidinones and lipopeptides, which significantly expanded the therapeutic options against resistant bacterial strains. Oxazolidinones, such as linezolid, act by inhibiting the initiation of bacterial protein synthesis through binding to the 50S ribosomal subunit, making them effective against Gram-positive organisms, including methicillin-resistant *Staphylococcus aureus* (MRSA) and vancomycin-resistant Enterococcus (VRE). Lipopeptides, like daptomycin, disrupt the bacterial cell membrane potential, leading to rapid depolarization and cell death. These agents are crucial in treating complicated skin and bloodstream infections caused by multidrug-resistant pathogens [7]. Despite the success of antibiotics, the overuse of these drugs has caused an increase in resistance to antibiotics, prompting the exploration of natural compounds with antibacterial effects as potential alternatives to traditional antibiotics. Additionally, historical records suggest that radiation therapy was once considered an effective treatment for infections before the widespread use of antibiotics, demonstrating how the field of treatments for bacterial infections has evolved over time [8].

Table 1. Evolution of antibiotics.

Year	Antibiotics	Chemical Structure	Ref.
1909	Arsphenamine (First sulpha drug)	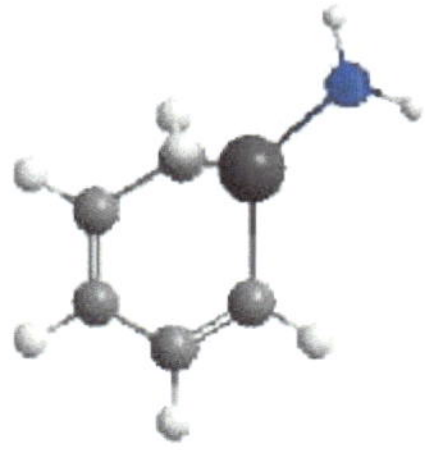 Arsaphenamine	[21]
1928	Penicillin (The most important drug of the last century)	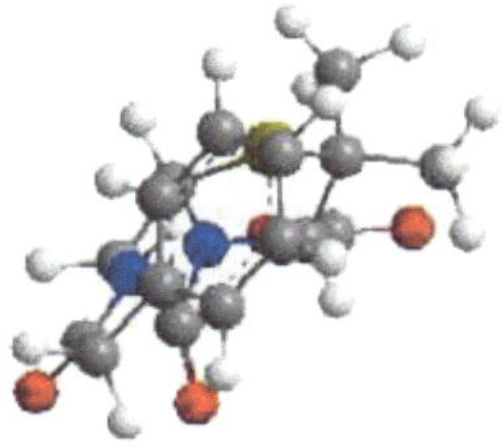 Penicillin	[22]
1932	Prontosil (The most important drug of the last century)	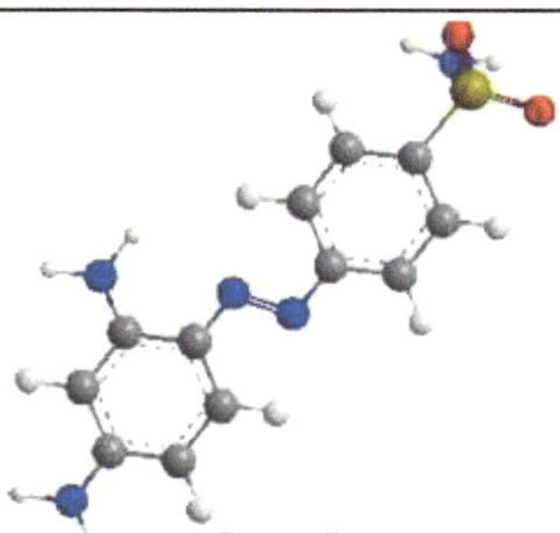 Prontosil	[23]
1943	Streptomycin (First aminoglycoside)	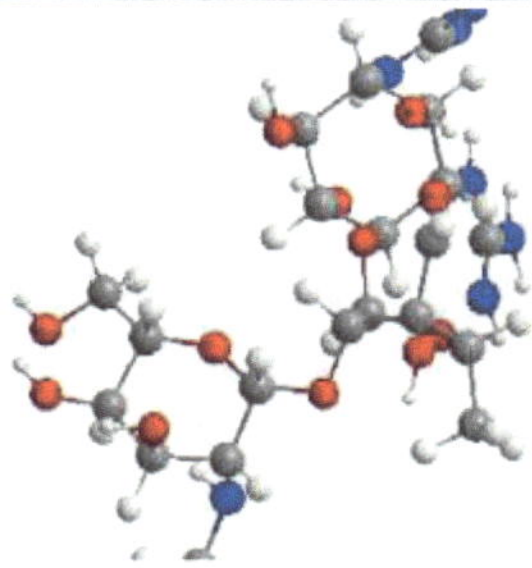 Streptomycin	[24]

(Table 1) cont.....

Year	Antibiotics	Chemical Structure	Ref.
1945	Cephalosporin P Cephalosporin N (First cephalosporins)	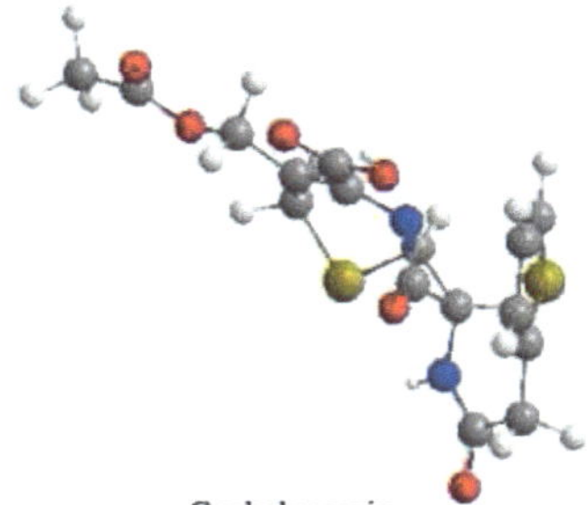 Cephalosporin	[25]
1950-1960	Tetracyclines, Amphenicols, Macrolides, Glycopeptides, Annamycin, Lacosamide, Streptogramins, and Cycloserine Sulfones, Nitrofurans, quinolones, Azoles, Phenazines, Ethambutol, Thioamides (Golden Age)	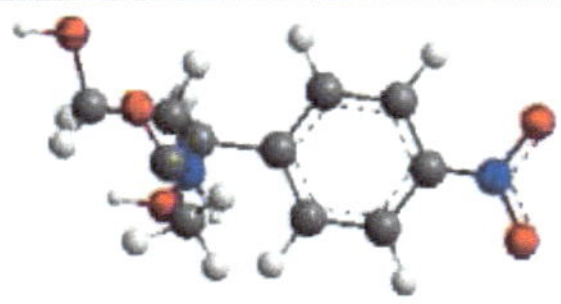 Amphenicol 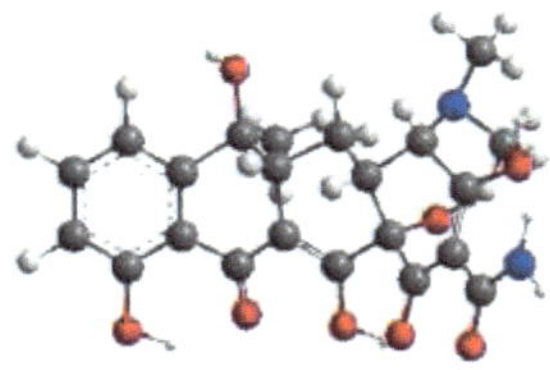 Tetracycline	[26]
1976-1979	Carbapenems Monobactams	-	[27, 28]
1980-2014	Lipopeptides Pleuromutilins Quinolones Linezolid Tedizolid (Oxazolidinone)	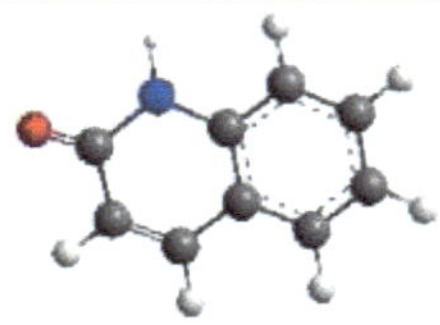 Quinolones	[29]

THE DISCOVERY OF ANTIBIOTICS

The 20th century saw a transformation in medicine with the exploration of antibiotics, with Alexander Fleming's accidental 1928 discovery of penicillin signaling a paradigm shift in managing bacterial illnesses. Since then, a large number of classes of antibiotics have been developed, each focusing on a distinct aspect of its metabolism or cellular structure of bacteria [9].

Alexander Fleming and Penicillin

The early 20th century marked a turning point in medical science with the advent of antibiotics, revolutionizing the treatment of bacterial infections. A pivotal moment occurred in 1928 when Alexander Fleming, a Scottish bacteriologist, observed that a mold (*Penicillium notatum*) had contaminated one of his Petri dishes containing Staphylococcus bacteria. Remarkably, bacterial growth was inhibited around the mold colony. This led to the isolation of penicillin, the first true antibiotic, which demonstrated potent antibacterial activity [10].

Fleming's discovery, though groundbreaking, initially lacked the technological means for mass production and purification. It was not until the late 1930s that a team at Oxford University, led by Howard Florey and Ernst Boris Chain, successfully developed methods for large-scale extraction and clinical testing of penicillin. Their collaborative efforts transformed Fleming's observation into a therapeutic reality, especially critical during World War II, when penicillin saved thousands of lives from infected wounds [11].

Penicillin's success catalyzed the antibiotic era, prompting the search for additional naturally derived antimicrobial agents [12]. The period that followed saw the discovery of streptomycin, tetracyclines, and chloramphenicol, which greatly expanded the arsenal against various bacterial pathogens [13].

The impact of Fleming's work earned him, along with Florey and Chain, the 1945 Nobel Prize in Physiology or Medicine [14]. His legacy extends beyond the discovery itself, as he was also among the first to warn about the potential for antimicrobial resistance (AMR), a concern that remains critical in modern medicine [15].

Early Antibiotic Development

The development of penicillin as a viable antibiotic gained momentum during World War II. Fleming's work was expanded and developed by a group of scientists at Oxford University under the direction of Ernst Chain and Howard Florey. They developed methods for mass-producing penicillin and conducted the first clinical trials. This collaborative effort between British and American scientists resulted in the large-scale production of penicillin by 1945 [16]. Fleming's role in antibiotic development extended beyond penicillin. Recent archival research has [17] uncovered Fleming's lesser-known work on other potential antibacterial substances, including lysozyme, which he discovered in 1922. While lysozyme proved less effective than penicillin against pathogenic bacteria, this work demonstrated Fleming's broader interest in natural antibacterial compounds. The impact of Fleming's discovery on modern medicine cannot be overstated. It not only saved countless lives but also spurred the search for other antibiotics. A comprehensive review [18] highlighted how Fleming's work laid the foundation for the discovery of numerous other antibiotics in the following decades, including streptomycin, tetracycline, and erythromycin. Along with Florey and Chain, Fleming received the 1945 Nobel Prize in medicine or physiology for the discovery of penicillin and its ability to treat a variety of infectious diseases. In his Nobel lecture, Fleming presciently warned about the potential for bacteria to develop resistance to antibiotics, a concern that has become increasingly relevant in modern times [19]. Recent historical analyses have also explored Fleming's role in promoting responsible antibiotic use. A 2023 study [20] examined Fleming's public statements and writings, revealing his early advocacy for the judicious use of antibiotics to prevent resistance development – a message that remains critically important in today's fight against antimicrobial resistance. Alexander Fleming's discovery of penicillin and his contributions to early antibiotic development revolutionized medicine and paved the way for modern antimicrobial therapy. His work continues to influence research and public health strategies in the ongoing battle against infectious diseases.

CLASSES OF ANTIBIOTICS

Beta-Lactams

Beta-lactams are a class of antibiotics that include penicillin, cephalosporins, monobactams, and carbapenems. Fig. (**1**) illustrates the major classes of antibiotics. A beta-lactam chain in their molecular structure is what distinguishes them. These antibiotics function by attaching to proteins that bind to penicillin (PBPs) and preventing the bacterial cell wall's peptidoglycan cross-links from forming, therefore suppressing the development of the bacterial cell wall.

Penicillin

Almost a century after Alexander Fleming's 1928 discovery, penicillin is still a mainstay of antibacterial treatment. Being the first antibiotic to be used in a clinical setting, it transformed medicine and opened the door for the creation of a wide range of other antibiotics. Because of their beta-lactam ring structure, penicillins are members of the beta-lactam class of antibiotics. Penicillins work against bacteria by preventing the synthesis of their cell walls. Penicillin-binding proteins (PBPs), which are enzymes necessary for the cross-linking of peptidoglycan in bacterial cell walls, are bound by them and subsequently rendered inactive. Cell lysis and death result from this disruption to the synthesis of the cell wall [30]. A 2021 study used cryo-electron microscopy to visualize the interaction between penicillin and PBPs at the molecular level. They discovered that penicillin binds covalently to the serine residue of PBPs' active site, resulting in a conformational shift that stops the enzyme from completing the peptidoglycan cross-linking process. Penicillins work best against gram-positive bacteria, such as enteric bacteria species, strains of Streptococcus, and Staphylococcus species (apart from those that are resistant to methicillin). Additionally, they exhibit efficacy against a few gram-negative bacteria, specifically species of Neisseria [31]. A study analyzed the current spectrum of activity of various penicillins against clinically relevant pathogens. They found that Benzylpenicillin (Penicillin G) remains highly effective against *Streptococcus pyogenes* and *Streptococcus pneumoniae*, with resistance rates below 1% globally. Ampicillin and amoxicillin show broader spectrum activity, including against some Enterobacterales, but resistance rates vary significantly by region. Piperacillin, often combined with the beta-lactamase inhibitor tazobactam, demonstrates activity against *Pseudomonas aeruginosa* and many *Enterobacterales* [32].

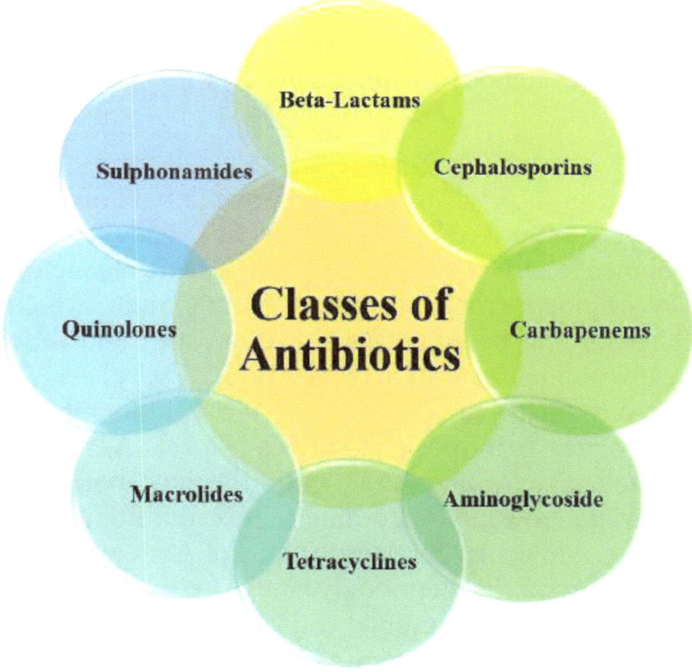

Fig. (1). Classes of antibiotics.

Case Studies

Despite the rise of antibiotic resistance, penicillin continues to play a crucial role in treating various bacterial infections. Recent studies have reaffirmed its importance in several key areas:

- A multicenter observational study involving 30,000 patients from 30 countries found that amoxicillin remains a highly effective first-line treatment for mild to moderate community-acquired pneumonia (CAP) in areas with low resistance. The study reported clinical cure rates of 85–90%, reaffirming its place in empiric therapy for respiratory tract infections. The findings support judicious use of beta-lactams in outpatient care [33].
- A study conducted a randomized controlled trial comparing flucloxacillin (a penicillinase-resistant penicillin) to newer antibiotics for the treatment of cellulitis. They found that flucloxacillin was non-inferior to more expensive alternatives, with similar cure rates and fewer adverse effects [34].
- The recommended course of therapy for syphilis is still Penicillin G. A systematic review of 25 studies confirmed its efficacy, with cure rates exceeding 95% for early syphilis [35].
- For susceptible strains of viridians group streptococci and *Streptococcus bovis*, penicillin G in combination with gentamicin remains a recommended regimen for infective endocarditis. A retrospective cohort study of 1,200 endocarditis cases found that this regimen was linked to decreased death rates for vulnerable organisms as compared to other treatments [36].

Cephalosporins

Since their discovery in the 1940s, cephalosporins, a type of β-lactam antibiotic, have been extensively employed in clinical practice. They have undergone many rounds of development to enhance their pharmacokinetic characteristics and range of activity. They originate from the fungus Acremonium, which was formerly known as Cephalosporium. Based on the time of creation and antibacterial action, cephalosporins are divided into five generations. Every generation has more gram-negative activity than the generation before it, although some generations after it also have better gram-positive coverage [37]. As with other β-lactam antibiotics, the mechanism of action (MOA) of cephalosporins is to prevent the formation of bacterial cell walls. According to research titled Old and New Beta-Lactamase Inhibitors: Molecular Structure, Mode of Action, and Therapeutic Use, these medications disrupt the peptidoglycan layer by attaching to penicillin-binding proteins (PBPs) in the microbial cell wall. Cytolysis and cell death result from this. The specificity of cephalosporins for bacterial cells and their inability to affect human cells (which lack a cell wall) contribute to their relatively low toxicity and wide therapeutic index [38].

Spectrum of Activity

The spectrum of activity of cephalosporins varies across generations:

The first-generation cephalosporins are mostly effective against some gram-negative and gram-positive bacteria. Better action against gram-negative bacteria while maintaining gram-positive coverage is the hallmark of second-generation cephalosporins. Third-generation medications are characterized by broader coverage of gram-negative bacteria, including, for certain agents, *Pseudomonas aeruginosa*. Broad-spectrum action against gram-positive and gram-negative bacteria, including certain resistant forms, characterizes fourth-generation cephalosporins. Methicillin-resistant *Staphylococcus aureus* (MRSA) is one of the multidrug-resistant (MDR) pathogens that fifth-generation cephalosporins are designed to fight. Research emphasizes the creation of siderophore-conjugated cephalosporins, which offer a novel method of combating bacterial resistance [39].

Clinical Applications

Cephalosporins are employed in numerous clinical settings for various bacterial infections. Their specific applications include:

Respiratory tract infections: A meta-analysis found that cephalosporins, particularly third-generation agents, effectively treat community-acquired pneumonia [40].

Urinary tract infections (UTIs): The paper discusses the role of various cephalosporins in managing both uncomplicated and complicated UTIs [41].

Skin and soft tissue infections: It emphasizes the importance of cephalosporins, especially first-generation agents, in treating these infections [42].

Intra-abdominal infections: The study demonstrates the effectiveness of third and fourth-generation cephalosporins in managing these complex infections [43].

Surgical prophylaxis: A systematic review confirms the continued efficacy of cephalosporins in preventing post-surgical infections [44].

Role in Specific Patient Populations

Cephalosporins play important roles in treating infections in various patient populations:

Paediatric patients: A Review highlights the importance of cephalosporins in managing infections in children, emphasizing their safety and efficacy in this population [45].

The paper " Use of Antibiotic Treatment in Pregnancy and the Risk of Several Neonatal Outcomes: A Population-Based Study: A Systematic Review and Meta-Analysis" provides evidence in favor of using specific cephalosporins during pregnancy when clinically indicated [46].

Elderly patients: The study "Review of antimicrobial use and considerations in the elderly population" discusses considerations for using cephalosporins in older adults, including dosage adjustments and monitoring for adverse effects [47].

The review of cephalosporins as key lead generation beta-lactam antibiotics examines the role of cephalosporins in managing infections in patients with compromised immune systems [48].

Carbapenems

A family of β-lactam antibiotics known as carbapenems is essential for treating severe bacterial infections, especially those brought on by organisms that are resistant to multiple drugs (MDR). They are useful in a variety of clinical contexts due to their stability against several β-lactamases and broad-spectrum action. Here is a detailed examination of their function in traditional treatment. Because of their broad-spectrum effectiveness against both Gram-positive and Gram-negative bacteria, including many MDR strains, carbapenems are frequently regarded as antibiotics of last resort. As per the publication "Carbapenems: Past, Present, and Future," carbapenems are recommended for treating a variety of serious infections, such as:

- Complex infections throughout the abdomen.
- Complex infections of the urinary tract.
- The nosocomial pneumonia.
- Bacteremia.
- Infections of the skin and soft tissues.
- Meningitis (On occasion).

The authors stress that since extended-spectrum beta-lactamase (ESBL)-producing Enterobacterales are resistant to several antibiotics, carbapenems are especially helpful in treating infections brought on by these bacteria [49].

Method of action: A 2022 publication offers a thorough description of the carbapenems' mode of action. Similar to other β-lactams, carbapenems attach to penicillin-binding proteins (PBPs) to impede the formation of cell walls. Nonetheless, their distinct molecular structure confers increased resistance to β-lactamases and enhances their ability to permeate Gram-negative bacteria's outer barrier. The scientists point out that PBP2, which is necessary for many bacteria to retain their rod-shaped structure, has a high affinity for carbapenems. This enhances their ability to combat a variety of infections and increases their bactericidal action [50].

Role in Empiric Therapy

The significance of carbapenems in the first empirical therapy of severe infections is shown by a 2020 study, especially in healthcare-associated settings. The authors argue that in situations where MDR pathogens are suspected, such as in patients with recent hospitalization or antibiotic exposure, empiric carbapenem therapy can be life-saving. However, they also stress the need for rapid de-escalation once culture results are available to prevent overuse and resistance development [51].

Aminoglycosides

A family of antibiotics known as aminoglycosides has been around for decades and is still quite effective in treating severe bacterial infections. Because of their broad-spectrum efficacy, aminoglycosides continue to be significant in traditional therapy even with the discovery of newer antibiotics, especially against Gram-negative bacteria [52].

Mechanism of Action and Spectrum of Activity

Aminoglycosides

"Mechanism of Action along with Antimicrobial Spectrum in the Era of Resistance" provides a detailed explanation of how aminoglycosides work. Aminoglycosides enter bacterial cells through an energy-related procedure that requires electron transport. Once inside, the bacterial ribosome's 30S subunit is bound specifically to the 16S rRNA component. This binding causes several effects. Misreading of the genetic code of aminoglycosides induces the incorporation of incorrect amino acids into growing peptide chains, resulting in premature termination of protein synthesis. They can cause ribosomes to halt translation prematurely.

Disruption of the Bacterial Cell Membrane

Some aminoglycosides can also affect membrane integrity. The review highlights that this multifaceted mechanism contributes to the bactericidal activity of aminoglycosides and helps explain their broad range of operations. The authors point out that because of their oxygen-dependent absorption mechanism, aminoglycosides are especially efficient against aerobic Gram-negative bacteria.

The paper also discusses the activity of aminoglycosides against specific pathogens. They are highly effective against Enterobacterales, such as *E. coli, Klebsiella pneumoniae*, and Enterobacter species. They exhibit potent activity against *Pseudomonas aeruginosa*, making them valuable for treating pseudomonal infections. They have been found to be active against *Acinetobacter baumannii*, an increasingly problematic nosocomial pathogen. They show limited activity against anaerobes due to the oxygen-dependent uptake mechanism. Varying degrees of action are observed with certain aminoglycosides (gentamicin, for example) against Gram-positive bacteria, showing good activity against *Staphylococcus aureus* [53].

Clinical Indications

Sepsis and Septic Shock

As part of empirical therapy, the guideline advises considering aminoglycosides for patients with suspected Gram-negative sepsis, especially in cases of healthcare-associated infections or in regions where the prevalence of multidrug-resistant (MDR) organisms is high. For synergistic effects, they recommend mixing an aminoglycoside with a β-lactam antibiotic [52].

Nosocomial Pneumonia

When *Pseudomonas aeruginosa* or MDR Gram-negative infections are detected, the authors advise using aminoglycosides in combination therapy for hospital-acquired and ventilator-associated pneumonia; they also mention that inhaled aminoglycosides may be considered an adjuvant therapy in some situations [54].

Complicated Urinary Tract Infections

The recommendation recommends aminoglycosides as an empirical treatment option for complex UTIs, particularly in regions with elevated prevalence of organisms that produce extended-spectrum β-lactamase (ESBL). In these situations, they highlight the significance of adjusting dosage following renal function [55].

Infective Endocarditis

For infective endocarditis caused by Enterococcus species, the authors recommend gentamicin in conjunction with a substance that activates the cell wall (like ampicillin) for synergistic bactericidal activity. They note that shorter courses of aminoglycosides (1-2 weeks) may be considered to minimize toxicity [56].

Tuberculosis

The guideline discusses the role of streptomycin in multidrug-resistant tuberculosis (MDR-TB) treatment regimens, noting its importance in some cases but also highlighting the increasing use of newer agents [57].

Specific Aminoglycoside Agents

This section elaborates on the characteristics and uses of common aminoglycoside agents:

Gentamicin

"The Use of Gentamicin to Treat Gram-negative Infections: A Retrospective Analysis" provides insights into the current use of gentamicin. The study analyzed data from 500 patients treated with gentamicin for various Gram-negative infections. Key findings are as follows. Gentamicin showed good efficacy against Enterobacterales, with clinical cure rates of 85% for urinary tract infections and 78% for bacteremia. It remained effective against many ESBL-producing organisms, with susceptibility rates of 72% in the study population. The authors found that once-daily dosing of gentamicin was as effective as multiple-daily dosing and was linked to a decreased incidence of nephrotoxicity (12% *vs.* 18%) [58].

Tobramycin

"Optimizing Therapy" focuses on the use of tobramycin, particularly in cystic fibrosis (CF) patients. Tobramycin has a superior activity against *P. aeruginosa* compared to other aminoglycosides, with MIC90 values typically 2-4 fold lower than gentamicin. The effectiveness of inhaled tobramycin in CF patients is shown by enhanced lung capacity and decreased exacerbation rates. The potential of tobramycin in treating biofilm-associated infections is supported by in vitro studies demonstrating its ability to penetrate *P. aeruginosa* biofilms [59].

Amikacin

"A Reserve Aminoglycoside for MDR Infections" positions amikacin as a valuable option for treating MDR Gram-negative infections. Amikacin's stability against many aminoglycoside-modifying enzymes makes it effective against some gentamicin-resistant strains. It has a role in treating diseases brought on by Enterobacterales that are resistant to carbapenem, often in combination with other antibiotics. Liposomal amikacin formulations have potential for inhaled therapy in non-tuberculous mycobacterial lung infections [60].

Tetracyclines

Tetracyclines are a type of antibiotic with a broad spectrum that work by attaching to the 30S ribosome and preventing the production of bacterial proteins. They are highly effective against infections caused by Mycoplasma, chlamydia, rickettsia, and both gram-positive and gram-negative bacteria. Tetracyclines have several clinical indications, such as complex skin and skin structure infections, complicated invasive stomach infections, Lyme disease, respiratory tract infections, and locally acquired pneumonia caused by bacterial infections with specific agents like doxycycline, tigecycline, eravacycline, and omadacycline being commonly used for these purposes. Additionally, tetracyclines have shown potential as antiviral agents by inducing disease tolerance against viral infections like influenza, suggesting a broader protective role beyond their antimicrobial effects.

Method of Action: Since the 1940s, tetracyclines, a type of broad-spectrum antibiotic, have been used in medicine. Their principal mode of action is to impede the production of bacterial proteins, which in turn produces bacteriostatic effects. The detailed molecular mechanisms by which tetracyclines exert their antibacterial activity have been elucidated through decades of research [61, 62].

Cellular Uptake

The first step in the action of tetracyclines involves their entry into bacterial cells. Passive diffusion takes place during this process across the cell membranes of gram-positive and gram-negative bacteria, as well as their outer membranes. Tetracyclines also use an energy-dependent transport mechanism in gram-negative organisms to build up inside the cell at concentrations much greater than those in the extracellular environment [63].

Binding to the Ribosome

Once within the cell of the bacteria, tetracyclines bind reversibly to the 30S component of the bacterial ribosome, specifically interacting with the ribosome's A site (aminoacyl site), where nucleotides in helices 31 and 34 form the main binding site, and where new aminoacyl-tRNA molecules normally bind during protein synthesis [64].

Inhibition of Protein Synthesis

Tetracyclines impede the connection between the aminoacyl-tRNA and the ribosomal acceptor site by binding to the A site. This interference prevents new amino acids from being added to the growing peptide chain, thereby stopping the manufacture of proteins. It is noteworthy that this inhibition is reversible, which is one of the factors that make these antibiotics bacteriostatic as opposed to bactericidal [65].

Magnesium Chelation

Tetracyclines also act as chelating agents, forming complexes with divalent metal ions, particularly magnesium (Mg^{2+}). This chelation contributes to their antimicrobial activity by allowing the structure to remain intact, as magnesium ions (Mg^{2+}) are essential for the stability of bacterial ribosomes and the function of various enzymatic reactions. By depleting available Mg^{2+}, tetracyclines further disrupt bacterial cellular processes [66].

Effects on Mitochondrial Protein Synthesis

It is worth noting that tetracyclines can also affect mitochondrial protein synthesis in eukaryotic cells, as mitochondrial ribosomes are similar to bacterial ribosomes. This effect is generally less pronounced than their impact on bacterial cells but can contribute to a few of the adverse effects noted during trial use [67].

Inhibition of Matrix Metalloproteinases

In addition to their antimicrobial effects, some tetracyclines, particularly doxycycline, have been found to inhibit matrix metalloproteinases (MMPs). This property is independent of their antimicrobial activity and has led to the development of chemically modified tetracyclines for non-antibiotic purposes, such as treating periodontal diseases and certain skin conditions [68].

Anti-Inflammatory and Immunomodulatory Effects

Recent research has revealed that tetracyclines possess anti-inflammatory and immunomodulatory properties. These effects are mediated through various mechanisms, including inhibition of neutrophil migration, reduction of pro-inflammatory cytokine production, and modulation of T-cell function. These properties contribute to their efficacy in treating certain inflammatory conditions and may enhance their overall therapeutic value [69].

Resistance Mechanisms

It is essential to comprehend the processes behind tetracycline resistance for their continued clinical use. Several resistance mechanisms have been identified.

Efflux pumps: Bacteria can develop energy-dependent efflux systems that actively pump tetracyclines out of the cell, reducing intracellular concentrations.

Ribosomal protection proteins: Some bacteria produce proteins that interact with the ribosome, causing conformational changes that prevent tetracycline binding or dislodge bound tetracycline molecules.

Enzymatic inactivation: Although less common, some bacteria possess enzymes capable of chemically modifying tetracyclines, rendering them inactive.

Target site mutations: Alterations in the ribosomal binding site can reduce the affinity of tetracyclines for their target, conferring resistance [70].

Synergistic Effects

Tetracyclines have been shown to exhibit synergistic effects when paired with certain other antibiotics. As an illustration, a mixture of tetracyclines with β-lactams or aminoglycosides can enhance their bactericidal activity against some organisms. This synergy is thought to result from the tetracyclines' ability to increase the permeability of the bacterial cell membrane, facilitating the entry of other antibiotics [71].

Clinical Indications

Tetracyclines have been a cornerstone of antimicrobial therapy for decades because of their advantageous pharmacokinetic characteristics and wide range of activities. A variety of bacterial illnesses are among their clinical indications. This chapter explores the primary clinical indications for tetracyclines, considering both traditional and emerging uses [72].

Respiratory Tract Infections

Tetracyclines—doxycycline in particular—are frequently used to treat community-acquired pneumonia (CAP). They work well against uncommon pathogens like *Legionella pneumophila*, *Chlamydophila pneumoniae*, and *Mycoplasma pneumoniae* [73]. For empirical outpatient therapy of CAP, doxycycline is suggested by the recommendations of the American Thoracic Society (ATS) and the Infectious Diseases Society of America (IDSA) as a substitute for macrolides [74]. Acute flare-ups of chronic bronchitis can also benefit from tetracyclines, especially if *Moraxella catarrhalis* or *Haemophilus influenzae* are probable culprits [75]

Sexually Transmitted Infections (STIs)

Doxycycline is a first-line treatment for chlamydial infections, including urethritis, cervicitis, and pelvic inflammatory disease caused by *Chlamydia trachomatis* [76]. It is also effective against *Ureaplasma urealyticum* and *Mycoplasma genitalium*. For syphilis, tetracyclines (particularly doxycycline) are suggested as a substitute for penicillin in people with penicillin allergy who are not pregnant [77].

Tick-Borne Diseases

The preferred medication for many diseases carried by ticks is doxycycline. Treatment for early localized or early disseminated Lyme disease caused by *Borrelia burgdorferi* is the recommended course of action [78]. For patients of any age with Rocky Mountain spotted fever, Doxycycline is the recommended medication, even in younger ones [79]. First-line therapy for human granulocytic anaplasmosis and ehrlichiosis is usually doxycycline [80].

Acne and Rosacea

In dermatology, tetracyclines, particularly doxycycline and minocycline, are frequently used to treat rosacea and acne vulgaris. Their antibacterial and anti-inflammatory qualities are responsible for their effectiveness [81]. Doxycycline at a low dosage has been authorized for the management of rosacea, maximizing its anti-inflammatory properties while reducing the likelihood of developing antibiotic resistance [82].

Malaria

Doxycycline is used for malaria prophylaxis in travelers to endemic areas. It is particularly useful in regions with chloroquine-resistant *Plasmodium falciparum*. Additionally, it can be used to treat severe malaria in conjunction with quinine [83].

Periodontal Diseases

Tetracyclines, especially doxycycline, are used in the management of periodontal diseases. Their effectiveness is due to both antimicrobial activity against oral pathogens and inhibition of matrix metalloproteinases involved in tissue destruction [84].

Rickettsial Infections

Tetracyclines are the preferred medication for treating rickettsial illnesses, such as epidemic typhus, scrub typhus, and Q fever, in addition to Rocky Mountain spotted fever [85].

Cholera

Although resistance to tetracyclines has become an issue in some areas, they can still be utilized as part of a cholera treatment regimen [86].

Atypical Mycobacterial Infections

Minocycline and doxycycline have activity against some atypical mycobacteria, including *Mycobacterium marinum* and *Mycobacterium fortuitum* [87].

Intestinal Amebiasis

Tetracyclines can be used as an alternative treatment for intestinal amebiasis, particularly in combination with other antiprotozoal agents [88].

Anthrax

Doxycycline is approved for the treatment of inhalational anthrax (post-exposure) and is part of the recommended regimen for cutaneous anthrax [89].

Helicobacter pylori Eradication

Tetracyclines, particularly tetracycline hydrochloride, are sometimes included in quadruple therapy regimens for *H. pylori* eradication, especially in areas with high clarithromycin resistance [90].

Ocular Infections

Tetracyclines are used in the treatment of various ocular infections, including trachoma caused by *Chlamydia trachomatis* and inclusion conjunctivitis [91].

Non-Infectious Indications

Tetracyclines, particularly doxycycline, have found use in several non-infectious conditions due to their anti-inflammatory and immunomodulatory properties.

Bullous Pemphigoid: Low-dose doxycycline has shown efficacy in managing this autoimmune blistering disease [92].

Sarcoidosis: Minocycline has been used as an alternative treatment in some cases of cutaneous sarcoidosis [93].

Rheumatoid Arthritis: Minocycline has demonstrated modest disease-modifying effects in early, seropositive rheumatoid arthritis [93].

Emerging and Investigational Uses

Recent research has explored new potential applications for tetracyclines.

COVID-19: Doxycycline has been investigated as a potential adjunctive therapy in COVID-19 due to its anti-inflammatory properties and possible antiviral effects [94].

Preclinical studies have suggested potential anticancer properties of some tetracyclines, particularly in combination with other therapies [95]. Minocycline has shown neuroprotective effects in animal models of various neurodegenerative diseases, although clinical trials have yielded mixed results [96].

Macrolides

The molecular structure of a family of antibiotics known as macrolides is typified by a large macrocyclic lactone ring. They work well against both gram-negative and gram-positive bacteria. Macrolides function by attaching to the 50S subunit of the bacterial ribosome and preventing the production of proteins in bacteria [97].

Mechanism of Action

One family of antibiotics called macrolides mainly prevents bacteria from synthesizing proteins. They attach reversibly to the bacterial ribosome's 50S subunit, particularly at the peptidyl transferase center or in close proximity to the peptide exit tunnel. Because of this interaction, nascent peptide chains cannot elongate, which inhibits bacterial growth and replication. Additional methods by which macrolides exert their antibacterial properties have been uncovered by a recent study.

Inhibition of quorum sensing: Macrolides can disrupt bacterial communication systems, potentially reducing virulence and biofilm formation.

Anti-inflammatory effects: Some macrolides have been shown to modulate the host immune response, which may contribute to their clinical efficacy.

Inhibition of bacterial virulence factors: Certain macrolides can interfere with the production or secretion of bacterial toxins and other virulence factors [98 - 100].

Spectrum of Activity

Macrolides are effective against a wide range of bacterial infections. Gram-positive bacteria include methicillin-susceptible types of *Staphylococcus aureus*, *Streptococcus pneumoniae*, and *Streptococcus pyogenes*. Atypical pathogens include *Legionella pneumophila*, *Chlamydophila pneumoniae*, and *Mycoplasma pneumoniae*. Some gram-negative microorganisms are *Haemophilus influenzae*, *Moraxella catarrhalis*, *Bordetella pertussis*. Intracellular pathogens include *Chlamydia trachomatis*, *Ureaplasma urealyticum*, and *Mycobacterium avium* complex (MAC). Recent studies have shown that the spectrum of activity can vary among different macrolides, with newer generations demonstrating enhanced activity against certain pathogens. For example, azithromycin has shown improved activity against some gram-negative bacteria compared to older macrolides. However, emerging resistance to macrolides has become a significant concern in recent years. Resistance mechanisms include target site modification (*e.g.*, methylation of the 23S rRNA), efflux pumps, and enzymatic inactivation of the drug [101 - 103].

Clinical Indications

The therapeutic indications for macrolides, which are used to treat a variety of bacterial illnesses, are constantly changing in response to new findings and recommendations. Here are a few important clinical indications:

- **Respiratory tract infections**, such as community-acquired pneumonia, pharyngitis, sinusitis, and acute exacerbations of chronic bronchitis.
- **Skin and soft tissue infections**, including cellulitis, impetigo, and erythrasma.
- **Sexually transmitted infections**, such as those caused by *Ureaplasma urealyticum* and *Chlamydia trachomatis*.
- **Gastrointestinal infections**, specifically for the eradication of *Helicobacter pylori,* when used as part of a combination therapy.
- **Prophylaxis in immunocompromised individuals**, particularly to prevent *Mycobacterium avium complex* (MAC) infections in patients with HIV.
- **Treatment of MAC lung disease**, which includes non-tuberculous mycobacterial infections.
- **Pertussis (whooping cough)**, where macrolides are used for both treatment and post-exposure prophylaxis.

Current research has also looked into the possibility of using macrolides to treat COVID-19. The existing data does not support the regular use of azithromycin for the treatment of COVID-19, despite initial investigations. Some macrolides have shown promise in managing conditions like cystic fibrosis and bronchiectasis due to their anti-inflammatory properties. Ongoing research explores macrolides' potential role in reducing inflammation associated with cardiovascular risk [104 - 106].

Specific Agents

The macrolide class includes several specific agents, with newer generations developed to address the limitations of earlier compounds. Key macrolides are included in Table **2** [107 - 110].

Table 2. List of Macrolids with specific use.

Name of macrolide	Comments
Erythromycin	The first macrolide antibiotic, still used but limited by gastrointestinal side effects and drug interactions.
Clarithromycin	Second-generation macrolide with improved oral bioavailability and fewer gastrointestinal side effects compared to erythromycin.
Azithromycin	Third-generation macrolide with an extended half-life, allowing for once-daily dosing and shorter treatment courses. It has an expanded gram-negative spectrum.
Roxithromycin	Second-generation macrolide with improved pharmacokinetics compared to erythromycin.
Telithromycin	A ketolide antibiotic (related to macrolides) developed to address macrolide resistance, but its use is limited due to potential hepatotoxicity.
Fidaxomicin	A narrow-spectrum macrolide primarily used for Clostridioides difficile infections. Recent developments and ongoing research on macrolide antibiotics.
Solithromycin	Solithromycin is a novel fluoroketolide that has activity against macrolide-resistant pathogens, although its development for systemic use has been halted due to hepatotoxicity concerns.
Nafithromycin	A novel lactone-ketolide hybrid in clinical development, showing promise against resistant respiratory pathogens.
Modithromycin	A new macrolide derivative in early clinical development, designed to overcome existing resistance mechanisms.

Quinolones

Quinolones, a type of synthetic broad-spectrum antibiotics that target bacterial DNA replication, are sometimes referred to as fluoroquinolones when they contain a fluorine atom. DNA gyrase (also known as topoisomerase II) and topoisomerase IV are two crucial bacterial enzymes that are mostly inhibited by them.

Mechanism of Action

DNA gyrase is principally in charge of inserting negative supercoils, which are essential for transcription, chromosomal segregation, and DNA replication into bacterial DNA. In contrast, topoisomerase IV is involved in the decatenation of daughter chromosomes subsequent to DNA replication. Quinolones cause cell death in bacteria by inhibiting these enzymes that are responsible for bacterial DNA synthesis. Several structural and biochemical studies have clarified the precise molecular interactions between quinolones and their target enzymes. Quinolones and the enzyme form a stable ternary complex that traps the enzyme on the DNA and prevents the replication fork from proceeding, which causes the accumulation of double-strand breaks in bacterial DNA, which in turn triggers the SOS response and ultimately results in cell death. Recent studies have shed light on the nature of these interactions. For example, a study on cryo-electron microscopy revealed the structural basis of quinolone action against Mycobacterium tuberculosis DNA gyrase [111]. They found that the drug binds to a pocket formed by the DNA-protein interface, stabilizing a pre-cleavage state of the enzyme-DNA complex. The bactericidal activity of quinolones is concentration-dependent, meaning that higher drug concentrations result in more rapid and complete killing of bacteria. This property has important implications for dosing strategies in clinical practice. Interestingly, the mechanism of action of quinolones also contributes to their potential for inducing bacterial resistance. The SOS response triggered by quinolone-induced DNA damage can lead to increased mutation rates, potentially facilitating the development of resistance mechanisms. Recent research has also uncovered secondary mechanisms of quinolone action.

For example, a study showed that some quinolones, especially those that target gram-negative bacteria, have the ability to damage bacterial cell membranes [112]. The creation of novel quinolone derivatives may benefit from this extra mechanism, which may also contribute to the antibiotics' broad-spectrum action. Moreover, it has been demonstrated that quinolones' interaction with bacterial Type II topoisomerases produces reactive oxygen species (ROS), which enhances their bactericidal effect. A group of scientists elucidated the molecular pathway of this ROS generation, involving the activation of the bacterial TCA cycle and subsequent overproduction of NADH [113].

Spectrum of Activity

Quinolones are known for their broad spectrum of antibacterial activity, which has contributed to their widespread use in clinical practice. The spectrum of activity varies somewhat among different quinolone agents, with newer generations generally exhibiting an expanded spectrum compared to earlier ones.

Gram-positive bacteria: Quinolones exhibit high efficacy against a wide range of gram-positive bacteria, such as *Enterococcus faecalis*, *Staphylococcus aureus* (including some strains resistant to methicillin), and *Streptococcus pneumoniae*. However, generally speaking, they are less effective against gram-positive bacteria than gram-negative ones. Molifloxacin and delafloxacin, two of the most recent quinolones, have enhanced efficacy against gram-positive bacteria.

Gram-negative bacteria: A variety of gram-negative bacteria can be effectively combated by quinolones. They have outstanding efficacy against *Proteus mirabilis*, *Klebsiella pneumoniae*, and *Escherichia coli*, among other Enterobacteriaceae. They are also effective against *Moraxella catarrhalis, Haemophilus influenzae*, and *Pseudomonas aeruginosa*. Certain quinolones, such as ciprofloxacin, have a very strong anti-*P. aeruginosa* effect.

Atypical pathogens: *Legionella pneumophila*, *Mycoplasma pneumoniae*, and *Chlamydophila pneumoniae* are examples of intracellular pathogens against which quinolones are effective. When these unusual organisms are involved in respiratory tract illnesses, this action is very crucial.

Anaerobic bacteria: The anti-anaerobic action of earlier quinolone generations was restricted. Anaerobic coverage has been enhanced by more recent drugs, such as delafloxacin and moxifloxacin, which also have efficacy against Bacteroides fragilis and other anaerobic species. *Mycobacterium tuberculosis* is one of the mycobacterial species against which some quinolones, especially those from later generations, have action. When treating TB, levofloxacin and doxifloxacin are frequently utilized as second-line medications. A recent thorough investigation [114] analyzed the in vitro activity of various quinolones against a large collection of clinical isolates. They discovered that more recent quinolones, such as finafloxacin and delafloxacin, have shown improved efficacy against gram-positive and gram-negative infections, including some strains that were resistant to several drugs. Still, there is reason for alarm over the rising incidence of quinolone resistance. An international surveillance investigation conducted by [115] reported on the trends in quinolone resistance among common bacterial pathogens. They found that resistance rates varied significantly by geographic region and bacterial species, with particularly high rates observed in some gram-negative organisms like *E. coli* and *K. pneumoniae* in certain parts of the world. Interestingly, recent research has also explored the potential antiviral activities of some quinolones. A study [116] demonstrated that certain quinolone compounds exhibited inhibitory effects against influenza viruses, opening up potential new applications for these drugs. The spectrum of activity of quinolones is also influenced by their pharmacokinetic properties. Most quinolones achieve high concentrations in tissues and body fluids, contributing to their effectiveness in various types of infections. A pharmacokinetic study [117] compared the tissue penetration of different quinolones, finding that newer agents like delafloxacin showed improved penetration into difficult-to-treat sites such as bone and joint tissues. Although quinolones have a wide range of effects, it is crucial to remember that using them should be done carefully to avoid encouraging resistance. In order to maintain quinolones' efficacy for more severe illnesses, several guidelines currently suggest saving them for circumstances where narrower-spectrum antibiotics are not appropriate.

Sulphonamides

Sulfonamides remain an important class of antibiotics in the conventional therapy of bacterial infections. Their mechanism of action and continued relevance in modern medicine are supported by recent research. Here is an overview of the role of sulfonamides in bacterial infection treatment, focusing on their mechanism of action [118].

Mechanism of Action

In bacteria's folic acid manufacturing pathway, sulfonamides function as competitive inhibitors of the enzyme dihydropteroate synthase (DHPS). The synthesis of tetrahydrofolic acid, a necessary cofactor for the biosynthesis of purines, pyrimidines, and certain amino acids, depends on this enzyme. Sulfonamides impede bacterial DNA synthesis and protein synthesis by blocking DHPS, which eventually results in the suppression and death of bacterial growth. New research has shed further light on this process in detail.

Structural basis [119]: A study used cryo-electron microscopy to elucidate the structural basis of sulfonamide binding to DHPS. They found that sulfonamides bind to a conserved pocket in DHPS, competing with the natural substrate para-aminobenzoic acid (PABA). This structural information provides a foundation for developing new sulfonamide derivatives with improved efficacy.

Synergistic effects: Sulfonamides are often used in combination with dihydrofolate reductase (DHFR) inhibitors, such as trimethoprim [120]. It has been shown that this combination of medications lowers the risk of resistance development and improves antibacterial activity.

Resistance mechanisms: Understanding resistance mechanisms is crucial for effective antibiotic use. Wang *et al.* (2022) highlighted various molecular mechanisms of sulfonamide resistance, including mutations in the folP gene encoding DHPS and the acquisition of alternative DHPS enzymes [121].

Spectrum activity

A study by Imène *et al.* (2023) investigated the efficacy of sulfonamides against intracellular bacterial pathogens, particularly *Legionella pneumophila* [122]. They found that certain sulfonamide derivatives showed enhanced intracellular penetration and activity against this pathogen, which is notorious for its ability to evade many antibiotics. This research opens up new possibilities for treating Legionnaires' disease and other intracellular bacterial infections. A study by Reeves *et al.* (2024) published a comprehensive meta-analysis on the effectiveness of sulfonamide-trimethoprim combinations in treating community-acquired pneumonia (CAP) [123]. Their findings reaffirmed the utility of these combinations as empiric therapy for CAP in regions with low resistance rates, particularly in outpatient settings. The study also highlighted the need for ongoing surveillance of resistance patterns to guide treatment decisions. Gattu *et al.* (2024) explored the potential of sulfonamides in combating biofilm-associated infections [124]. Using advanced imaging techniques and molecular biology methods, they demonstrated that certain sulfonamide derivatives could disrupt bacterial biofilms of *Pseudomonas aeruginosa* and *Staphylococcus epidermidis*. This research suggests a potential new application for sulfonamides in treating chronic, biofilm-associated infections. Sarenje *et al.* (2024) suggest that the management of gonorrhoeal infections may be improved by this work, which adds to our understanding of antibiotic resistance mechanisms and identifies novel mutations in the folP gene associated with high-level sulfonamide resistance [125]. A rapid molecular test for detecting these mutations was developed. A large-scale genomic analysis of sulfonamide resistance in *Neisseria gonorrhoeae* was carried out. A study by Pathak *et al.* (2023) investigated the synergistic effects of sulphonamides with various natural compounds [126]. They found that certain plant-derived flavonoids significantly enhanced the ability of the substances to inhibit the growth of *Acinetobacter baumannii* strains that are resistant to several drugs. The findings of this study provide new avenues for combination therapy aimed at extending the half-life of sulphonamides against infections with resistance. Elawady *et al.* (2024) examined the *in vitro* activity of trimethoprim-sulfamethoxazole against clinical isolates of multidrug-resistant Gram-negative bacteria [127]. They found that it maintained good activity against many extended-spectrum beta-lactamase (ESBL) producing Enterobacteriaceae. Catania *et al.* (2004) tested sulfonamide efficacy against different bacterial infections, showing that they are still useful against some drug-resistant strains, especially when used in conjunction with other antibiotics [128]. A 2024 surveillance study by Wu *et al.* (2024) assessed the global patterns of sulfonamide susceptibility among common respiratory pathogens [129]. They noted regional variations in susceptibility rates and emphasized the importance of local antibiograms in guiding therapy.

MECHANISMS OF ACTION

Inhibition of Cell Wall Synthesis

The capacity of bacteria to become resistant to antimicrobial drugs makes treating bacterial illnesses more difficult. The primary mechanism of action of antimicrobial medicines is frequently used to classify them for usage in the treatment of bacterial infections. Mechanisms of action include [1]: suppression of protein synthesis [2], interference with cell wall production [3], interference with nucleic acid synthesis, and [4] inhibition of cell membrane function. Thus, the targets of antibacterial medications include the creation of proteins, nucleic acids, cell walls, membranes, and biological metabolic compounds, as indicated by their mode of action. The mechanisms of antibiotic action are summarized in Table **3** and Fig.(**2**). Peptidoglycan makes up the majority of the bacterial cell wall, which is necessary for both cell integrity and survival. It maintains cell shape and guards against osmotic pressure. Gram-negative bacteria have a thinner peptidoglycan layer encased in an outer membrane; Gram-positive bacteria, however, have a thicker covering. Antibiotics that prevent the production of cell walls usually disrupt the last steps in the construction of peptidoglycans. They perform various actions, including inhibition of transpeptidation or transglycosylation processes, inhibition of peptidoglycan precursor production, and prevention of precursor transport across the cell membrane. Scientists identified a new potential target in cell wall synthesis - the lipid II lipase [130]. They developed a small-molecule inhibitor showing promise against methicillin-resistant Staphylococcus aureus (MRSA). Ding *et al.* (2024) demonstrated synergistic effects between beta-lactams and outer membrane-permeabilizing peptides against multidrug-resistant Gram-negative bacteria, revitalizing the use of some beta-lactams [131].

Table 3. The manner in which certain antibiotic classes work [145].

Mechanism of action	Aims	Medication class	Particular medication example
Break down the membranes.	Lipid-polysaccharides	Polymyxins	Colistin and polymyxin B
Blocking the creation of proteins.	Peptidoglycan subunit 30s subunit	Glycopeptides, tetracyclines, and aminoglycosides	The medications streptomycin, gentamicin, neomycin, tetracycline, and doxycycline
	Subunit of the 50s	Chloramphenicol, oxazolidinones, and macrolides	Linezolid, chloramphenicol, azithromycin, and erythromycin

(Table 3) cont.....

Mechanism of action	Aims	Medication class	Particular medication example
Anti-metabolites	Enzymes for folic acid production	Trimethoprim and sulfonamides	Trimethoprim, Sulfamethoxazole, and Dapsone
Blocking the production of nucleic acids	RNA and DNA	Fluoroquinolones with rifamycin	Rifampin, ciprofloxacin, and ofloxacin
Inhibition of the formation of cell walls	Protein that binds penicillin	β-lactam antibiotics	Amoxicillin, cephalosporin C, and pPenicillin G

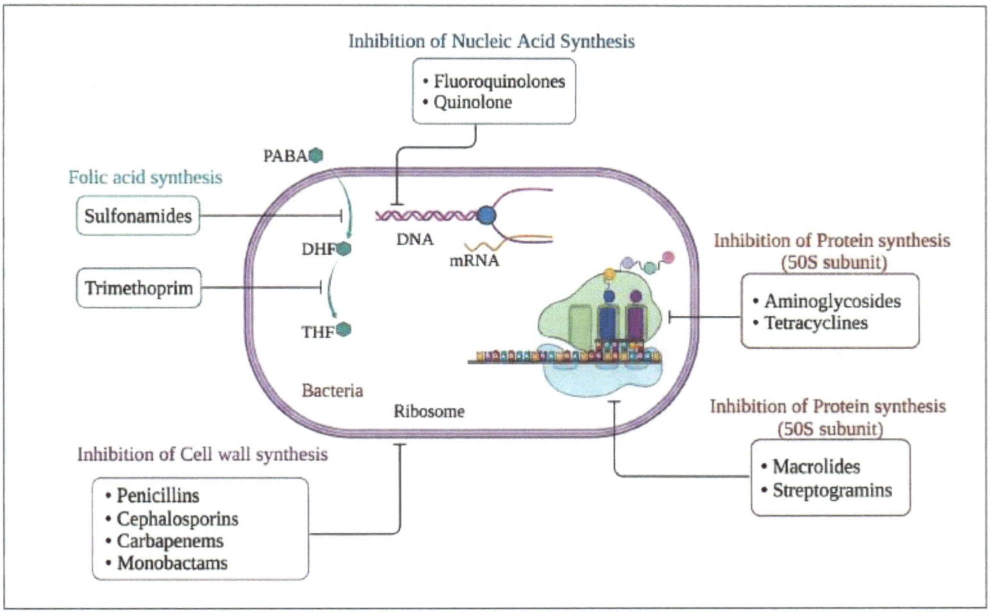

Fig. (2). Mechanism of action of antibiotics.

Inhibition of Protein Synthesis

The production of proteins in bacteria occurs on 70S ribosomes, which consist of 30S and 50S subunits. The process involves initiation, elongation, and termination phases, each presenting targets for antibiotic action. Aminoglycosides, such as gentamicin and tobramycin, inhibit protein synthesis by binding to the 16S rRNA of the 30S ribosomal subunit, which disrupts the decoding process, leading to misreading of the genetic code and premature termination of translation. A study used cryo-EM to reveal how aminoglycosides induce conformational changes in the decoding center, explaining their dual effects of misreading and translation inhibition [132]. Tetracyclines impede the ribosomal acceptor site from being occupied by aminoacyl-tRNA.Recent work by Barrenechea *et al.* (2021) identified novel binding sites for tetracycline derivatives, potentially overcoming existing resistance mechanisms [133].

Inhibition of 50S Ribosomal Subunit: Macrolides (*e.g.*, Erythromycin, Azithromycin) bind to the 23S rRNA of the 50S subunit, blocking the exit tunnel. A study by Thorat *et al.* (2024) demonstrated how macrolides selectively inhibit the synthesis of specific proteins, explaining their anti-inflammatory properties [134]. Chloramphenicol inhibits peptidyl transferase activity. Recent research by Wang *et al.* (2024) revealed how chloramphenicol analogs can overcome efflux-mediated binding to the P site of the 50S subunit, preventing formation of the initiation complex [135]. A structural study by Merazka *et al.* (2023) provided insights into the binding mechanism of new oxazolidinone derivatives, guiding the development of next-generation compounds [136].

Inhibition of Nucleic Acid Synthesis

The inhibition of the production of nucleic acids is a crucial mechanism in antibiotic therapy, focusing on DNA replication mechanisms and RNA transcription in bacteria. This approach is effective because it interferes with fundamental cellular processes essential for bacterial survival and reproduction. Let's explore this mechanism in detail. The mechanisms of nucleic acid synthesis inhibition are listed below:

Fluoroquinolones (*e.g.*, Ciprofloxacin, Levofloxacin) that inhibit DNA gyrase and topoisomerase IV: These enzymes are necessary for DNA supercoiling and chromosomal segregation; they bind to these proteins and form a ternary complex with them. Single-molecule techniques visualize how fluoroquinolones trap gyrase on DNA, providing insights into their bactericidal action [137]. A study by Powell *et al.* (2024) identified a new class of gyrase inhibitors that bind to a different site than fluoroquinolones, potentially overcoming existing resistance mechanisms [138].

Inhibition of RNA Synthesis: Rifamycins (*e.g.*, Rifampicin) bind to bacterial RNA polymerase, inhibiting transcription initiation. A recent cryo-EM study by Hamouche *et al.* (2021) revealed the precise binding mechanism of rifamycins and how mutations confer resistance [139]. Fidaxomicin inhibits bacterial RNA polymerase through a mechanism distinct from rifamycins. A study by Cao *et al.* (2022) demonstrated how fidaxomicin's unique binding site contributes to its narrow spectrum and reduced resistance development [140].

Disruption of Cell Membrane Function

The membrane of a cell is an essential component of bacterial cells, serving as a protective barrier and regulating the flow of substances in and out of the cell. Disrupting this membrane is a key strategy in many conventional therapies for bacterial infections. This approach has proven effective because compromising the integrity of the cell membrane can lead to bacterial cell death or increased susceptibility to other antimicrobial agents. Antimicrobial peptides are an important class of membrane-disrupting agents used in treating bacterial infections. These naturally occurring molecules form a component of the innate immune systemand have been the subject of extensive research for their potential as therapeutic agents. AMPs typically work by interacting with the bacterial cell membrane, leading to pore formation or membrane destabilization. This action can result in cell lysis or the loss of critical ions and metabolites, ultimately causing bacterial death. A study reviewed the therapeutic potential of AMPs, highlighting their excellent all-around effectiveness against both Gram-positive and Gram-negative bacteria. The proposed researchers noted that AMPs could potentially overcome antibiotic resistance mechanisms due to their unique mode of action, targeting the cell membrane. Lipopeptides are another class of compounds that disrupt bacterial cell membranes. One of the most well-known examples is daptomycin, a cyclic lipopeptide antibiotic used to treat infections caused by Gram-positive bacteria. Daptomycin works by inserting its lipid tail into the bacterial cell membrane, causing rapid depolarization and the efflux of potassium ions [141]. This leads to the inhibition of various cellular processes and ultimately results in cell death. A comprehensive review by Oberholzer *et al.* (2005) discussed the mechanism of action of daptomycin and its effectiveness against multidrug-resistant pathogens [142]. The authors emphasized the importance of membrane disruption as a strategy to combat antibiotic-resistant bacteria. Polymyxins are a group of polypeptide antibiotics that target the cell membrane of Gram-negative bacteria. They work by interacting with the lipopolysaccharide (LPS) constituent of the membrane outside, leading to increased permeability and eventually cell death. Colistin (polymyxin E) has gained renewed interest in recent years as a last-resort antibiotic for multidrug-resistant Gram-negative infections. A study by Manioglu *et al.* (2022) on many plant-derived compounds demonstrated promise in breaking down bacterial cell membranes. Essential oils and their constituents, such as terpenes and phenolics, have been investigated for their antimicrobial properties, and research has shed light on the molecular underpinnings of polymyxin activity and highlighted their potential in fighting antibiotic-resistant pathogens [143]. A review by Yousefi *et al.* (2022) discussed the mechanisms by which essential oils disrupt bacterial membranes [144]. The authors noted that these compounds could increase membrane permeability, leading to the leakage of ions and other cellular contents.

CLINICAL APPLICATIONS

Conventional therapy for bacterial infections involves various approaches, each playing a crucial role in different clinical scenarios. Empiric therapy, targeted therapy, and prophylactic use are three key strategies employed by clinicians to combat bacterial infections effectively. Fig. (**3**) outlines the clinical application strategies used in conventional therapy. Understanding the role of each approach is essential for optimal patient care and antibiotic stewardship.

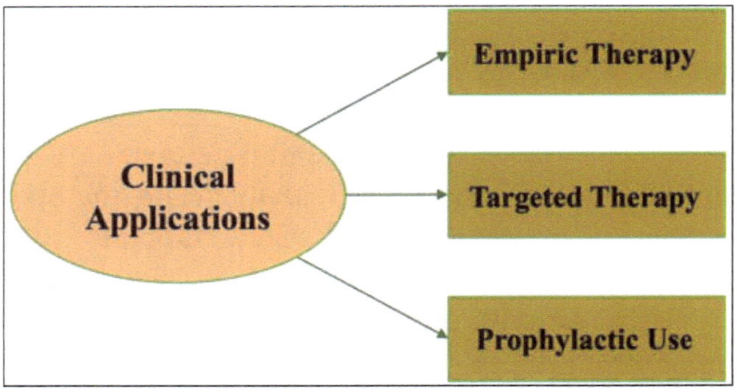

Fig. (3). Clinical applications.

Empiric therapy

Empiric therapy involves initiating antibiotic treatment based on clinical presentation and pathogen identification before obtaining definitive microbiological results. This approach is crucial in scenarios where delaying treatment could lead to severe consequences. Clinical Application: Empiric therapy is commonly used in sepsis and septic shock, community-acquired pneumonia, meningitis, and febrile neutropenia. A landmark study by Reeves *et al.* (2024) demonstrated the importance of early empiric antibiotic administration in septic shock [146]. They found that an hourly delay in the delivery of antibiotics was linked to a 7.6% reduction in survival on average. Broad-spectrum antibiotics are frequently advised by guidelines for empirical treatment in order to treat the most likely infections. For example, the Infectious Diseases Society of America (IDSA) recommends empiric treatment for community-acquired pneumonia, depending on patient risk factors and trends of local antibiotic resistance [147].

Targeted Therapy

Targeted therapy refers to the selection of antibiotics based on identified pathogens and their susceptibility profiles, usually after microbiological confirmation. It allows clinicians to tailor therapy, minimize side effects, and reduce resistance development. For example, using MALDI-TOF MS for rapid pathogen identification can significantly shorten the time to targeted treatment and improve clinical outcomes [148]. This contrasts with empiric therapy, which is initiated before laboratory results are available and often involves broad-spectrum agents [149].

Targeted Therapy *vs.* Conventional Therapy

Targeted therapy involves the administration of antibiotics based on the specific identification of the causative bacterial pathogen and its antibiotic susceptibility profile. This approach contrasts with conventional empiric therapy, where treatment is initiated based on clinical judgment and probable pathogens before laboratory confirmation is available. In targeted therapy, clinicians utilize microbiological culture results, rapid diagnostics (such as PCR or MALDI-TOF MS), and sensitivity testing to guide antibiotic selection. This precision significantly reduces unnecessary antibiotic exposure, minimizes the risk of adverse effects, and plays a crucial role in combating antimicrobial resistance (AMR). For example, in bloodstream infections, studies have shown that shifting from broad-spectrum empiric therapy to targeted therapy—once culture results are available—can decrease mortality rates, lower treatment costs, and prevent selection pressure for resistant organisms. In contrast, empiric therapy, although essential in critical situations like sepsis or meningitis, carries a higher risk of overuse of broad-spectrum antibiotics. While it ensures timely intervention, especially in life-threatening infections, it must be followed by de-escalation based on pathogen identification to avoid resistance development.

Therefore, targeted therapy is a key component of antibiotic stewardship programs, ensuring optimal use of antimicrobials. It aligns with modern clinical goals, including effective treatment, prevention of resistance, and preservation of microbiota. While empiric therapy remains necessary in many acute settings, its careful transition to targeted therapy ensures better patient and public health outcomes.

CHALLENGES IN CONVENTIONAL THERAPY

One of the biggest problems in treating bacterial illnesses is still antibiotic resistance. Declared a global health emergency by the World Health Organization, it poses a danger to the successful prevention and treatment of an ever-widening spectrum of illnesses.

Recent Developments: A comprehensive review demonstrated an increase in methicillin-resistant Staphylococcus aureus (MRSA), carbapenem-resistant

Enterobacteriaceae (CRE), and extensively drug-resistant (XDR) TB [150]. The U.S. experiences about 2.8 million antibiotic-resistant illnesses annually, leading to over 35,000 fatalities, according to the 2019 CDC Antibiotic Resistance Threats Report (CDC, 2019). Resistance mechanisms include altered antibiotic targets, decreased permeability, and enhanced efflux, as well as the enzymatic breakdown of antibiotics (such as beta-lactamases). A study by Vintila *et al.* (2023) found that the prevalence of MDR pathogens in intensive care units across Europe has increased significantly over the past decade, with particular concern for *Acinetobacter baumannii* and *Pseudomonas aeruginosa* [151]. While antibiotics have revolutionized medicine, they can also cause significant adverse effects and toxicity, presenting challenges in patient management. Common adverse effects were gastrointestinal disturbances, allergic reactions, nephrotoxicity, hepatotoxicity, and ototoxicity. A large-scale study by Yu *et al.* (2024) discovered that 20% of hospitalized patients had at least one significant medication event related to an antibiotic, with hematologic, renal, and gastrointestinal issues being the most frequent [152].

Specific concerns like C. difficile infections: A systematic review by Wang *et al.* (2024) highlighted the strong association between antibiotic use and *C. difficile* infections, emphasizing the need for judicious antibiotic prescribing [153]. Recent research has shown that antibiotics can permanently impact the gut microbiota. A study found that while most gut bacteria recovered after antibiotic treatment, some remained depleted for months, potentially increasing susceptibility to other infections [154].

Antibiotic-induced liver injury: A review by Román-Sagüillo *et al.* (2024) noted that antibiotics are among the most frequent causes of medication-induced liver damage, with amoxicillin-clavulanate being a prominent offender [155]. A meta-analysis by Yang *et al.* (2024) showed that therapeutic drug monitoring of vancomycin significantly reduced the incidence of nephrotoxicity [156].

Personalized dosing: Emerging research is exploring the use of pharmacogenomics to guide antibiotic dosing and reduce toxicity [157]. While controversial, some studies suggest that probiotics may help prevent antibiotic-associated diarrhea and *C. difficile* infections based on drug interactions [158]. Antibiotics can interact with numerous other medications, potentially leading to reduced efficacy, increased toxicity, or altered pharmacokinetics of either the antibiotic or the interacting drug.

Significant Interactions like Warfarin: Many antibiotics can increase the anticoagulant effect of warfarin. A study [159] discovered that the risk of serious bleeding episodes was considerably elevated when antibiotics and warfarin were administered together.

Oral contraceptives: The efficacy of some antibiotics may be compromised. However, a systematic review by Vega *et al.* (2023) concluded that most antibiotics do not affect hormonal contraception, with rifampin being a notable exception [160]. Proton pump inhibitors can affect the absorption of certain antibiotics. A study by Schumacher *et al.* (2024) discovered that using proton pump inhibitors concurrently greatly decreased the effectiveness of *Helicobacter pylori* eradication treatment.

Statins [161]. The risk of statin-induced myopathy may be elevated by macrolide antibiotics. A population-based cohort study by Wei *et al.* (2023) found an increased risk of rhabdomyolysis when clarithromycin was co-prescribed with statins [162].

STRATEGIES TO COMBAT RESISTANCE

The creation of novel antibiotics is vital in the battle against antimicrobial resistance. However, this process faces significant challenges, including high development costs and regulatory hurdles. Recent developments are as follows:

Teixobactin: Discovered in 2015, this compound shows potential against drug-resistant types of Gram-positive microbes. A study by [163] demonstrated its efficacy in animal models of MRSA infection.

Murepavadin: It is a novel outer membrane protein-targeting antibiotic for Pseudomonas aeruginosa. However [164], a study reported that phase III trials were halted due to nephrotoxicity concerns.

Lefamulin: It is a pleuromutilin antibiotic approved in 2019 for community-acquired bacterial pneumonia [165]. A research reported its non-inferiority to moxifloxacin in clinical trials. Programs for antibiotic stewardship, or ASPs, are organized efforts aimed at enhancing and monitoring the responsible use of antibiotics. Important elements include action, drug skills, responsibility, commitment from leadership, tracking, reporting, and education. A systematic review [166] found that ASPs can effectively reduce antibiotic use and improve patient outcomes. Specific strategies include prospective audit and feedback. A study [167] showed that this approach reduced antibiotic use by 14% in a pediatric hospital setting. Rapid diagnostic testing demonstrated that rapid pathogen identification led to faster targeted therapy and improved outcomes in bloodstream infections [168]. For clinical decision support systems, a meta-analysis by Tokgöz (2024) found that computerized decision support can significantly improve antibiotic prescribing practices [169]. As antibiotic resistance grows, alternative therapies are being explored to complement or replace conventional antibiotics. Similar to phages, bacteria-specific viruses are used in bacteriophage therapy. A case report by Schmalstig (2024) described the successful use of phage therapy in a person with an illness caused by multidrug resistance [170]. Antimicrobial peptides (AMPs) are naturally occurring molecules that can disrupt bacterial membranes. A review by Mulukutla *et al.* (2024) highlighted the potential of AMPs as alternatives to conventional antibiotics, noting their broad-spectrum activity and low propensity for resistance development [171]. Immunomodulatory approaches enhance the host immune response to fight infections. A study by Hedges *et al.* (2023) demonstrated that immunostimulation with a TLR4 agonist improved outcomes in a mouse model of pneumonia [172]. Antivirulence strategies are therapeutic approaches that target bacterial virulence factors rather than growth. A review by Ford *et al.* (2021) discussed various antivirulence approaches, including quorum-sensing inhibitors and toxin neutralizers [173]. Combining multiple antibiotics or an antibiotic with a non-antibiotic agent can enhance efficacy and potentially slow the development of resistance. Combinations of beta-lactam/beta-lactamase inhibitors are as follows:

Ceftazidime-avibactam: This combination is licensed for the management of infections caused by carbapenem-resistant enterobacterales (CRE). A meta-analysis by Baig *et al.* (2023) showed its superiority over colistin-based regimens for CRE infections.

Meropenem-vaborbactam: It is another combination effective against CRE [174]. Herald *et al.* (2023) reported its efficacy in an advanced infection of the urinary tract phase 3 study [175].

Antibiotic-Antibiotic Combinations: A systematic review [176] found that combination therapy could be effective for certain MDR infections, particularly in critically ill patients. However, they cautioned against routine use due to the potential for increased toxicity. Antibiotic-Adjuvant Combinations: Antibiotic + Efflux pump inhibitor: A study [177] demonstrated that combining levofloxacin with an efflux pump inhibitor restored its activity against resistant *P. aeruginosa* strains.

Antibiotic + Potentiator [178]: A study identified a compound that potentiated the activity of tetracycline against resistant *E. coli* by targeting a metabolic pathway.

FUTURE DIRECTIONS

The discovery of traditional antibiotics has been struggling to keep pace with the emergence of resistant bacteria. However, recent innovations are offering new hope in the fight against antimicrobial resistance. A groundbreaking study [179] on cells used a deep learning approach to identify a novel, broad-spectrum antibiotic named halicin. This compound showed efficacy against multidrug-resistant pathogens, including *Acinetobacter baumannii* and *Clostridioides difficile*. Another promising application is the application of AI to predict resistance to antibiotics. A study by Tan *et al.* (2024) showed how computer intelligence algorithms can utilize genetic data to predict antibiotic resistance, which might lead to more focused antibiotic use [180].

Novel Screening Methods: Innovative screening methods are uncovering antibiotics from previously untapped sources. Srivastava *et al.* (2022) discussed the potential of mining the human microbiome for new antimicrobials [181]. They highlighted the discovery of lugdunin, a novel antibiotic produced by nasal bacteria that shows activity against MRSA. Synthetic biology is being applied to engineer novel antibiotics. A review by Zhang *et al.* (2024) explored the potential of using synthetic biology to create new antimicrobial compounds and to modify existing ones for improved efficacy [182]. Nanoparticles offer new possibilities for antibiotic delivery and efficacy. A study by Albandar *et al.* (2024) demonstrated that vancomycin-loaded nanoparticles showed enhanced efficacy against MRSA biofilms compared to free vancomycin [183].

Role of Genomics and Personalized Medicine: The integration of genomics and personalized medicine approaches is poised to change the way bacterial infections are identified and treated. Next-generation sequencing (NGS) technologies are enabling faster and more accurate pathogen identification. A study by Wang *et al.* (2024) demonstrated the use of metagenomic NGS for rapid diagnosis of neurological infections, leading to timely and targeted antibiotic therapy [184]. Genomic data can be used to predict antibiotic susceptibility, potentially reducing the time to effective therapy. According to a large-scale study by Zhou *et al.* (2024), microbiologists used machine learning models trained on bacterial genome sequences to predict antibiotic resistance with high accuracy [185]. Understanding the host response to infection can guide treatment decisions [186]. A host gene expression signature can distinguish bacterial from viral infections, potentially reducing unnecessary antibiotic use.

Pharmacogenomics: Genetic variations can affect antibiotic metabolism and efficacy. A review discussed the impact of pharmacogenomics on antibiotic therapy, highlighting the potential for personalized dosing strategies [187]. Novel approaches beyond traditional antibiotics are showing promise in treating bacterial infections. Phage therapy is experiencing a renaissance, particularly for multidrug-resistant infections. A case report highlighted how a patient with cystic fibrosis was successfully treated for a multidrug-resistant Mycobacterium abscessus infection using engineered bacteriophages [188]. Despite the success of this treatment, there are still obstacles to overcome, such as potential phage resistance and regulatory barriers, but these are being addressed by developments in phage building and delivery techniques. A review discussed recent progress and future directions in phage therapy.

CRISPR-Cas Antimicrobials: CRISPR-Cas systems are being explored as programmable antimicrobials [189]. A study demonstrated the use of CRISPR-Cas9 to selectively kill antibiotic-resistant bacteria (190) using a mouse model of *Staphylococcus aureus*.

Antimicrobial Peptides (AMPs): AMPs offer a potential alternative to traditional antibiotics. A comprehensive review highlighted the diverse mechanisms of action of AMPs and their potential as therapeutics [191]. The authors discussed ongoing clinical trials and the challenges in AMP development, including stability and delivery issues.

Immunomodulatory Approaches: Harnessing the host immune response is an emerging strategy for treating bacterial infections. A study demonstrated that an immunostimulant with a TLR4 agonist improved outcomes in a mouse model of pneumonia [192].

Antivirulence Strategies: Targeting bacterial virulence factors rather than bacterial growth is a promising approach to combat resistance. A review discussed various antivirulence strategies, including quorum-sensing inhibitors and toxin neutralizers [193].

CONCLUSION

This chapter underscores the essential role of conventional antibiotics in treating bacterial infections, highlighting their mechanisms of action and clinical effectiveness. Aminoglycosides like gentamicin are particularly effective against aerobic Gram-negative bacteria, while cephalosporins inhibit bacterial cell wall synthesis, leading to cell lysis. Carbapenems, known for their broad-spectrum activity, are vital in managing infections caused by multidrug-resistant (MDR) pathogens. Alongside these conventional agents, the chapter also addresses the growing challenge of antimicrobial resistance (AMR), which complicates treatment outcomes and necessitates a reevaluation of antibiotic use. In response, alternative therapies such as phage therapy and metal-based antimicrobials are gaining attention as adjuncts to traditional antibiotics. Furthermore, the importance of judicious empiric therapy is emphasized, especially in healthcare-associated settings where MDR organisms are prevalent. Early initiation of empiric treatment should be promptly refined through culture-guided de-escalation to optimize therapeutic outcomes while minimizing resistance development.

REFERENCES

[1] Pancu DF, Scurtu A, Macasoi IG, *et al.* Antibiotics: Conventional therapy and natural compounds with antibacterial activity—a pharmaco-toxicological screening. Antibiotics (Basel) 2021; 10(4): 401.https://pubmed.ncbi.nlm.nih.gov/33917092/ [http://dx.doi.org/10.3390/antibiotics10040401] [PMID: 33917092]

[2] Alaoui Mdarhri H, Benmessaoud R, Yacoubi H, *et al.* Alternatives Therapeutic Approaches to Conventional Antibiotics: Advantages, Limitations and Potential Application in Medicine. Antibiotics (Basel) 2022; 11(12): 1826.https://pubmed.ncbi.nlm.nih.gov/36551487/ [http://dx.doi.org/10.3390/antibiotics11121826] [PMID: 36551487]

[3] Chaves AD, Kilbourne ED, Tompsett RR, Woodward TE. Therapy of Infections. Bull N Y Acad Med 2021; 34(2): 183-215.https://link.springer.com/chapter/10.1007/978-3-030-65225-8_14 [Internet].

[4] Yazici H, Alpaslan E, Bhardwaj G, Webster TJ. Conventional and nano-based approaches to prevent bacterial infection. Biomedical Nanomaterials: From design to implementation 2016 Jan 1 195-220.

[5] Ligon BL. Sir Alexander Fleming: Scottish researcher who discovered penicillin. Semin Pediatr Infect Dis 2004; 15(1): 58-64. [http://dx.doi.org/10.1053/j.spid.2004.02.002] [PMID: 15175996]

[6] Gulyás E, Horváth IL, Engh MA, *et al.* Assessment of the practical impact of adjusting beta-lactam dosages based on therapeutic drug monitoring in critically ill adult patients: a systematic review and meta-analysis of randomized clinical trials and observational studies. Sci Rep 2024; 14(1): 7793.https://www.nature.com/articles/s41598-024-58200-w [http://dx.doi.org/10.1038/s41598-024-58200-w] [PMID: 38565898]

[7] Mousavifar L, Roy R. Alternative therapeutic strategies to fight bacterial infections. Frontiers in Drug, Chemistry and Clinical Research 2019; 2(1). [http://dx.doi.org/10.15761/FDCCR.1000115]

[8] Roentgen therapy for infections: an historical review - PubMed [Internet]. [cited 2024 Aug 5] Available from:https://pubmed.ncbi.nlm.nih.gov/1750226/

[9] Hutchings MI, Truman AW, Wilkinson B. Antibiotics: past, present and future. Curr Opin Microbiol 2019; 51: 72-80.https://pubmed.ncbi.nlm.nih.gov/31733401/ [http://dx.doi.org/10.1016/j.mib.2019.10.008] [PMID: 31733401]

[10] Uddin TM, Chakraborty AJ, Khusro A, Zidan BRM, Mitra S, Emran T, *et al.* Antibiotic resistance in microbes: History, mechanisms, therapeutic strategies and future prospects. J Infect Public Health [Internet] 14(12): 1750-66.https://pubmed.ncbi.nlm.nih.gov/34756812/ 2021 Dec 1 [cited 2024 Aug 6]

[11] Downes KJ, Hayes M, Fitzgerald JC, *et al.* Mechanisms of antimicrobial-induced nephrotoxicity in children. J Antimicrob Chemother 2020; 75(1): 1-13. [http://dx.doi.org/10.1093/jac/dkz325] [PMID: 31369087]

[12] Volume 21 | Nature Reviews Microbiology [Internet]. [cited 2024 Aug 6] Available from: https://www.nature.com/nrmicro/volumes/21

[13] Shilpa Basak N, Meena SS. Microbial biodegradation of plastics: Challenges, opportunities, and a critical perspective. Front Environ Sci Eng [Internet] 2022 Dec 1 [cited 2024 Aug 6]; 16(12). Available from: /pmc/articles/PMC9295099/

[14] Trends in Microbiology | Journal | ScienceDirect.com by Elsevier [Internet]. [cited 2024 Aug 6] Available from: https://www.sciencedirect.com/journal/trends-in-microbiology

[15] Lobanovska M, Pilla G. Focus: Drug development: Penicillin's discovery and antibiotic resistance: Lessons for the future? Yale J Biol Med [Internet] 2017 Mar 1 [cited 2024 Aug 6]; 90(1): 135. Available from: /pmc/articles/PMC5369031/

[16] Twenty years of Nature Reviews Microbiology. Nat Rev Microbiol 2023; 21(10): 621. Available from:https://pubmed.ncbi.nlm.nih.gov/37700057/
[http://dx.doi.org/10.1038/s41579-023-00962-7] [PMID: 37700057]

[17] Boyd NK, Teng C, Frei CR. Brief overview of approaches and challenges in new antibiotic development: a focus on drug repurposing. Front Cell Infect Microbiol 2021; 11: 684515-5.
[http://dx.doi.org/10.3389/fcimb.2021.684515]

[18] Crunkhorn S. Explainable deep learning discovers novel antibiotic. Nat Rev Drug Discov 2024; 23(2): 107.
[PMID: 38216772]

[19] Aminov RI, Mackie RI. Evolution and ecology of antibiotic resistance genes. FEMS Microbiol Lett 2007; 271(2): 147-61.
[http://dx.doi.org/10.1111/j.1574-6968.2007.00757.x] [PMID: 17490428]

[20] Muteeb G, Rehman MT, Shahwan M, Aatif M. Origin of antibiotics and antibiotic resistance, and their impacts on drug development: A narrative review. Pharmaceuticals [Internet] 2023 Nov 1 [cited 2024 Aug 6]; 16(11). Available from:/pmc/articles/PMC10675245/
[http://dx.doi.org/10.3390/ph16111615]

[21] Williams KJ. The introduction of 'chemotherapy' using arsphenamine – the first magic bullet. J R Soc Med [Internet] 2009 Aug 8 [cited 2024 Aug 31] 102(8): 343. Available from: /pmc/articles/PMC2726818/

[22] Lalchhandama K. Reappraising Fleming's snot and mould. Sci Vis 2020; 20(1): 29-42.
[http://dx.doi.org/10.33493/scivis.20.01.03]

[23] Haller JS. The First Miracle Drugs: How the Sulfa Drugs Transformed Medicine. J Hist Med Allied Sci 2007; 63(1): 119-21. [Internet].
[http://dx.doi.org/10.1093/jhmas/jrm035]

[24] Quinn GA, Banat AM, Abdelhameed AM, Banat IM. Streptomyces from traditional medicine: sources of new innovations in antibiotic discovery J Med Microbiol [Internet] 2020 [cited 2024 Aug 31] 69(8): 1040. Available from:/pmc/articles/PMC7642979/

[25] Bo G. Giuseppe Brotzu and the discovery of cephalosporins. Clin Microbiol Infect 2000; 6(S3) (Suppl. 3): 6-8.
[http://dx.doi.org/10.1111/j.1469-0691.2000.tb02032.x] [PMID: 11449655]

[26] Pancu DF, Scurtu A, Macasoi IG, *et al.* Antibiotics: Conventional therapy and natural compounds with antibacterial activity—a pharmaco-toxicological screening. Antibiotics [Internet] 2021 Apr 1 [cited 2024 Aug 31] 10(4). Available from:/pmc/articles/PMC8744278/

[27] Armstrong T, Fenn SJ, Hardie KR. JMM Profile: Carbapenems: a broad-spectrum antibiotic J Med Microbiol [Internet] 2021 [cited 2024 Aug 31]; 70(12): 1462. Available from:/pmc/articles/PMC8744278/

[28] Sykes RB, Bonner DP. Aztreonam: The first monobactam. Am J Med 1985; 78(2): 2-10.https://pubmed.ncbi.nlm.nih.gov/3871589/
[http://dx.doi.org/10.1016/0002-9343(85)90196-2] [PMID: 3871589]

[29] Fernandes GFS, Scarim CB, Kim SH, Wu J, Castagnolo D. Oxazolidinones as versatile scaffolds in medicinal chemistry. RSC Med Chem [Internet] 2023 May 5 [cited 2024 Aug 31] 14(5): 823. Available from:/pmc/articles/PMC10211318/

[30] Lobanovska M, Pilla G. Focus: Drug Development: Penicillin's Discovery and Antibiotic Resistance: Lessons for the Future? Yale J Biol Med [Internet] 2017 Mar 1 [cited 2024 Aug 6] 90(1): 135. Available from:/pmc/articles/PMC5369031/

[31] Martins BA, Deffune E, Oliveira ON Jr, Moraes ML. Penicillin-binding proteins (PBPs) determine antibiotic action in Langmuir monolayers as nanoarchitectonics mimetic membranes of methicillin-resistant *Staphylococcus aureus*. Colloids Surf B Biointerfaces 2022; 214: 112447. [http://dx.doi.org/10.1016/j.colsurfb.2022.112447] [PMID: 35334310]

[32] Farooq S, Nissa MU, Saba NU, *et al.* Evaluation of Penicillins minimum inhibitory concentration against clinically isolated *Streptococcus pyogenes*. Int J Health Sci (Qassim) [Internet] 2023 May 25 [cited 2024 Aug 6] 7(S1): 2673-85. Available from:https://sciencescholar.us/journal/index.php/ijhs/article/view/14564

[33] Bennett D, Cunney RM, Meehan M, Mulhall R, Corcoran M, Broughton K, *et al.* Trends in invasive bacterial diseases during the first 2 years of the COVID-19 pandemic: analyses of prospective surveillance data from 30 countries and territories in the IRIS Consortium. Articles Lancet Digit Health [Internet] 2023 [cited 2024 Aug 7] 5: 582-93. Available from: www.thelancet.com/

[34] Quirke M, O'Sullivan R, Mccabe A, Ahmed J, Wakai A. Are two penicillins better than one? A systematic review of oral flucloxacillin and penicillin V *versus* oral flucloxacillin alone for the emergency department treatment of cellulitis. Eur J Emerg Med [Internet] 2014 [cited 2024 Aug 7] 21(3): 170-4. Available from: https://pubmed.ncbi.nlm.nih.gov/23542420/ [http://dx.doi.org/10.1097/MEJ.0b013e328360d980] [PMID: 23542420]

[35] Clement ME, Okeke NL, Hicks CB. Treatment of Syphilis A Systematic Review. JAMA [Internet] 2014 Nov 11 [cited 2024 Aug 7]; 3(12): 18-905. Available from: /pmc/articles/PMC6690208/

[36] Pericàs JM, Nathavitharana R, Garcia-de-la-Mària C, *et al.* Endocarditis caused by highly penicillin-resistant viridans group streptococci: Still room for vancomycin-based regimens. Antimicrob Agents Chemother [Internet] 2019 [cited 2024 Aug 7] 63(8): e00516-19. Available from:https://pubmed.ncbi.nlm.nih.gov/31182540/ [http://dx.doi.org/10.1128/AAC.00516-19] [PMID: 31182540]

[37] Lin X, Kück U. Cephalosporins as key lead generation beta-lactam antibiotics. Appl Microbiol Biotechnol [Internet] 2022 Dec 1 [cited 2024 Aug 7] 106(24): 8007. Available from:/pmc/articles/PMC9712332/ [http://dx.doi.org/10.1007/s00253-022-12272-8]

[38] Carcione D, Siracusa C, Sulejmani A, Leoni V, Intra J. Old and New Beta-Lactamase Inhibitors: Molecular Structure, Mechanism of Action, and Clinical Use. Antibiotics (Basel) 2021; 10(8): 995.https://pubmed.ncbi.nlm.nih.gov/34439045/ [http://dx.doi.org/10.3390/antibiotics10080995] [PMID: 34439045]

[39] Chaudhry SB, Veve MP, Wagner JL. Cephalosporins: A Focus on Side Chains and β-Lactam Cross-Reactivity. Pharmacy: Journal of Pharmacy Education and Practice [Internet] 2019 Jul 29 [cited 2024 Aug 7] 7(3): 103. Available from:/pmc/articles/PMC6789778/ [http://dx.doi.org/10.3390/pharmacy7030103]

[40] Lupia T, Corcione S, Pinna SM, de Rosa FG. New cephalosporins for the treatment of pneumonia in internal medicine wards. J Thorac Dis [Internet] 2020 Jul 1 [cited 2024 Aug 7]; 12(7): 37-47. Available from:/pmc/articles/PMC7399401/

[41] Bradley JS. Urinary Tract Infections Treated by Third-Generation Cephalosporins. Pediatrics [Internet] 2022 Jul 1 [cited 2024 Aug 7] 150(1). Available from:/pediatrics/article/150/1/e2022056219/188321/Urinary-Tract-Infections-Treated-by-Third [http://dx.doi.org/10.1542/peds.2022-056219]

[42] Burnham JP, Kirby JP, Kollef MH. Diagnosis and management of skin and soft tissue infections in the intensive care unit: a review. Intensive Care Med [Internet] 2016 Dec 1 [cited 2024 Aug 7] 42(12): 1899. Available from:/pmc/articles/PMC6276373/

[43] Kong W, Deng T, Li S, Shu Y, Wu Y. Efficacy, safety, and tolerability of antimicrobial agents for complicated intra-abdominal infection: a systematic review and network meta-analysis. BMC Infect Dis 2023; 23(1): 256.https://bmcinfectdis.biomedcentral.com/articles/10.1186/s12879-023-08209-9 [http://dx.doi.org/10.1186/s12879-023-08209-9] [PMID: 37085768]

[44] Geroulanos S, Marathias K, Kriaras J, Kadas B. Cephalosporins in surgical prophylaxis. J Chemother [Internet] 2001 [cited 2024 Aug 7]; (1): 23-6. 13 Spec No 1 Available from: https://pubmed.ncbi.nlm.nih.gov/11936371/

[45] Harrison CJ, Bratcher D. CephalosporinsA Review. Pediatr Rev [Internet] 2008 Aug 1 [cited 2024 Aug 7]; 29(8): 264-73. Available from: /pediatricsinreview/article/29/8/264/62769/CephalosporinsA-Review

[46] Cantarutti A, Rea F, Franchi M, Beccalli B, Locatelli A, Corrao G. Use of antibiotic treatment in pregnancy and the risk of several neonatal outcomes: A population-based study. Int J Environ Res Public Health [Internet] 2021 Dec 1 [cited 2024 Aug 7] 18(23). Available from: /pmc/articles/PMC8657211/ [http://dx.doi.org/10.3390/ijerph182312621]

[47] Giarratano A, Green SEL, Nicolau DP. Review of antimicrobial use and considerations in the elderly population. Clin Interv Aging [Internet] 2018 Apr 17 [cited 2024 Aug 7] 13(657). Available from: /pmc/articles/PMC5909780/ [http://dx.doi.org/10.2147/CIA.S133640]

[48] Lupia T, Corcione S, Mornese Pinna S, De Rosa FG. New cephalosporins for the treatment of pneumonia in internal medicine wards. Journal of Thoracic Disease 2020; 12(7): 3747-63. [http://dx.doi.org/10.21037/jtd-20-417]

[49] Papp-Wallace KM, Endimiani A, Taracila MA, Bonomo RA. Carbapenems: past, present, and future. Antimicrob Agents Chemother 2011; 55(11): 4943-60.https://pubmed.ncbi.nlm.nih.gov/21859938/ [http://dx.doi.org/10.1128/AAC.00296-11] [PMID: 21859938]

[50] Pervez MT, Hasnain MJU, Abbas SH, Moustafa MF, Aslam N, Shah SSM. A Comprehensive Review of Performance of Next-Generation Sequencing Platforms. Biomed Res Int [Internet] 2022 [cited 2024 Aug 7]; 2022. Available from:https://pubmed.ncbi.nlm.nih.gov/36212714/ [http://dx.doi.org/10.1155/2022/3457806]

[51] Strich JR, Heil EL, Masur H. Considerations for empiric antimicrobial therapy in sepsis and septic shock in an era of antimicrobial resistance J Infect Dis [Internet] 2020 Aug 8 [cited 2024 Aug 7] 222((Suppl 2)): S119. Available from:/pmc/articles/PMC7372215/

[52] Guillamet MCV, Damulira C, Atkinson A, Fraser VJ, Micek S, Kollef MH. Addition of aminoglycosides reduces recurrence of infections with multidrug-resistant Gram-negative bacilli in patients with sepsis and septic shock. Int J Antimicrob Agents 2023; 62(4): 106913. [http://dx.doi.org/10.1016/j.ijantimicag.2023.106913] [PMID: 37422096]

[53] Serio AW, Magalhães ML, Blanchard JS, Connolly LE. Aminoglycosides: Mechanisms of Action and Resistance. Antimicrobial Drug Resistance [Internet] 2017 [cited 2024 Aug 10]; 213-9. Available from:https://link.springer.com/chapter/10.1007/978-3-319-46718-4_14

[54] Hammoudi Halat D, Ayoub Moubareck C. Hospital-acquired and ventilator-associated pneumonia caused by multidrug-resistant Gram-negative pathogens: Understanding epidemiology, resistance patterns, and implications with COVID-19 F1000Research 2024 12:92 [Internet] 2024 Mar 25 [cited 2024 Aug 25] 12(92). Available from: https://f1000research.com/articles/12-92

[55] Bouwman K, George M. Clinical outcomes in patients who received a one-time aminoglycoside dose for extended-spectrum beta-lactamase-producing enterobacterales or pseudomonas aeruginosa cystitis. Antibiotics 2024, Vol 13, Page 552 [Internet]. 2024 Jun 13 [cited 2024 Aug 25] 13(6): 552. Available from: https://www.mdpi.com/2079-6382/13/6/552/htm [http://dx.doi.org/10.3390/antibiotics13060552]

[56] Caliman-Sturdza OA, Caliman-Sturdza OA. Enteroccocus and Endocarditis. 2024 Jun 11 [cited 2024 Aug 25] Available from: https://www.intechopen.com/online-first/89491 [http://dx.doi.org/10.5772/intechopen.114918]

[57] Cohen KA, Stott KE, Munsamy V, Manson AL, Earl AM, Pym AS. Evidence for expanding the role of streptomycin in the management of drug-resistant mycobacterium tuberculosis. Antimicrob Agents Chemother 2020; 64(9): e00860-20.https://journals.asm.org/doi/10.1128/aac.00860-20 [http://dx.doi.org/10.1128/AAC.00860-20] [PMID: 32540971]

[58] Kutob LF, Justo JA, Bookstaver PB, Kohn J, Albrecht H, Al-Hasan MN. Effectiveness of oral antibiotics for definitive therapy of Gram-negative bloodstream infections. Int J Antimicrob Agents 2016; 48(5): 498-503. [http://dx.doi.org/10.1016/j.ijantimicag.2016.07.013] [PMID: 27590704]

[59] Kanj SS, Bassetti M, Kiratisin P, *et al.* Clinical data from studies involving novel antibiotics to treat multidrug-resistant Gram-negative bacterial infections. Int J Antimicrob Agents 2022; 60(3): 106633. [http://dx.doi.org/10.1016/j.ijantimicag.2022.106633] [PMID: 35787918]

[60] Siegel SAR, Griffith DE, Philley JV, *et al.* Open-Label Trial of Amikacin Liposome Inhalation Suspension in Mycobacterium abscessus Lung Disease. Chest 2023; 164(4): 846-59. Available from: http://journal.chestnet.org/article/S0012369223008073/fulltext [http://dx.doi.org/10.1016/j.chest.2023.05.036] [PMID: 37419144]

[61] Grossman TH. Tetracycline Antibiotics and Resistance. Cold Spring Harb Perspect Med 2016; 6(4): a025387. Available from: https://pubmed.ncbi.nlm.nih.gov/26989065/ [http://dx.doi.org/10.1101/cshperspect.a025387] [PMID: 26989065]

[62] Gaur S, Bal AM. Tetracyclines. Comprehensive Pharmacology 2022; 7: 136-53. [http://dx.doi.org/10.1016/B978-0-12-820472-6.00185-7]

[63] Warner AJ, Hathaway-Schrader JD, Lubker R, Davies C, Novince CM. Tetracyclines and bone: Unclear actions with potentially lasting effects. Bone 2022; 159: 116377. [http://dx.doi.org/10.1016/j.bone.2022.116377] [PMID: 35248788]

[64] Khusainov I, Romanov N, Goemans C, Turoňová B, Zimmerli CE, Welsch S, *et al.* Bactericidal effect of tetracycline in *E. coli* strain ED1a may be associated with ribosome dysfunction. Nature Communications 2024 15:1 [Internet] 2024 Jun 5 [cited 2024 Aug 25] 15(1): 1-15. Available from: https://www.nature.com/articles/s41467-024-49084-5

[65] Barrenechea V, Vargas-Reyes M, Quiliano M, Milón P. A complementary mechanism of bacterial mRNA translation inhibition by tetracyclines. Front Microbiol 2021; 12: 682682. [http://dx.doi.org/10.3389/fmicb.2021.682682] [PMID: 34262544]

[66] Xia M, Fu S, Liu B. Discovery, development and syntheses of tetracycline antibiotics: derivation from natural products and application for human health. Scientia Sinica Chimica [Internet] 2023 Feb 27 [cited 2024 Aug 25] 53(3): 485-502. Available from:https://www.sciengine.com/10.1360/SSC-2022-0205 [http://dx.doi.org/10.1360/SSC-2022-0205]

[67] Ronayne CT, Jackson TD, Bennett CF, Perry EA, Kantorovic N, Puigserver P. Tetracyclines activate mitoribosome quality control and reduce ER stress to promote cell survival. EMBO Rep [Internet] 2023 Oct 11 [cited 2024 Aug 25] Available from: https://www.embopress.org/doi/10.15252/embr.202357228 [http://dx.doi.org/10.15252/embr.202357228]

[68] Dean RS, Kahat DH, Graden NR, DePhillipo NN, LaPrade RF, Laprade RF. Doxycycline improves tendon and cartilage pathologies in preclinical studies: current concepts. J ISAKOS 2020; 5(3): 144-9.http://www.jisakos.com/article/S205977542100119X/fulltext [Internet]. [http://dx.doi.org/10.1136/jisakos-2020-000451]

[69] Rassouli A, Shihmani B, Mehrzad J, Shokrpoor S. The immunomodulatory effect of minocycline on

gene expression of inflammation related cytokines in lipopolysaccharide-treated human peripheral blood mononuclear cells. Anim Biotechnol 2023; 34(7): 2159-65. Available from: https://www.tandfonline.com/doi/abs/10.1080/10495398.2022.2077743 [http://dx.doi.org/10.1080/10495398.2022.2077743] [PMID: 35622407]

[70] Gasparrini AJ, Markley JL, Kumar H, Wang B, Fang L, Irum S, *et al.* Tetracycline-inactivating enzymes from environmental, human commensal, and pathogenic bacteria cause broad-spectrum tetracycline resistance. Communications Biology 2020 3:1 [Internet] 2020 May 15 [cited 2024 Aug 25] 3(1): 1-12. Available from: https://www.nature.com/articles/s42003-020-0966-5 [http://dx.doi.org/10.1038/s42003-020-0966-5]

[71] Osei-Owusu H, Rondevaldova J, Houdkova M, *et al.* Evaluation of *in vitro* synergistic effects of tetracycline with alkaloid-related compounds against diarrhoeic bacteria. Int J Mol Sci 2024; 25(11): 6038.https://www.mdpi.com/1422-0067/25/11/6038/htm [http://dx.doi.org/10.3390/ijms25116038] [PMID: 38892226]

[72] Kounatidis D, Dalamaga M, Grivakou E, Karampela I, Koufopoulos P, Dalopoulos V, *et al.* Third-Generation Tetracyclines: Current Knowledge and Therapeutic Potential. Biomolecules 2024; 14: 783. [Internet]. 2024 Jun 30 [cited 2024 Aug 25] Available from: https://www.mdpi.com/2218-273X/14/7/783/htm

[73] Mandell LA, Wunderink RG, Anzueto A, Bartlett JG, Campbell GD, Dean NC, *et al.* Infectious Diseases Society of America/American Thoracic Society consensus guidelines on the management of community-acquired pneumonia in adults. Clin Infect Dis [Internet] 2007 Mar 1 [cited 2024 Aug 10] 44(Suppl 2(Suppl 2)) Available from: https://pubmed.ncbi.nlm.nih.gov/17278083/

[74] Ramirez JA, Musher DM, Evans SE, *et al.* Treatment of Community-Acquired Pneumonia in Immunocompromised Adults. Chest 2020; 158(5): 1896-911. Available from:https://pubmed.ncbi.nlm.nih.gov/32561442/ [http://dx.doi.org/10.1016/j.chest.2020.05.598] [PMID: 32561442]

[75] Sethi S, Murphy TF. Bacterial Infection in Chronic Obstructive Pulmonary Disease in 2000: a State-of-the-Art Review Clin Microbiol Rev [Internet] 2001 [cited 2024 Aug 10] 14(2): 336. Available from:/pmc/articles/PMC88978/

[76] Sexually transmitted diseases treatment guidelines PubMed [Internet] [cited 2024 Aug 10] 2015. Available from: https://pubmed.ncbi.nlm.nih.gov/26042815/

[77] Clement ME, Okeke NL, Hicks CB. Treatment of Syphilis. JAMA 2014; 312(18): 1905-17. Available from:https://pubmed.ncbi.nlm.nih.gov/25387188/ [http://dx.doi.org/10.1001/jama.2014.13259] [PMID: 25387188]

[78] Wormser GP, Dattwyler RJ, Shapiro ED, *et al.* The clinical assessment, treatment, and prevention of lyme disease, human granulocytic anaplasmosis, and babesiosis: clinical practice guidelines by the Infectious Diseases Society of America. Clin Infect Dis 2006; 43(9): 1089-134. Available from: https://pubmed.ncbi.nlm.nih.gov/17029130/ [http://dx.doi.org/10.1086/508667] [PMID: 17029130]

[79] Biggs HM, Behravesh CB, Bradley KK, *et al.* Diagnosis and management of tickborne rickettsial diseases: Rocky mountain spotted fever and other spotted fever group rickettsioses, ehrlichioses, and anaplasmosis — United States. MMWR Recomm Rep 2016; 65(2): 1-44.https://pubmed.ncbi.nlm.nih.gov/27172113/ [http://dx.doi.org/10.15585/mmwr.rr6502a1] [PMID: 27172113]

[80] Bakken JS, Dumler JS. Human granulocytic anaplasmosis. Infect Dis Clin North Am 2015; 29(2): 341-55.https://pubmed.ncbi.nlm.nih.gov/25999228/ [http://dx.doi.org/10.1016/j.idc.2015.02.007] [PMID: 25999228]

[81] Zaenglein AL, Pathy AL, Schlosser BJ, *et al.* Guidelines of care for the management of acne vulgaris. J Am Acad Dermatol 2016; 74(5): 945-973.e33. Available from: https://pubmed.ncbi.nlm.nih.gov/26897386/

[http://dx.doi.org/10.1016/j.jaad.2015.12.037] [PMID: 26897386]

[82] Del Rosso JQ, Webster GF, Jackson M, *et al.* Two randomized phase III clinical trials evaluating anti-inflammatory dose doxycycline (40-mg doxycycline, USP capsules) administered once daily for treatment of rosacea. J Am Acad Dermatol 2007; 56(5): 791-802. Available from: https://pubmed.ncbi.nlm.nih.gov/17367893/ [http://dx.doi.org/10.1016/j.jaad.2006.11.021] [PMID: 17367893]

[83] Tan KR, Magill AJ, Parise ME, Arguin PM. Doxycycline for malaria chemoprophylaxis and treatment: report from the CDC expert meeting on malaria chemoprophylaxis. Am J Trop Med Hyg 2011; 84(4): 517-31. Available from:https://pubmed.ncbi.nlm.nih.gov/21460003/ [http://dx.doi.org/10.4269/ajtmh.2011.10-0285] [PMID: 21460003]

[84] Raoult D, Roux V. Rickettsioses as paradigms of new or emerging infectious diseases. Clin Microbiol Rev 1997; 10(4): 694-719. Available from: https://pubmed.ncbi.nlm.nih.gov/9336669/ [http://dx.doi.org/10.1128/CMR.10.4.694] [PMID: 9336669]

[85] Ariza J, Bosilkovski M, Cascio A, Colmenero JD, Corbel MJ, Falagas ME. Perspectives for the treatment of brucellosis in the 21st century: the Ioannina recommendations. PLoS Med 2007; 4(12): e317. Available from:https://pubmed.ncbi.nlm.nih.gov/18162038/ [http://dx.doi.org/10.1371/journal.pmed.0040317] [PMID: 18162038]

[86] Sack DA, Sack RB, Nair GB, Siddique AK. Cholera. Lancet 2004; 363(9404): 223-33. Available from:https://pubmed.ncbi.nlm.nih.gov/14738797/ [http://dx.doi.org/10.1016/S0140-6736(03)15328-7] [PMID: 14738797]

[87] Brown-Elliott BA, Philley JV. Rapidly Growing Mycobacteria. Microbiol Spectr 2017; 5(1): 5.1.02. Available from: https://pubmed.ncbi.nlm.nih.gov/28084211/ [http://dx.doi.org/10.1128/microbiolspec.TNMI7-0027-2016] [PMID: 28084211]

[88] Loftus EV Jr. Management of extraintestinal manifestations and other complications of inflammatory bowel disease. Curr Gastroenterol Rep 2004; 6(6): 506-13. Available from: https://pubmed.ncbi.nlm.nih.gov/15527681/ [http://dx.doi.org/10.1007/s11894-004-0073-7] [PMID: 15527681]

[89] Malfertheiner P, Megraud F, O'Morain CA, *et al.* Management of *Helicobacter pylori* infection—the Maastricht V/Florence Consensus Report. Gut 2017; 66(1): 6-30. Available from: https://pubmed.ncbi.nlm.nih.gov/27707777/ [http://dx.doi.org/10.1136/gutjnl-2016-312288] [PMID: 27707777]

[90] Yanoff M, Duker JS, Zeitz O, Myron Yanoff and, Jay S. Duker: Ophthalmology, Fifth Edition. Graefe's Archive for Clinical and Experimental Ophthalmology 2019 258:2 [Internet] 2019 Nov 25 [cited 2024 Aug 10] 258(2): 459-9. Available from: https://link.springer.com/article/10.1007/s00417-019-04489-7

[91] Williams HC, Wojnarowska F, Kirtschig G, *et al.* Doxycycline versus prednisolone as an initial treatment strategy for bullous pemphigoid: a pragmatic, non-inferiority, randomised controlled trial. Lancet 2017; 389(10079): 1630-8. Available from: https://pubmed.ncbi.nlm.nih.gov/28279484/ [http://dx.doi.org/10.1016/S0140-6736(17)30560-3] [PMID: 28279484]

[92] Bachelez H, Senet P, Cadranel J, Kaoukhov A, Dubertret L. The use of tetracyclines for the treatment of sarcoidosis. Arch Dermatol 2001; 137(1): 69-73. Available from: https://pubmed.ncbi.nlm.nih.gov/11176663/ [http://dx.doi.org/10.1001/archderm.137.1.69] [PMID: 11176663]

[93] O'Dell JR, Leff R, Paulsen G, *et al.* Treatment of rheumatoid arthritis with methotrexate and hydroxychloroquine, methotrexate and sulfasalazine, or a combination of the three medications: Results of a two-year, randomized, double-blind, placebo-controlled trial. Arthritis Rheum 2002; 46(5): 1164-70. [http://dx.doi.org/10.1002/art.10228] [PMID: 12115219]

[94] Yates PA, Newman SA, Oshry LJ, Glassman RH, Leone AM, Reichel E. Doxycycline treatment of

high-risk COVID-19-positive patients with comorbid pulmonary disease. Ther Adv Respir Dis 2020; 14: 1753466620951053. Available from: https://pubmed.ncbi.nlm.nih.gov/32873175/ [http://dx.doi.org/10.1177/1753466620951053] [PMID: 32873175]

[95] Lamb R, Ozsvari B, Lisanti CL, *et al.* Antibiotics that target mitochondria effectively eradicate cancer stem cells, across multiple tumor types: Treating cancer like an infectious disease. Oncotarget 2015; 6(7): 4569-84. Available from: https://pubmed.ncbi.nlm.nih.gov/25625193/ [http://dx.doi.org/10.18632/oncotarget.3174] [PMID: 25625193]

[96] Dutta K, Basu A. Use of minocycline in viral infections. Indian J Med Res [Internet] 2011 May [cited 2024 Aug 10] 1335 : 467. Available from: /pmc/articles/PMC3121275/

[97] Dinos GP. The macrolide antibiotic renaissance. Br J Pharmacol [Internet] 2017 [cited 2024 Aug 16] 174(18): 2967. Available from: /pmc/articles/PMC5573421/ [http://dx.doi.org/10.1111/bph.13936]

[98] Kanoh S, Rubin BK. Mechanisms of action and clinical application of macrolides as immunomodulatory medications. Clin Microbiol Rev [Internet] [cited 2024 Aug 14] 2010; 23(3): 590. Available from: /pmc/articles/PMC2901655/ [http://dx.doi.org/10.1128/CMR.00078-09]

[99] Parnham MJ, Haber VE, Giamarellos-Bourboulis EJ, Perletti G, Verleden GM, Vos R. Azithromycin: Mechanisms of action and their relevance for clinical applications. Pharmacol Ther 2014; 143(2): 225-45. [http://dx.doi.org/10.1016/j.pharmthera.2014.03.003] [PMID: 24631273]

[100] Dinos GP. The macrolide antibiotic renaissance. Br J Pharmacol 2017; 174(18): 2967-83. Available from: https://onlinelibrary.wiley.com/doi/full/10.1111/bph.13936 [http://dx.doi.org/10.1111/bph.13936] [PMID: 28664582]

[101] Gomes C, Martínez-Puchol S, Palma N, *et al.* Macrolide resistance mechanisms in *Enterobacteriaceae* : Focus on azithromycin. Crit Rev Microbiol 2017; 43(1): 1-30. [http://dx.doi.org/10.3109/1040841X.2015.1136261] [PMID: 27786586]

[102] Malhotra-Kumar S, Lammens C, Coenen S, Van Herck K, Goossens H. Effect of azithromycin and clarithromycin therapy on pharyngeal carriage of macrolide-resistant streptococci in healthy volunteers: a randomised, double-blind, placebo-controlled study. Lancet 2007; 369(9560): 482-90. [http://dx.doi.org/10.1016/S0140-6736(07)60235-9] [PMID: 17292768]

[103] Muñoz JL, García-Molina F, Varón R, Rodriguez-Lopez JN, García-Cánovas F, Tudela J. Calculating molar absorptivities for quinones: Application to the measurement of tyrosinase activity. Anal Biochem 2006; 351(1): 128-38. Available from:https://pubmed.ncbi.nlm.nih.gov/16476401/ [http://dx.doi.org/10.1016/j.ab.2006.01.011] [PMID: 16476401]

[104] Abaleke E, Abbas M, Abbasi S, *et al.* Azithromycin in patients admitted to hospital with COVID-19 (RECOVERY): a randomised, controlled, open-label, platform trial. Lancet [Internet] 2021 Feb 13 [cited 2024 Aug 16] 397(10274): 605. Available from:/pmc/articles/PMC7884931/

[105] Daley CL, Iaccarino JM, Lange C, *et al.* Treatment of nontuberculous mycobacterial pulmonary disease: an official ATS/ERS/ESCMID/IDSA clinical practice guideline. Eur Respir J 2020; 56(1): 2000535. Available from: https://pubmed.ncbi.nlm.nih.gov/32636299/ [http://dx.doi.org/10.1183/13993003.00535-2020] [PMID: 32636299]

[106] Metlay JP, Waterer GW, Long AC, Anzueto A, Brozek J, Crothers K, *et al.* Diagnosis and treatment of adults with community-acquired pneumonia. An official clinical practice guideline of the American thoracic society and infectious diseases society of America Am J Respir Crit Care Med [Internet] 2019 Oct 10 [cited 2024 Aug 16] 200(7) Available from: /pmc/articles/PMC6812437/

[107] Karlowsky JA, Hackel MA, McLeod SM, Miller AA. *In Vitro* Activity of Sulbactam-Durlobactam against Global Isolates of *Acinetobacter baumannii-calcoaceticus* Complex Collected from 2016 to 2021. Antimicrob Agents Chemother 2022; 66(9): e00781-22. Available from: https://pubmed.ncbi.nlm.nih.gov/36005804/

[http://dx.doi.org/10.1128/aac.00781-22] [PMID: 36005804]

[108] Flamm RK, Farrell DJ, Rhomberg PR, Scangarella-Oman NE, Sader HS. Gepotidacin (GSK2140944) *In Vitro* Activity against Gram-Positive and Gram-Negative Bacteria. Antimicrob Agents Chemother 2017; 61(7): e00468-17. Available from: https://pubmed.ncbi.nlm.nih.gov/28483959/ [http://dx.doi.org/10.1128/AAC.00468-17] [PMID: 28483959]

[109] Fernandes P, Martens E, Bertrand D, Pereira D. The solithromycin journey—It is all in the chemistry. Bioorg Med Chem 2016; 24(24): 6420-8. [http://dx.doi.org/10.1016/j.bmc.2016.08.035] [PMID: 27595539]

[110] Blondeau JM. Immunomodulatory effects of macrolides considering evidence from human and veterinary medicine. Microorganisms 2022; 10(12). [http://dx.doi.org/10.3390/microorganisms10122438]

[111] Mustaev A, Malik M, Zhao X, *et al.* Fluoroquinolone-Gyrase-DNA Complexes: Two modes of drug binding*. J Biol Chem [Internet] 2014 May 5 [cited 2024 Aug 16] 289(18): 12300. Available from: /pmc/articles/PMC4007428/

[112] Tang K, Zhao H. Quinolone Antibiotics: Resistance and Therapy Infect Drug Resist [Internet] 2023 [cited 2024 Aug 16] 16(811) Available from: /pmc/articles/PMC9926991/

[113] Nowakowska J, Radomska D, Czarnomysy R, Marciniec K. Recent Development of Fluoroquinolone Derivatives as Anticancer Agents. Molecules. 2024 27; 29(15): 3538. [http://dx.doi.org/10.3390/molecules29153538]

[114] Hooper DC, Jacoby GA. Mechanisms of drug resistance: quinolone resistance. Ann N Y Acad Sci [Internet] 2015 Sep 1 [cited 2024 Aug 20] 1354(1): 12. Available from: /pmc/articles/PMC4626314/ [http://dx.doi.org/10.1111/nyas.12830]

[115] Zhu Y, Huang WE, Yang Q. Clinical Perspective of Antimicrobial Resistance in Bacteria. Infect Drug Resist [Internet] 2022 [cited 2024 Aug 20]; 15735. Available from: /pmc/articles/PMC8899096/ [http://dx.doi.org/10.2147/IDR.S345574]

[116] Li M, Wang Y, Jin J, Dou J, Guo Q, Ke X, *et al.* Inhibitory Activity of Honeysuckle Extracts against Influenza A Virus *In Vitro* and *In Vivo*. Virol Sin [Internet] 2021 Jun 1 [cited 2024 Aug 20] 36(3): 490. Available from: /pmc/articles/PMC8257810/ [http://dx.doi.org/10.1007/s12250-020-00302-6]

[117] Wise R, Lister D, McNulty CAM, Griggs D, Andrews JM. The comparative pharmacokinetics and tissue penetration of four quinolones including intravenously administered enoxacin. Infection [Internet] 1986 May [cited 2024 Aug 20]; 14(Suppl 3) (3 Supplement). Available from: https://pubmed.ncbi.nlm.nih.gov/3463542/ [http://dx.doi.org/10.1007/BF01667843]

[118] Uddin TM, Chakraborty AJ, Khusro A, *et al.* Antibiotic resistance in microbes: History, mechanisms, therapeutic strategies and future prospects. J Infect Public Health 2021; 14(12): 1750-66. [http://dx.doi.org/10.1016/j.jiph.2021.10.020] [PMID: 34756812]

[119] Ovung A, Bhattacharyya J. Sulfonamide drugs: structure, antibacterial property, toxicity, and biophysical interactions. Biophys Rev [Internet] 2021 Apr 1 [cited 2024 Aug 21] 13(2): 259. Available from: /pmc/articles/PMC8046889/ [http://dx.doi.org/10.1007/s12551-021-00795-9]

[120] Pereira LM, Baroni L, Yatsuda AP. A transgenic Neospora caninum strain based on mutations of the dihydrofolate reductase-thymidylate synthase gene. Exp Parasitol 2014; 138(1): 40-7. [http://dx.doi.org/10.1016/j.exppara.2014.01.004] [PMID: 24440296]

[121] Wang N, Luo J, Deng F, Huang Y, Zhou H. Antibiotic combination therapy: A strategy to overcome bacterial resistance to aminoglycoside antibiotics. Front Pharmacol [Internet] 2022 Feb 23 [cited 2024 Aug 21] 13. Available from: /pmc/articles/PMC8905495/ [http://dx.doi.org/10.3389/fphar.2022.839808]

[122] Imène B, Akram MM, Eddine MS, *et al.* Antibacterial, cytotoxic and genotoxic assessment of new sulfonamide derivatives. Chem Biodivers 2023; 20(9): e202300505. Available from: https://onlinelibrary.wiley.com/doi/full/10.1002/cbdv.202300505 [http://dx.doi.org/10.1002/cbdv.202300505] [PMID: 37532674]

[123] Wang M, Zhang J, Wang X, *et al.* Comparison of initial empirical antibiotic regimens in severe community-acquired pneumonia: a network meta-analysis. BMC Pulmonary Medicine 2025; 25(1): 246-6.
[http://dx.doi.org/10.1186/s12890-025-03695-w]

[124] Gattu R, Ramesh SS, Ramesh S. Role of small molecules and nanoparticles in effective inhibition of microbial biofilms: A ray of hope in combating microbial resistance. Microb Pathog 2024; 188: 106543.
[http://dx.doi.org/10.1016/j.micpath.2024.106543] [PMID: 38219923]

[125] Sarenje KL, van Zwetselaar M, Kumburu H, *et al.* Antimicrobial resistance and heterogeneity of Neisseria gonorrhoeae isolated from patients attending sexually transmitted infection clinics in Lusaka, Zambia. BMC Genomics 2024; 25(1): 290. Available from: https://bmcgenomics.biomedcentral.com/articles/10.1186/s12864-024-10155-y [http://dx.doi.org/10.1186/s12864-024-10155-y] [PMID: 38500064]

[126] Pathak D, Mazumder A. Potential of flavonoids as promising phytotherapeutic agents to combat multidrug-resistant infections. Curr Pharm Biotechnol 2024; 25(13): 1664-92. Available from: https://www.eurekaselect.com/article/136345
[http://dx.doi.org/10.2174/0113892010271172231108190233] [PMID: 38031767]

[127] Elawady BA, Mahmoud NR, Badawi HES, Badr AEE, Gohar NM. Antimicrobial activity of cefepime-tazobactam combination against extended spectrum beta-lactamase and/or AmpC beta-lactamase- producing gram-negative bacilli. BMC Infect Dis 2024; 24(1): 434. Available from: https://bmcinfectdis.biomedcentral.com/articles/10.1186/s12879-024-09296-y
[http://dx.doi.org/10.1186/s12879-024-09296-y] [PMID: 38654148]

[128] Catania AM, Stella MC, Cimino F, Zoppi S, Grego E. Sulfonamide resistance evaluation in five animal species and first report of sul4 in companion animals. Vet Microbiol 2024; 296: 110170.
[http://dx.doi.org/10.1016/j.vetmic.2024.110170] [PMID: 39029236]

[129] Wu Y, Zhou J, Shu T, Li W, Shang S, Du L. Epidemiological study of post-pandemic pediatric common respiratory pathogens using multiplex detection. Virol J 2024; 21(1): 168. Available from: https://virologyj.biomedcentral.com/articles/10.1186/s12985-024-02441-8
[http://dx.doi.org/10.1186/s12985-024-02441-8] [PMID: 39080730]

[130] Allison DG, Lambert PA. Modes of action of antibacterial agents. Molecular Medical Microbiology, Third Edition 2024 Jan 1 597-614.
[http://dx.doi.org/10.1016/B978-0-12-818619-0.00133-7]

[131] Ding T, Guo Z, Fang L, *et al.* Synergistic antibacterial effects of closantel and its enantiomers in combination with colistin against multidrug resistant gram-negative bacteria. Front Microbiol 2024; 15: 1374910.
[http://dx.doi.org/10.3389/fmicb.2024.1374910] [PMID: 38765678]

[132] Liang X, Cheng A, Ma C, Gao N. Bacterial protein synthesis. Molecular Medical Microbiology, Third Edition 2024 Jan 1 257-75.
[http://dx.doi.org/10.1016/B978-0-12-818619-0.00134-9]

[133] Barrenechea V, Vargas-Reyes M, Quiliano M, Milón P. A complementary mechanism of bacterial mRNA translation inhibition by tetracyclines. Front Microbiol [Internet] 2021 Jun 28 [cited 2024 Aug 21] 12 Available from: /pmc/articles/PMC8273347/
[http://dx.doi.org/10.3389/fmicb.2021.682682]

[134] Thorat VM, Bharambe MM, Thorat VM, Bharambe MM. Macrolide's anti-inflammatory effects on acute and subacute inflammation (azithromycin, clarithromycin, and roxithromycin). Available from:

https://services.igi-global.com/resolvedoi/resolve.aspx?doi=104018/979-8-3693-1301-5.ch018 Available from: www.igi-global.com/gateway/chapter/330413

[135] Wang X, Sun J, Nie Z, *et al.* Effect of Chloramphenicol as Antibiotic on the Structure and Function of Pepsin and Its Mechanism of Action. Chem Biodivers 2024; 21(2): e202301554. Available from: https://onlinelibrary.wiley.com/doi/full/10.1002/cbdv.202301554 [http://dx.doi.org/10.1002/cbdv.202301554] [PMID: 38128109]

[136] Merazka H, Bouchoucha A, Nessaib M, *et al.* Novel oxazolidinone zinc(II) complexes as antibacterial and anti-SARS-CoV-2 agents: synthesis, characterization, DFT calculations, ADMET, *in silico* molecular docking and biological activities. J Coord Chem 2023; 76(5-6): 798-829. Available from:https://www.tandfonline.com/doi/abs/10.1080/00958972.2023.2204512 [Internet]. [http://dx.doi.org/10.1080/00958972.2023.2204512]

[137] Wang X, Liu D, Li Y, Zhang D. Comparative analysis of antibiotics: Inhibition of protein synthesis versus DNA synthesis. Theoretical and Natural Science [Internet] 2024 Jul 26 [cited 2024 Aug 21] 44: 57-63. Available from: https://www.ewadirect.com/proceedings/tns/article/view/14327

[138] Powell JW, Mann CA, Toth PD, *et al.* Development of novel bacterial topoisomerase inhibitors assisted by computational screening. ACS Med Chem Lett [Internet] 2024 Aug 8 [cited 2024 Aug 21] Available from: https://pubs.acs.org/doi/abs/10.1021/acsmedchemlett.4c00162 [http://dx.doi.org/10.1021/acsmedchemlett.4c00162]

[139] Hamouche L, Poljak L, Carpousis AJ. Ribosomal RNA degradation induced by the bacterial RNA polymerase inhibitor rifampicin. RNA 2021; 27(8): 946-58. Available from: http://rnajournal.cshlp.org/content/27/8/946.full [http://dx.doi.org/10.1261/rna.078776.121] [PMID: 34099575]

[140] Cao X, Boyaci H, Chen J, Bao Y, Landick R, Campbell EA. Basis of narrow-spectrum activity of fidaxomicin on Clostridioides difficile. Nature 2022 604:7906 [Internet] 2022 Apr 6 [cited 2024 Aug 21] 604(7906): 541-5. Available from: https://www.nature.com/articles/s41586-022-04545-z [http://dx.doi.org/10.1038/s41586-022-04545-z]

[141] Dombach JL, Christensen GL, Allgood SC, Quintana JL, Detweiler CS. Inhibition of multiple staphylococcal growth states by a small molecule that disrupts membrane fluidity and voltage. bioRxiv 2024; 2024.01.17.576101. Internet Available from: https://www.biorxiv.org/content/10.1101/2024.01.17.576101v1

[142] Oberholzer CM, Caserta MT. Antimicrobial Update. Pediatr Infect Dis J 2005; 24(10): 919-20. Available from: https://journals.lww.com/pidj/fulltext/2005/10000/antimicrobial_update__daptomycin.13.aspx [http://dx.doi.org/10.1097/01.inf.0000181741.59226.a0] [PMID: 16220092]

[143] Manioglu S, Modaresi SM, Ritzmann N, Thoma J, Overall SA, Harms A, *et al.* Antibiotic polymyxin arranges lipopolysaccharide into crystalline structures to solidify the bacterial membrane. Nature Communications 2022 13:1 [Internet] 2022 Oct 21 [cited 2024 Aug 21] 13(1): 1-12. Available from: https://www.nature.com/articles/s41467-022-33838-0 [http://dx.doi.org/10.1038/s41467-022-33838-0]

[144] Yousefi S, Weisany W, Hosseini SE, Ghasemlou M. Mechanisms of nanoencapsulation to boost the antimicrobial efficacy of essential oils: A review. Food Hydrocoll 2024; 150: 109655. [http://dx.doi.org/10.1016/j.foodhyd.2023.109655]

[145] Kapoor G, Saigal S, Elongavan A. Action and resistance mechanisms of antibiotics: A guide for clinicians. J Anaesthesiol Clin Pharmacol 2017; 33(3): 300-5. Available from: https://journals.lww.com/joacp/fulltext/2017/33030/action_and_resistance_mechanisms_of_antibiotics__a.4.aspx [http://dx.doi.org/10.4103/joacp.JOACP_349_15] [PMID: 29109626]

[146] Reeves SD, Hartmann AP, Tedder AC, *et al.* Comparison of empiric antibiotic treatment regimens for

hospitalized, non-severe community-acquired pneumonia: A retrospective, multicenter cohort study. Clin Ther 2024; 46(4): 338-44. Available from: http://www.clinicaltherapeutics.com/article/S0149291824000201/fulltext [http://dx.doi.org/10.1016/j.clinthera.2024.01.009] [PMID: 38403509]

[147] Tomaszewski D, Guzek A, Rybicki Z. The empiric antimicrobial therapy: the comparison of initial choice with the results of microbiological investigations. an observational study. The Polish Journal of Aviation Medicine, Bioengineering and Psychology [Internet] 2023 Mar 18 [cited 2024 Aug 22] 29(1): 5-10. Available from: http://pjambp.com/view/abstract/id/16387

[148] Pandey N, Singh K, Kushwaha SP, Kumar A, *et al.* Targeted Drug Delivery to Combat Antibacterial Drug Resistance. In A. Grewal, A. Dhingra, K. Nepali, G. Deswal, & A. Srivastav (Eds.), Contemporary Approaches to Mitigating Antibacterial Drug Resistance pp. 250-267. https://services.igi-global.com/resolvedoi/resolve.aspx?doi=104018/979-8-3693-1540-8.ch0101AD Jan 1 [cited 2024 Aug 22]; [Internet] Available from: www.igi-global.com/gateway/chapter/343382 [http://dx.doi.org/10.4018/979-8-3693-1540-8.ch010]

[149] Moore BA, Barnett JE. Prophylactic Antibiotics. Case Studies in Clinical Psychological Science: Bridging the Gap from Science to Practice 2024; 1-7. [Internet] [cited 2024 Aug 22]. Available from: https://academic.oup.com/book/57303/chapter/461784914

[150] Abebe A, Birhanu A. Methicillin resistant *Staphylococcus aureus*: Molecular mechanisms underlying drug resistance development and novel strategies to combat. Infect Drug Resist 2023; 16: 7641-62. Available from: https://www.dovepress.com/methicillin-resistant-staphylococcus-aureus-molec-lar-mechanisms-under-peer-reviewed-fulltext-article-IDR [http://dx.doi.org/10.2147/IDR.S428103] [PMID: 38111667]

[151] Vintila BI, Arseniu AM, Butuca A, Sava M, Bîrluțiu V, Rus LL, *et al.* Adverse drug reactions relevant to drug resistance and ineffectiveness associated with meropenem, linezolid, and colistin: An analysis based on spontaneous reports from the European pharmacovigilance database. Antibiotics 2023; 12: 918.12(5): 918. [Internet] May 16 [cited 2024 Aug 22]. Available from: https://www.mdpi.com/2079-6382/12/5/918/htm

[152] Yu X, Zhou X, Li M, Zhao Y. Hematological adverse events associated with anti-MRSA agents: a real-world analysis based on FAERS. Expert Opin Drug Saf [Internet] 2024. Jan 27 [cited 2024 Aug 22]. Available from:https://www.tandfonline.com/doi/abs/10.1080/14740338.2024.2309225 [http://dx.doi.org/10.1080/14740338.2024.2309225]

[153] Wang L, Cao Y, Lou E, Zhao X, Chen X. The role of gut fungi in Clostridioides difficile infection. Biomed J 2024; 47(3): 100686. [http://dx.doi.org/10.1016/j.bj.2023.100686] [PMID: 38086471]

[154] Liu P, Zhang Y, Zhang Z, *et al.* Antibiotic-induced dysbiosis of the gut microbiota impairs gene expression in gut-liver axis of mice. Genes (Basel) 2023; 14(7): 1423. Available from: https://www.mdpi.com/2073-4425/14/7/1423/htm [http://dx.doi.org/10.3390/genes14071423] [PMID: 37510327]

[155] Román-Sagüillo S, Quiñones Castro R, Juárez-Fernández M, *et al.* Idiosyncratic Drug-Induced Liver Injury and Amoxicillin–Clavulanate: Spotlight on Gut Microbiota, Fecal Metabolome and Bile Acid Profile in Patients. Int J Mol Sci 2024; 25(13): 6863. Available from:https://www.mdpi.com/1422-0067/25/13/6863/htm [http://dx.doi.org/10.3390/ijms25136863] [PMID: 38999973]

[156] Yang JJ, Brett J, Sordo A, *et al.* The Influence of a Therapeutic Drug Monitoring Service on Vancomycin-Associated Nephrotoxicity. J Clin Pharmacol 2024; 64(1): 19-29. Available from: https://onlinelibrary.wiley.com/doi/full/10.1002/jcph.2363 [http://dx.doi.org/10.1002/jcph.2363] [PMID: 37779493]

[157] Dey S, Das S. The Impact of Probiotics Co-administration with Antibiotics on Health. Radinka journal of health science [Internet] 2024; 1(4): 123-30. 2024 Apr 30 [cited 2024 Aug 22]. Available from: https://rjupublisher.com/ojs/index.php/RJHS/article/view/237

[http://dx.doi.org/10.56778/rjhs.v1i4.237]

[158] Talukder A, Neog N, Goswami C, Kalita C. Current trajectory and prospective potential of pharmacogenomics in personalized medicines Futuristic Trends in Pharmacy & Nursing Volume 3 Book 3 2024 Mar 5 313-25.

[159] Vega AJ, Smith C, Matejowsky HG, Thornhill KJ, Borne GE, Mosieri CN, *et al.* Warfarin and Antibiotics: Drug Interactions and Clinical Considerations Life 2023 13: 1661. [Internet] 2023 Jul 30 [cited 2024 Aug 22]. Available from: https://www.mdpi.com/2075-1729/13/8/1661/htm

[160] Simmons KB, Haddad LB, Nanda K, Curtis KM. Drug interactions between rifamycin antibiotics and hormonal contraception: a systematic review. BJOG 2018; 125(7): 804-11. Available from: https://onlinelibrary.wiley.com/doi/full/10.1111/1471-0528.15027 [http://dx.doi.org/10.1111/1471-0528.15027] [PMID: 29130574]

[161] Schumacher J, Müller P, Sulzer J, Faber F, Molitor B, Maier L. Proton-pump inhibitors increase C. difficile infection risk by altering pH rather than by affecting the gut microbiome based on a bioreactor model. bioRxiv 2024; 7. Internet Available from:https://www.biorxiv.org/content/10.1101/2024.07.10.602898v1

[162] Wei C, Yin W, He Z, Wu B. Reporting of drug-induced myopathies associated with the combination of statins and daptomycin: A disproportionality analysis using the US food and drug administration adverse event reporting system. J Clin Med 2023; 12(10): 3548. Available from: https://www.mdpi.com/2077-0383/12/10/3548/htm [http://dx.doi.org/10.3390/jcm12103548] [PMID: 37240654]

[163] Qi YK, Tang X, Wei NN, Pang CJ, Du SS, Wang K. Discovery, synthesis, and optimization of teixobactin, a novel antibiotic without detectable bacterial resistance. J Pept Sci 2022; 28(11): e3428. Available from: https://onlinelibrary.wiley.com/doi/full/10.1002/psc.3428 [http://dx.doi.org/10.1002/psc.3428] [PMID: 35610021]

[164] Wei X, Gao J, Xu C, *et al.* Murepavadin induces envelope stress response and enhances the killing efficacies of β-lactam antibiotics by impairing the outer membrane integrity of *Pseudomonas aeruginosa.* Microbiol Spectr 2023; 11(5): e01257-23. Available from:https://journals.asm.org/doi/10.1128/spectrum.01257-23 [http://dx.doi.org/10.1128/spectrum.01257-23] [PMID: 37668398]

[165] Chen F, Dong Q, Hong W, Zhao J, Li Y. Moxifloxacin monotherapy for treatment of uncomplicated pelvic inflammatory disease: A systematic review and meta-analysis with trial sequential analysis of randomized controlled trials. Pharmacoepidemiol Drug Saf 2023; 32(11): 1189-99. Available from: https://onlinelibrary.wiley.com/doi/full/10.1002/pds.5677 [http://dx.doi.org/10.1002/pds.5677] [PMID: 37655831]

[166] Ryder JH, Preusker J, Watkins AB, *et al.* In-depth assessment of critical access hospital stewardship program adherence to the CDC Core Elements in Iowa and Nebraska. Infect Control Hosp Epidemiol 2024; 45(1): 123-6. Available from: https://www.cambridge.org/core/journals/infection-control-and-hospi-al-epidemiology/article/abs/indepth-assessment-of-critical-access-hospital-stew-rdship-program-adherence-to-the-cdc-core-elements-i--iowa-and-nebraska/531C5493D7F66FE624110263DD40D78E [http://dx.doi.org/10.1017/ice.2023.179] [PMID: 37534519]

[167] McCulloh RJ, Kerns E, Flores R, *et al.* A national quality improvement collaborative to improve antibiotic use in pediatric infections. Pediatrics [Internet] 2024 May 1 [cited 2024 Aug 24] 153(5). Available from: /pediatrics/article/153/5/e2023062246/197166/A-National-Quality-Improvem-nt-Collaborative-to [http://dx.doi.org/10.1542/peds.2023-062246]

[168] Peri AM, Chatfield MD, Ling W, Furuya-Kanamori L, Harris PNA, Paterson DL. Rapid diagnostic tests and antimicrobial stewardship programs for the management of bloodstream infection: What is their relative contribution to improving clinical outcomes? a systematic review and network meta-

analysis. Clin Infect Dis 2024; 79(2): 502-15.
[http://dx.doi.org/10.1093/cid/ciae234] [PMID: 38676943]

[169] Tokgöz P, Krayter S, Hafner J, Dockweiler C. Decision support systems for antibiotic prescription in hospitals: a survey with hospital managers on factors for implementation. BMC Med Inform Decis Mak 2024; 24(1): 96. Available from: https://bmcmedinformdecismak.biomedcentral.com/articles/10.1186/s12911-024-02490-7
[http://dx.doi.org/10.1186/s12911-024-02490-7] [PMID: 38622595]

[170] Schmalstig AA, Wiggins A, Badillo D, Wetzel KS, Hatfull GF, Braunstein M. Bacteriophage infection and killing of intracellular *Mycobacterium abscessus*. MBio 2024; 15(1): e02924-23. Available from: https://journals.asm.org/doi/10.1128/mbio.02924-23
[http://dx.doi.org/10.1128/mbio.02924-23] [PMID: 38059609]

[171] Mulukutla A, Shreshtha R, Kumar Deb V, Chatterjee P, Jain U, Chauhan N. Recent advances in antimicrobial peptide-based therapy. Bioorg Chem 2024; 145: 107151.
[http://dx.doi.org/10.1016/j.bioorg.2024.107151] [PMID: 38359706]

[172] Hedges JF, Snyder DT, Robison A, *et al.* A TLR4 agonist liposome formulation effectively stimulates innate immunity and enhances protection from bacterial infection. Innate Immun 2023; 29(3-4): 45-57. Available from: https://journals.sagepub.com/doi/10.1177/17534259231168725
[http://dx.doi.org/10.1177/17534259231168725] [PMID: 37083049]

[173] Ford CA, Hurford IM, Cassat JE. Antivirulence strategies for the treatment of *Staphylococcus aureus* infections: A mini review. Front Microbiol 2021; 11: 632706. Available from: www.frontiersin.org
[http://dx.doi.org/10.3389/fmicb.2020.632706] [PMID: 33519793]

[174] Baig M, Rahim S, Naseem Khan R, Memon DD, Ansari ZA, Athar Khan M. Efficacy of Intravenous Colistin Monotherapy Versus Colistin Combined With Meropenem in Patients With Multidrug-Resistant Infections: A Retrospective Observational Study. Cureus 2023; 15(10): e47342.
Available from: https://www.cureus.com/articles/194456-efficacy-of-intravenous-colistin-monotherapy-versus-colistin-combined-with-meropenem-in-patients-with-multidrug-resistant-infections-a-retrospective-observational-study
[http://dx.doi.org/10.7759/cureus.47342] [PMID: 38022127]

[175] Herald F, Burgos RM. Clinical evaluation of meropenem-vaborbactam combination for the treatment of urinary tract infection: Evidence to date. Infect Drug Resist 2023; 16: 555-68. Available from: https://www.dovepress.com/clinical-evaluation-of-meropenem-vaborbactam-combination--or-the-treat-peer-reviewed-fulltext-article-IDR
[http://dx.doi.org/10.2147/IDR.S187360] [PMID: 36726388]

[176] Halim J, Carr RA, Fliorent R, *et al.* Combinations of antibiotics effective against extensively- and pandrug-resistant *Acinetobacter baumannii* patient isolates. Microorganisms 2024; 12(7): 1353. Available from: https://www.mdpi.com/2076-2607/12/7/1353/htm
[http://dx.doi.org/10.3390/microorganisms12071353] [PMID: 39065123]

[177] Sheikhy M, Karbasizade V, Ghanadian M, Fazeli H. Evaluation of chlorogenic acid and carnosol for anti-efflux pump and anti-biofilm activities against extensively drug-resistant strains of Staphylococcus aureus and Pseudomonas aeruginosa. Papp-Wallace KM, editor Microbiol Spectr [Internet] 2024 Jul 24 [cited 2024 Aug 25] Available from:https://journals.asm.org/doi/10.1128/spectrum.03934-23
[http://dx.doi.org/10.1128/spectrum.03934-23]

[178] Sun F, Zhang L, Ma X, Ali T, Wu Y, Li L. A promising metabolite, 9-aminominocycline, restores the sensitivity of tigecycline against *tet*(X4)-positive *Escherichia coli.* Front Microbiol 2024; 15: 1432320.
[http://dx.doi.org/10.3389/fmicb.2024.1432320] [PMID: 39044954]

[179] Chinnaiyan K, Mugundhan SL, Narayanasamy D, Mohan M. Revolutionizing Healthcare and Drug Discovery: The Impact of Artificial Intelligence on Pharmaceutical Development. Curr Drug Ther 2024; 19: 1-16. Available from: https://www.eurekaselect.com/article/141789 [Internet].

[http://dx.doi.org/10.2174/0115748855313948240711043701]

[180] Tan Y, Le Scornet A, Yap MNF, Zhang D. Machine learning-based classification reveals distinct clusters of non-coding genomic allelic variations associated with Erm-mediated antibiotic resistance. mSystems [Internet] 2024. Jul 2 [cited 2024 Aug 25]. Available from: https://journals.asm.org/doi/10.1128/msystems.00430-24

[181] Srivastava N, Sarethy IP, Jeevanandam J, Danquah M. Emerging strategies for microbial screening of novel chemotherapeutics. J Mol Struct 2022; 1255: 132419. [http://dx.doi.org/10.1016/j.molstruc.2022.132419]

[182] Zhang X. Applications of synthetic biology in drug discovery. BIO Web Conf [Internet] 2024 May 31 [cited 2024 Aug 25] 111(02012). Available from: https://www.bio-conferences.org/articles/bioconf/abs/2024/30/bioconf_icbb2024_02012/bioconf_icbb2024_02012.html [http://dx.doi.org/10.1051/bioconf/202411102012]

[183] Albandar I, Jabbar SK, Ibrahim TK, Radhi OA, Mbalaha ZS. Advances of Nanotechnology in Eradication Bacterial Infectious Diseases: A Recent Review. Kirkuk Journal of Science [Internet] 2024 Jun 1 [cited 2024 Aug 25] 19(2): 34-6.2024. Available from: https://kujss.uokirkuk.edu.iq/article_183629.html [http://dx.doi.org/10.32894/kujss.2024.145530.1131]

[184] Wang X, Xu H, Qin L, *et al.* Metagenomic next-generation sequencing of cerebrospinal fluid reveals etiological and microbiological features in patients with various central nervous system infections. FASEB J 2024; 38(14): e23812. Available from:https://onlinelibrary.wiley.com/doi/full/10.1096/fj.202400792R [http://dx.doi.org/10.1096/fj.202400792R] [PMID: 39041354]

[185] Zhou X, Yang M, Chen F, *et al.* Prediction of antimicrobial resistance in *Klebsiella pneumoniae* using genomic and metagenomic next-generation sequencing data. J Antimicrob Chemother 2024; 79(10): 2509-17. [http://dx.doi.org/10.1093/jac/dkae248] [PMID: 39028665]

[186] Schlapbach LJ, Ganesamoorthy D, Wilson C, *et al.* Host gene expression signatures to identify infection type and organ dysfunction in children evaluated for sepsis: a multicentre cohort study. Lancet Child Adolesc Health 2024; 8(5): 325-38. Available from:http://www.thelancet.com/article/S2352464224000178/fulltext [http://dx.doi.org/10.1016/S2352-4642(24)00017-8] [PMID: 38513681]

[187] S MrRK, G MsS, Singh MrA, Ilango DrK. Pharmacogenomics-a genome based drug tailoring. Futuristic Trends in Pharmacy & Nursing Volume 2 Book 25 256-65. 2023 Nov 30

[188] Molina WPC, Riofrio MDP, Espinosa PMJ, Jurado MAS. Phage therapy against multiresistant bacteria Interamerican Journal of Health Sciences [Internet] 4: 91.(91) 2024 Jul 22 [cited 2024 Aug 25] Available from: https://ijhsc.uai.edu.ar/index.php/ijhsc/article/view/91/499

[189] Caillet C, Stofberg ML, Muleya V, Shonhai A, Zininga T. Host cell stress response as a predictor of COVID-19 infectivity and disease progression. Front Mol Biosci 2022; 9: 938099. [http://dx.doi.org/10.3389/fmolb.2022.938099] [PMID: 36032680]

[190] Sheng Y. Application of CRISPR technology in the prevention and control of bacterial drug resistance. [Internet] 2024 Jan 8 [cited 2024 Aug 25] 129224: 342-5. Available from: https://www.spiedigitallibrary.org/conference-proceedings--f-spie/12924/129241E/Application-of-CRISPR-technology-in-the-preven-ion-and-control-of/10.1117/12.3012860.full [http://dx.doi.org/10.1117/12.3012860]

[191] Maresca M, Lee BJ, Sabatier JM, Satchanska G, Davidova S, Gergova A. Diversity and mechanisms of action of plant, animal, and human antimicrobial peptides Antibiotics 2024, Vol 13, Page 202 [Internet] 2024 Feb 21 [cited 2024 Aug 25] 2024; 13(3): 202. Available from: https://www.mdpi.com/2079-6382/13/3/202/htm

[192] Chauhan RS, Malik YS, Saminathan M, Tripathi BN. . Immunomodulation. Essentials of Veterinary Immunology and Immunopathology [Internet] 2024 [cited 2024 Aug 25] 143-68. Available from: https://link.springer.com/chapter/10.1007/978-981-99-2718-0_6

[193] Julyantoro PGS, Bossier P, Defoirdt T. Minireview on sustainable antivirulence strategy for aquaculture Jurnal Riset Akuakultur [Internet] 2024 Jul 5 [cited 2024 Aug 25] 19(2): 157-76. Available from: http://ejournal-balitbang.kkp.go.id/index.php/jra/article/view/14352

CHAPTER 4

Challenges and Classical Strategies for Bacterial Infections

Arun K. Mishra[1,*], **Harpreet Singh**[2], **S.K. Paliwal**[3] and **Ajay Kumar Yadav**[4]

[1] *SOS School of Pharmacy, IFTM University, Moradabad-244102, India*

[2] *School of Pharmaceutical Sciences, IFTM University, Moradabad-2444102, India*

[3] *Department of Pharmacy, Banasthali Vidyapith, Banasthali-304022, India*

[4] *School of Pharmaceutical Sciences, CSJM University, Kanpur-208024, India*

Abstract: Conventional therapy, specifically the administration of antibiotics, plays a vital role in combating bacterial infections. The significance of this approach lies in its ability to efficiently eradicate bacteria from the body, prevent infection dissemination, and reduce the likelihood of complications or mortality. Antibiotics are specifically formulated to selectively attack bacteria, either by directly causing their death (bactericidal) or by impeding their growth and ability to reproduce (bacteriostatic). This approach's focused nature makes antibiotics highly effective in treating bacterial infections. Antibiotics are categorised into distinct classes that function through diverse mechanisms, including disruption of the bacterial cell wall, inhibition of protein synthesis, or interference with DNA replication. This particular type of variety enables customised treatment based on the specific type of bacteria and the location of the infection. Antibiotics rapidly eradicate bacteria, thereby mitigating the transmission of infectious diseases to others. It is especially crucial in extremely contagious diseases, such as bacterial meningitis, tuberculosis, or specific sexually transmitted infections. Unaddressed bacterial infections have the potential to disseminate throughout the body, resulting in serious complications such as sepsis, organ impairment, or long-term illness. Traditional treatment methods help to control the infection, thereby decreasing the likelihood of such consequences.

Keywords: Antibiotics, Bacteria, Conventional therapy, Infections.

INTRODUCTION

Bacterial infections such as sepsis, bacterial pneumonia, and meningitis can pose a serious risk to one's life [1]. Antibiotics can be crucial in these instances, as they swiftly eradicate the bacteria responsible for the infection, potentially saving lives [2]. The advent of antibiotics in the 20th century significantly diminished the

* **Corresponding author Arun K. Mishra:** SOS School of Pharmacy, IFTM University, Moradabad-244102, India; E-mail: arun_azam@rediffmail.com

Mukesh Kumar Singh, Gurdeep Singh, Amrendra Pratap Yadav & Papiya Bigoniya (Eds.)

mortality rates linked to bacterial infections, which had previously been a prominent global cause of death [3]. Appropriate use of antibiotics guarantees the eradication of all the bacteria responsible for the infection. Insufficient administration or improper use of antibiotics can lead to the survival of bacteria that are resistant to the drugs. These bacteria can then reproduce and cause more severe infections that are more difficult to treat [4]. When conventional therapy is prescribed and followed correctly, it reduces this risk to a minimum. Conventional therapy is a component of larger initiatives aimed at encouraging responsible antibiotic use, thereby mitigating the emergence of antibiotic-resistant bacteria, which pose a growing public health risk [5]. Antibiotics expedite the healing process by efficiently combating bacterial infections, resulting in a shorter duration of illness and alleviating associated discomfort [6]. Certain bacterial infections, if not treated, can result in long-term health conditions. Untreated strep throat can result in the development of rheumatic fever, a condition that can cause long-term heart damage [7]. Antibiotics aid in the prevention of such complications. In the field of public health, conventional therapy is critical for managing outbreaks of bacterial infections. Healthcare providers can mitigate broader community transmission by providing treatment to affected individuals. The availability and use of antibiotics have had a significant impact on global health, enhancing both life span and quality of life through the management and eradication of previously devastating infections [8]. Conventional therapy, specifically antibiotics, is crucial for efficiently eradicating bacteria, halting the transmission of infections, preserving lives, and expediting the healing process. Additionally, it plays a vital role in combating antibiotic resistance, which is essential for preserving the efficacy of these life-saving therapies for future generations [9]. The use of conventional therapy in treating bacterial infections has led to significant improvements in patient outcomes, decreased mortality rates, and effectively tackled issues such as antibiotic resistance. Bacterial infections are pathogenic conditions resulting from the invasion, replication, and subsequent harm inflicted by detrimental bacteria on bodily tissues [4]. Bacteria are minuscule, unicellular organisms that inhabit diverse environments, such as soil, water, and the human body. Although numerous bacteria are innocuous or even advantageous, certain ones can induce illnesses upon infiltrating the body [10].

IMPORTANCE OF CONVENTIONAL THERAPY IN BACTERIA-BORNE INFECTIONS

The present chapter highlights the crucial role of antibiotics in the treatment of bacterial infections, which are considered a standard form of therapy (Fig. **1**). Antibiotics, which are fundamental in traditional treatment, are specifically formulated to exterminate bacteria or impede their proliferation [9]. These treatments specifically attack the bacterial cells, making them extremely efficient in addressing various bacterial infections, ranging from minor skin infections to severe conditions such as sepsis and meningitis [9].

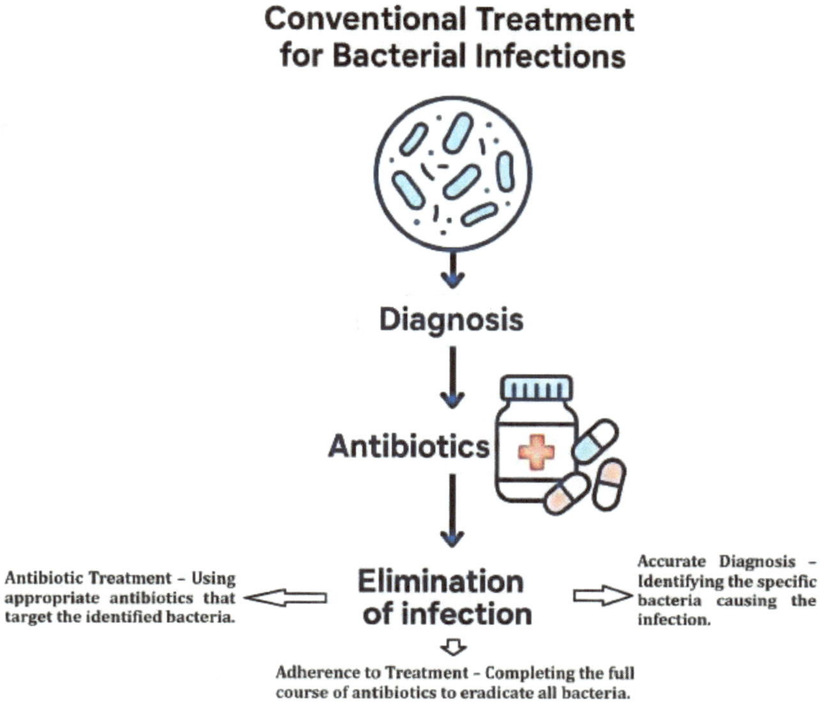

Fig. (1). Elimination of bacteria-borne infections.

Conventional antibiotics have undergone thorough research and testing, resulting in consistent and predictable results when used to treat bacterial infections. The predictability is crucial in clinical settings, as it guarantees that patients are administered treatments with a high probability of success [11]. Unaddressed bacterial infections can result in grave complications, such as the dissemination of the infection to other body regions (such as bacteremia or sepsis), long-term health problems, or even mortality [12]. Conventional therapy effectively eradicates the infection, thereby minimising the likelihood of such consequences. Untreated bacterial infections, including bacterial pneumonia, tuberculosis, and bacterial meningitis, have the potential to be lethal if not promptly treated with antibiotics. Conventional therapy is crucial for preserving lives, especially in cases of severe or rapidly advancing infections [2].

Certain bacterial infections, such as tuberculosis or bacterial meningitis, have a high level of contagiousness. Conventional therapy plays a crucial role in preventing the transmission of infections to others and safeguarding public health by effectively treating infected individuals. The extensive utilisation of antibiotics in the past has effectively managed bacterial outbreaks and mitigated diseases that previously caused widespread epidemics [13].

Despite the increasing issue of antibiotic resistance, traditional therapy remains essential in the management and treatment of infections caused by bacteria that are resistant to antibiotics. Conventional treatment strategies are continuously adjusting to the difficulties presented by resistant strains through the creation of new antibiotics and the implementation of combination therapies [14].

Conventional therapy involves following specific guidelines for the proper use of antibiotics, which is crucial in preventing the emergence of resistance. Accurate identification, appropriate amount, and optimal length of therapy contribute to the maintenance of antibiotics' efficacy. Conventional therapy efficiently eliminates bacterial infections, leading to faster recovery and reducing the length of illness and the resulting physical and emotional strain on the patient [15].

Untreated bacterial infections can result in chronic conditions or permanent damage. Untreated streptococcal infections can result in the development of rheumatic fever, which has the potential to cause irreversible damage to the heart. Antibiotic treatment aids in the prevention of these enduring consequences [16]. Antibiotic therapy is the established and widely accepted approach for treating bacterial infections, serving as the fundamental basis of contemporary medical practice. It has revolutionized the capacity of healthcare providers to address infections that were previously deemed lethal [17]. The extensive accessibility and utilisation of antibiotics have significantly enhanced worldwide health, resulting in a reduction in death rates and an improvement in life expectancy through the efficient management of bacterial illnesses [18]. Conventional therapy may be supplemented with additional treatments, such as surgery, immunotherapy, or supportive care, to effectively address complicated or severe bacterial infections. This comprehensive approach guarantees that every aspect of the infection is taken into account, resulting in improved outcomes [19]. Conventional therapy is based on rigorous research, clinical trials, and evidence-based guidelines, which guarantee that the treatments offered are firmly rooted in scientific knowledge and have been demonstrated to be effective. Conventional therapy is crucial for treating bacterial infections because it effectively eliminates bacteria, prevents complications, reduces the transmission of infectious diseases, manages antibiotic resistance, and aids in the recovery process. It is the fundamental basis for modern medicine's capacity to combat bacterial infections and safeguard public health [20].

HOW BACTERIAL INFECTIONS OCCUR

Bacteria can enter the human body through various routes. One common pathway is the respiratory tract, where airborne bacteria are inhaled. The gastrointestinal tract serves as another entry point, typically through the consumption of contaminated food or water. Additionally, bacteria can penetrate the body *via* breaks in the skin, such as cuts, wounds, or insect bites. The genitourinary tract is also a potential route of entry, often through sexual contact or due to inadequate hygiene. Once inside the body, bacteria may attach to host tissues, begin to multiply, and subsequently colonise the affected area. If not effectively eliminated by the host immune system, they may spread to other regions and cause infection.

Many pathogenic bacteria produce toxins, which are harmful substances that damage tissues and organs. These toxins can lead to various symptoms, including inflammation, fever, and tissue destruction. In response to bacterial invasion, the immune system mounts a defence to eliminate the pathogens. This immune response may manifest through symptoms such as pus formation, fever, swelling, and other signs of inflammation [21 - 25].

Types of Bacterial Infections

Bacterial infections can affect almost every part of the human body, presenting with a wide range of clinical manifestations. In the respiratory system, bacteria can cause infections such as pneumonia, tuberculosis, and streptococcal pharyngitis (commonly known as strep throat). These conditions often result in symptoms like cough, chest pain, difficulty breathing, and sore throat.

The skin is also a frequent site of bacterial invasion. Infections such as cellulitis, impetigo, and abscesses are commonly encountered. These may present with redness, swelling, pain, and the formation of pus. In the gastrointestinal tract, bacterial infections typically result from the ingestion of contaminated food or water. Conditions such as food poisoning, gastritis, and cholera lead to symptoms like nausea, vomiting, abdominal cramps, and diarrhea.

Urinary tract infections (UTIs), including cystitis and pyelonephritis, are common, especially among women. These infections can cause painful urination, frequent urges to urinate, fever, and lower abdominal pain. In the genitourinary system, several sexually transmitted infections (STIs) are caused by bacteria, including gonorrhea, syphilis, and chlamydia. These infections may initially be asymptomatic but can lead to serious complications if left untreated.

The central nervous system can also be affected by bacterial infections, with meningitis and brain abscesses being among the most serious. These conditions can lead to high fever, severe headache, neck stiffness, confusion, and even seizures. Infections of the bones and joints, such as osteomyelitis and septic arthritis, typically result from bacteria spreading through the bloodstream or entering through a wound, leading to pain, swelling, and reduced mobility.

When bacteria enter the bloodstream, they can cause bacteremia and, in severe cases, sepsis—a life-threatening condition characterized by systemic inflammation, fever, rapid heart rate, and organ dysfunction. Lastly, bacteria can infect the ears and eyes, causing conditions like otitis media (middle ear infection) and conjunctivitis (commonly known as pink eye), both of which are particularly common in children and can cause discomfort, redness, and discharge [26 - 30].

Symptoms of Bacterial Infections

The symptoms of bacterial infections are dependent upon the type of bacteria and the affected area. However, common signs include fatigue, fever, and a rash. Other typical symptoms are inflammation and pain at the infection site, the presence of pus or discharge, and redness and swelling. For gastrointestinal infections, symptoms may include nausea, vomiting, and diarrhea. Respiratory infections often cause coughing, sneezing, and difficulty breathing [31 - 33].

Diagnosis

The diagnosis of bacterial infections typically begins with a physical examination, during which a healthcare provider carefully evaluates the affected area and assesses the patient's symptoms. This initial assessment helps in identifying the likely site and nature of the infection.

To confirm the diagnosis and determine the exact cause, various laboratory tests are conducted. These may include blood tests, urine tests, or the collection of samples from the affected area for culture. In a bacterial culture, the collected sample is placed in a controlled environment to encourage the growth of bacteria, allowing for the identification of the specific pathogen responsible for the infection.

In certain cases, imaging techniques such as X-rays, computed tomography (CT) scans, or magnetic resonance imaging (MRI) may be used. These tools help evaluate the extent and severity of the infection, particularly when it affects internal organs, bones, joints, or deep tissues. Together, these diagnostic methods provide a comprehensive understanding of the infection, guiding appropriate treatment strategies [34, 35].

Therapy

Antibiotics are the primary treatment for bacterial infections. Antibiotics function by either destroying bacteria or impeding their proliferation. Pain relief, hydration, and rest may comprise supportive care. Surgical intervention may be required in certain instances to remove infected tissue or drain abscesses [36].

Preventative Measures

The prevention of bacterial infections relies heavily on maintaining proper hygiene. This includes thorough and regular hand washing, proper wound care to prevent bacterial entry through cuts or abrasions, and safe food handling practices to avoid the ingestion of contaminated food and water. These simple yet effective measures play a crucial role in reducing the risk of infection in both community and healthcare settings. Vaccination also serves as a powerful preventive tool. Vaccines are available for several serious bacterial infections, such as pneumonia, meningitis, and tuberculosis. Immunization not only protects individuals but also contributes to community-wide immunity, thereby limiting the spread of these diseases.

Adopting safe practices is equally important in preventing certain types of infections. For instance, the use of condoms significantly reduces the risk of sexually transmitted bacterial infections, including gonorrhea, syphilis, and chlamydia. Avoiding close contact with individuals known to be infected can further help in limiting the transmission of contagious bacterial diseases.

The prevention of complications arising from bacterial infections is largely dependent on early diagnosis and prompt treatment. Bacterial infections can vary widely in severity, ranging from mild and self-limiting to life-threatening conditions. The cornerstone of treatment is the use of antibiotics—medications specifically designed to kill bacteria or inhibit their growth. The appropriate selection and timely administration of antibiotics are critical not only for effective treatment but also for preventing the development of antibiotic resistance [37].

COMMON USES AND TYPES OF ANTIBIOTICS

Antibiotics are classified into several groups based on their chemical structure and mechanism of action. Among these, macrolides such as clarithromycin, azithromycin, and erythromycin are widely used. These antibiotics function by inhibiting bacterial protein synthesis and are primarily employed in the treatment of skin infections, respiratory tract infections, and sexually transmitted infections.

Another important group is the glycopeptides, with vancomycin and teicoplanin being notable examples. These antibiotics inhibit bacterial cell wall synthesis and are particularly effective against Gram-positive organisms. They are commonly used in the management of methicillin-resistant *Staphylococcus aureus* (MRSA) and other resistant infections.

Cephalosporins, such as ceftriaxone, cephalexin, and cefuroxime, also act by inhibiting bacterial cell wall synthesis, similar to penicillins. However, they offer a broader spectrum of activity and are frequently prescribed for respiratory tract infections, skin infections, and urinary tract infections.

The oxazolidinone class, represented by linezolid, works by inhibiting protein synthesis and is reserved for serious Gram-positive infections, including MRSA and vancomycin-resistant enterococci (VRE).

Aminoglycosides, such as tobramycin, gentamicin, and amikacin, are powerful antibiotics that also inhibit protein synthesis. These are often used to treat severe infections caused by Gram-negative bacteria, including sepsis and hospital-acquired infections.

Fluoroquinolones, including moxifloxacin, levofloxacin, and ciprofloxacin, act by preventing bacterial DNA replication. These broad-spectrum antibiotics are effective in treating a range of infections, including those affecting the gastrointestinal tract, respiratory system, and urinary tract.

Tetracyclines, such as doxycycline, minocycline, and tetracycline, function by binding to bacterial ribosomes and inhibiting protein synthesis. They are used in the treatment of respiratory infections, chlamydia, Lyme disease, and acne.

The sulfonamides, often combined with trimethoprim (as in sulfamethoxazole), inhibit the bacterial synthesis of folic acid. These are commonly used to treat bronchitis, urinary tract infections, and certain forms of pneumonia.

Penicillins, including amoxicillin and ampicillin, are among the oldest and most widely used antibiotics. They work by inhibiting bacterial cell wall synthesis and are effective in treating conditions such as strep throat, pneumonia, ear infections, and syphilis.

Metronidazole is another important antibiotic that inhibits bacterial DNA synthesis. It is particularly effective against anaerobic bacteria and certain protozoa, and is commonly used for gastrointestinal infections, including those caused by *Clostridium difficile.*

Finally, carbapenems such as imipenem, meropenem, and ertapenem are broad-spectrum antibiotics that inhibit cell wall synthesis. Due to their potency and wide range of activity, they are typically reserved for the treatment of severe or high-risk bacterial infections, especially those caused by multidrug-resistant organisms [38 - 48].

Treatment Recommendations

An essential component of effective antibiotic treatment is culture and sensitivity testing, which is performed to identify the specific bacterial pathogen responsible for the infection and to determine the most effective antibiotic for treatment. This targeted approach helps ensure the appropriate use of antibiotics and improves clinical outcomes.

The duration of antibiotic therapy can vary considerably depending on the type and severity of the infection. While some infections may respond to a short course of a few days, others—particularly more severe or deep-seated infections—may require treatment for several weeks. Adherence to the prescribed duration is crucial to fully eradicate the infection and prevent recurrence.

One of the major challenges in modern medicine is antibiotic resistance, which arises primarily from the overuse or inappropriate use of antibiotics. When antibiotics are misused—for example, taken unnecessarily or not completed as prescribed—bacteria can evolve mechanisms to survive future treatments, rendering common antibiotics ineffective. This poses a serious threat to public health and limits treatment options for resistant infections.

In addition to antibiotic therapy, supportive care is often necessary to manage symptoms and promote recovery. Pain management using analgesics may be required to alleviate discomfort associated with the infection. Adequate hydration is also vital, as maintaining fluid balance helps the body function properly and supports immune response. In some cases, surgical intervention may be necessary—for example, to drain abscesses, remove infected tissue, or manage complications that cannot be resolved through medication alone [49, 50].

MEDICAL TREATMENTS THAT ARE EMPLOYED TO TREAT INFECTIONS CAUSED BY BACTERIA

The medical treatments employed to combat infections caused by bacteria are the primary focus when conventional therapy is discussed in the context of bacterial infections [9].

Bacterial Infection Diagnosis

The symptoms of bacterial infections vary depending on the site of infection. Common manifestations include fever, fatigue, pain, inflammation, and the formation of pus. These symptoms can differ based on whether the infection affects the respiratory tract, urinary system, skin, or other body areas.

Diagnosis of bacterial infections is confirmed through laboratory investigations. These may include cultures of blood, urine, or other bodily fluids to identify the causative bacteria, as well as blood tests to assess the body's response to infection. In some cases, imaging techniques such as X-rays or CT scans are also employed to evaluate the extent and severity of the infection. Accurate identification of the specific bacteria is essential for selecting the most appropriate and effective treatment [51].

Conventional Treatment for Bacterial Infections

Antibiotics remain the primary treatment modality for bacterial infections. These drugs function by either killing the bacteria directly (bactericidal) or by inhibiting their growth (bacteriostatic). The choice of an appropriate antibiotic depends on several factors, including the type of bacteria causing the infection, the site of infection, the patient's medical history, and the presence of any antibiotic resistance. Antibiotics can be broadly categorized into broad-spectrum and narrow-spectrum agents. Broad-spectrum antibiotics are capable of targeting a wide range of bacterial species and are typically used when the causative bacteria have not yet been identified or when an infection is suspected to involve multiple types of bacteria. In contrast, narrow-spectrum antibiotics are specifically designed to target particular bacterial species and are preferred once the responsible bacteria have been identified and their antibiotic sensitivities have been established.

The duration of antibiotic therapy varies depending on the severity and nature of the infection. It is crucial that patients complete the entire prescribed course of antibiotics to ensure complete eradication of the bacteria and to minimize the risk of developing antibiotic resistance [9].

Resistance to Antibiotics

One of the most significant challenges in the treatment of bacterial infections is the escalating rate of antibiotic resistance. This phenomenon occurs when bacteria develop the ability to survive exposure to antibiotics that would normally eliminate them. The emergence and spread of resistant strains reduce the effectiveness of available treatments and complicate infection management.

To combat antibiotic resistance, healthcare providers employ various strategies. These include combination therapies, which involve the use of multiple antibiotics simultaneously to overcome resistant bacteria. Adjusting antibiotic dosages based on the severity and nature of the infection can also enhance treatment outcomes. In addition to pharmacological approaches, infection prevention measures such as vaccination programs and the promotion of proper hygiene practices play a critical role in limiting the spread of resistant bacteria and reducing the overall incidence of bacterial infections [52].

Supportive Care

In addition to antibiotic therapy, symptomatic treatment is often necessary to provide relief and support the patient's recovery. Supportive care typically includes the administration of fluids to maintain adequate hydration, as well as the use of pain relievers and fever reducers to alleviate discomfort and control elevated body temperature.

In cases of severe bacterial infections, hospitalization may be required. This allows for the administration of intravenous antibiotics, which can achieve higher and more consistent drug levels in the bloodstream. Hospitalization also facilitates close monitoring of the patient's condition and timely management of any complications that may arise during the course of treatment [53].

Preventive Measures

Vaccination plays a crucial role in the prevention of certain bacterial infections. For example, infections such as tetanus, caused by *Clostridium tetani*, and *pneumonia*, caused by *Streptococcus pneumoniae*, can be effectively prevented through immunization. These vaccines have significantly reduced the incidence and severity of these diseases worldwide. In addition to vaccination, maintaining proper hygiene practices is essential for reducing the risk of bacterial infections. Regular handwashing, appropriate wound care, and adherence to food safety measures are fundamental strategies that help limit bacterial transmission and infection.

Another important approach to controlling bacterial infections and combating antibiotic resistance is the implementation of antibiotic stewardship programs. These programs aim to optimize the use of antibiotics by ensuring that patients receive the correct antibiotic, at the right dose, and for the appropriate duration. Through such measures, antibiotic stewardship helps minimize the development of resistant bacterial strains while promoting effective treatment outcomes [54 - 56].

Long-Term Management

Certain bacterial infections, particularly those caused by antibiotic-resistant strains, have a tendency to recur. Therefore, ongoing monitoring and follow-up care are essential to detect any signs of reinfection at an early stage. Timely identification of recurrence allows for prompt intervention, which is crucial to preventing further complications.

In some cases, antibiotic treatment can disrupt the body's natural microbial flora, especially in the gastrointestinal tract. To restore a healthy balance of bacteria, probiotics may be prescribed. These beneficial microorganisms help re-establish normal flora, reducing the risk of complications such as antibiotic-associated diarrhea.

Antibiotics remain the cornerstone of bacterial infection treatment, with their effectiveness largely dependent on accurate diagnosis and sensitivity testing. However, antibiotic resistance poses a significant challenge to successful therapy. Addressing this issue requires a multifaceted approach, including the implementation of preventive strategies, careful antibiotic prescribing practices, and strict adherence to prescribed treatment regimens. These measures are vital to achieving favourable clinical outcomes and limiting the spread of resistant bacteria [57 - 60].

DEVELOPMENTS IN THE FIELD OF NEW ANTIBIOTICS

The discovery and development of novel antibiotic classes have significantly expanded the arsenal of treatment options available, particularly for combating drug-resistant bacteria. For example, lipopeptides such as daptomycin and oxazolidinones like linezolid have been developed specifically to target Gram-positive infections that are resistant to conventional antibiotics. These new classes offer promising alternatives in the fight against resistant pathogens. Combination therapies have also played a crucial role in enhancing antibiotic effectiveness. By simultaneously targeting multiple bacterial mechanisms, these therapies reduce the likelihood of resistance development while improving clinical outcomes. A notable example is the combination of β-lactam antibiotics and β-lactamase inhibitors, such as amoxicillin combined with clavulanic acid, which protects the antibiotic from degradation by bacterial enzymes, thereby restoring its efficacy.

Advancements in rapid diagnostic technologies have revolutionized the identification of bacterial pathogens and their resistance profiles. Techniques like polymerase chain reaction (PCR) and next-generation sequencing enable timely and accurate detection, reducing reliance on broad-spectrum antibiotics and minimizing the risk of resistance. This facilitates more precise and targeted antibiotic therapy tailored to the specific infection.

Personalized medicine is becoming increasingly feasible in the field of infectious diseases. By considering factors such as the patient's genetics, microbiome composition, and the specific bacterial strain involved, pharmacogenomics allows for the customization of antibiotic treatments. This approach helps ensure that patients receive the most effective therapy with the least toxicity.

To optimize antibiotic use and combat resistance, many healthcare systems have implemented antibiotic stewardship programs. These initiatives provide guidelines for appropriate prescribing, monitor antibiotic consumption, and promote education among healthcare professionals and the public about the risks associated with antibiotic overuse and misuse. A key strategy within these programs is de-escalation, which involves starting treatment with broad-spectrum antibiotics and then narrowing therapy based on identified pathogens, thereby reducing resistance development and adverse effects.

In addition to antibiotics, adjunctive therapies are gaining attention. The use of probiotics alongside antibiotics is an emerging approach aimed at maintaining or restoring a healthy gut microbiome. Probiotics may prevent the overgrowth of resistant bacteria such as *Clostridioides difficile* and help mitigate antibiotic-associated side effects like diarrhoea. Another area of progress is the use of immunomodulators—drugs that modulate the immune response to enhance the body's ability to fight bacterial infections. These agents are particularly beneficial in immunocompromised patients or those suffering from severe infections [61 - 70].

Conventional therapy, primarily through the use of antibiotics, plays a vital role in combating bacterial infections by effectively eradicating pathogenic bacteria, preventing their dissemination, and reducing the risk of serious complications or mortality. Antibiotics are specifically designed to target bacterial cells either by directly causing their death (bactericidal) or by inhibiting their growth and ability to reproduce (bacteriostatic). They are classified into various groups that operate through different mechanisms, such as disrupting the bacterial cell wall, inhibiting protein synthesis, or interfering with DNA replication, which allows for tailored treatment depending on the specific bacteria and infection site. The advent of antibiotics in the 20th century significantly reduced mortality associated with bacterial diseases like pneumonia, meningitis, and sepsis, revolutionizing healthcare and public health outcomes worldwide. Proper and responsible use of antibiotics ensures the complete eradication of bacteria, minimizing the emergence of resistant strains, which has become an increasing concern. Inappropriate use or insufficient dosing can lead to the survival of resistant bacteria, resulting in more severe and difficult-to-treat infections. Therefore, adherence to clinical guidelines, accurate pathogen identification, and optimal therapy duration are crucial in preserving antibiotic efficacy. Traditional antibiotics have undergone extensive research and clinical testing, providing predictable and reliable results in treating a wide range of bacterial infections, from minor skin conditions to life-threatening diseases. They also play an essential role in preventing the spread of contagious diseases such as tuberculosis and bacterial meningitis, thereby safeguarding public health. Despite the rising challenge of antibiotic resistance, ongoing efforts include the development of new antibiotics and combination therapies to combat resistant strains. For instance, newer formulations like beta-lactamase inhibitors (*e.g.*, piperacillin-tazobactam), advanced agents such as linezolid and carbapenems, and innovative approaches like phage therapy, antimicrobial peptides, and nanotechnology are at the forefront of recent developments. These advances aim to address resistance, enhance treatment efficacy, and reduce side effects. Research by various authors emphasizes the importance of combination therapies to overcome resistance, the use of genomic tools to identify new bacterial targets, and the development of rapid diagnostic techniques for timely and precise treatment. Examples of practical applications include the utilization of ceftazidime-avibactam against multidrug-resistant bacteria, phage therapy in resistant wound infections, and nanoparticle-based drug delivery systems [71, 72]. These developments highlight a multidisciplinary approach to ensuring the continued effectiveness of antibacterial therapies, preserving public health, and improving patient outcomes.

Drug Delivery Systems, Nanotechnology, and Emerging Therapies

Innovations in drug delivery systems and nanotechnology have significantly transformed the landscape of bacterial infection treatment. Nanotechnology involves the manipulation and application of materials at the nanoscale, typically between 1 and 100 nanometers. At this scale, materials can exhibit unique physical, chemical, and biological properties, making them highly useful in medical applications, especially for targeted drug delivery. One of the most promising advancements is targeted drug delivery, made possible through nanotechnology. By designing nanoparticles that can recognize infection-specific markers or respond to local environmental conditions such as pH or temperature, nanotechnology enables the selective delivery of antibiotics to infected tissues while sparing healthy cells. These systems enhance the drug's efficacy while reducing systemic side effects. Controlled-release mechanisms further improve treatment precision, ensuring that the antibiotic is released at the optimal rate and concentration where it is needed most.

Another critical application of nanotechnology in infectious disease treatment involves the disruption of biofilms. Biofilms are protective layers formed by bacterial communities that render many infections—especially chronic or device-associated ones—highly resistant to conventional antibiotics. New drug delivery platforms capable of penetrating or disrupting these biofilms have led to improved outcomes in managing persistent infections associated with catheters, implants, and other medical devices.

Alongside these technological developments, bacteriophage therapy—also known as phage therapy—is re-emerging as a potential solution to the growing crisis of antibiotic resistance. Bacteriophages are viruses that specifically infect and destroy bacteria. Unlike broad-spectrum antibiotics, they can be engineered to selectively target particular bacterial strains, making them an attractive alternative or complement to traditional antibiotic therapies. Although not yet a standard clinical practice, phage therapy is receiving increasing attention in research and clinical trials, especially for the treatment of multidrug-resistant infections where conventional antibiotics fail. Together, these advances in drug delivery, nanomedicine, and biologically targeted treatments are shaping the future of antimicrobial therapy, offering new hope in the fight against resistant bacterial infections [73 - 75].

Emerging Strategies in the Fight Against Bacterial Infections

Recent advancements in biomedical science have introduced several innovative approaches for combating bacterial infections, especially in the context of rising antibiotic resistance. One such development is the use of monoclonal antibodies, which are laboratory-engineered molecules designed to target specific components of bacteria. These antibodies can neutralize toxins produced by pathogens or bacteria for destruction by the host's immune system. They have shown particular promise in treating severe infections caused by bacteria like Staphylococcus aureus, where traditional antibiotic therapies may be less effective or compromised due to resistance.

In parallel, the creation of novel vaccines has played a critical role in reducing the incidence of serious bacterial diseases. Vaccines targeting pathogens responsible for conditions such as pneumococcal pneumonia, meningitis, and whooping cough have significantly decreased the burden of these illnesses. By preventing infections before they occur, vaccines reduce the reliance on antibiotics and contribute to the broader effort to curb antimicrobial resistance.

Another promising area of research is resistance control through gene editing. The CRISPR-C as system, originally discovered as a natural defense mechanism in bacteria, is now being explored for its potential to target and eliminate antibiotic resistance genes within bacterial populations. By editing or disrupting these genes, researchers aim to restore bacterial susceptibility to existing antibiotics, thereby enhancing the effectiveness of current treatment options and reversing the spread of resistance.

These emerging strategies—ranging from immunotherapy and vaccine development to genetic interventions—represent the future of bacterial infection control. They offer hope for overcoming the limitations of conventional antibiotic therapy and addressing the growing global challenge of antibiotic resistance [76 - 78].

CHALLENGES

Traditional methods for controlling bacterial infections, including antibiotic utilization, encounter many obstacles in contemporary times. A significant concern is the increase in antibiotic resistance resulting from the overutilization and improper application of these medications. This has rendered numerous previously effective antibiotics outdated, complicating treatment significantly. Moreover, the advancement of novel antibiotics has markedly decelerated, resulting in a restricted repertoire against resistant microorganisms.

Conventional antibiotics frequently exhibit a lack of specificity, affecting both harmful and helpful bacteria, thereby disrupting the microbiome and potentially resulting in secondary infections or other consequences. Furthermore, specific bacterial infections, particularly those induced by biofilm-forming or intracellular pathogens, are intrinsically challenging to manage with traditional methods. Biofilms offer a protective barrier, but intracellular bacteria circumvent immune responses and pharmacological interventions.

The worldwide proliferation of multidrug-resistant bacteria exacerbates infection control, especially in resource-constrained environments. Inadequate diagnostic tools further facilitate improper antibiotic utilization, intensifying resistance.

Innovative techniques, including targeted drug delivery systems, antimicrobial peptides, and combination medicines, are being investigated to address these issues. Addressing these concerns necessitates synchronized worldwide initiatives in research, monitoring, and education.

CONCLUSION

Conventional therapy for bacterial infections has made significant progress through the introduction of novel antibiotics, targeted therapies, enhanced diagnostics, antibiotic stewardship programs, and innovative methods such as bacteriophage therapy, monoclonal antibodies, and nanotechnology. These technological advancements have enhanced the efficacy of medical treatments, tackled the issue of antibiotic resistance, and improved patient outcomes.

ACKNOWLEDGEMENT

The authors are thankful to the management of IFTM University for ultramodern library facilities.

REFERENCES

[1] Palazzi DL, Klein JO, Baker CJ. Bacterial sepsis and meningitis. Infectious diseases of the fetus and newborn infant. Elsevier 2006; pp. 247-95. https://linkinghub.elsevier.com/retrieve/pii/B0721605370500086 Internet [http://dx.doi.org/10.1016/B0-72-160537-0/50008-6]

[2] Hauser AR, Mecsas J, Moir DT. Antibiotics: New Therapeutic Approaches for Bacterial Infections. Clin Infect Dis. (1)89-95. 2016 Jul 1.

[3] Chopra I, Hodgson J, Metcalf B, Poste G. The search for antimicrobial agents effective against bacteria resistant to multiple antibiotics. Antimicrob Agents Chemother 1997; 41(3): 497-503. [http://dx.doi.org/10.1128/AAC.41.3.497] [PMID: 9055982]

[4] Patini R, Mangino G, Martellacci L, Quaranta G, Masucci L, Gallenzi P. The effect of different antibiotic regimens on bacterial resistance: A systematic review. Antibiotics (Basel) 2020; 9(1): 22. [http://dx.doi.org/10.3390/antibiotics9010022] [PMID: 31936186]

[5] Thappeta KRV, Vikhe YS, Yong AMH, Chan-Park MB, Kline KA. Combined Efficacy of an Antimicrobial Cationic Peptide Polymer with Conventional Antibiotics to Combat Multidrug-Resistant Pathogens. ACS Infect Dis 2020; 6(5): 1228-37. [http://dx.doi.org/10.1021/acsinfecdis.0c00016] [PMID: 32138506]

[6] Caldwell MD. Bacteria and Antibiotics in Wound Healing. Surg Clin North Am 2020; 100(4): 757-76. [http://dx.doi.org/10.1016/j.suc.2020.05.007] [PMID: 32681875]

[7] Franczyk B, Gluba-Brzózka A, Rysz-Górzyńska M, Rysz J. The Role of Inflammation and Oxidative Stress in Rheumatic Heart Disease. Int J Mol Sci 2022; 23(24): 15812. [http://dx.doi.org/10.3390/ijms232415812] [PMID: 36555452]

[8] Klein EY, Van Boeckel TP, Martinez EM, *et al.* Global increase and geographic convergence in antibiotic consumption between 2000 and 2015. Proc Natl Acad Sci USA 2018; 115(15): E3463-70. Available from:https://pnas.org/doi/full/10.1073/pnas.1717295115 [http://dx.doi.org/10.1073/pnas.1717295115] [PMID: 29581252]

[9] Paterson IK, Hoyle A, Ochoa G, Baker-Austin C, Taylor NGH. Optimising Antibiotic Usage to Treat Bacterial Infections. Sci Rep 2016; 6(1): 37853. [http://dx.doi.org/10.1038/srep37853] [PMID: 27892497]

[10] Turnbaugh PJ, Stintzi A. Human Health and Disease in a Microbial World. Front Microbio [Internet] 2011 [cited 2024 Aug 3] 2. Available from:http://journal.frontiersin.org/article/10.3389/fmicb.2011.00190/abstract [http://dx.doi.org/10.3389/fmicb.2011.00190]

[11] Howard-Anderson J, Dai W, Yahav D, *et al.* A Desirability of Outcome Ranking Analysis of a Randomized Clinical Trial Comparing Seven *Versus* Fourteen Days of Antibiotics for Uncomplicated Gram-Negative Bloodstream Infection. Open Forum Infect Dis 2022; 9(6): ofac140. [http://dx.doi.org/10.1093/ofid/ofac140] [PMID: 35615299]

[12] Tapper H, Herwald H. Modulation of hemostatic mechanisms in bacterial infectious diseases. Blood 2000; 96(7): 2329-37. [http://dx.doi.org/10.1182/blood.V96.7.2329] [PMID: 11001879]

[13] Fox GJ, Dobler CC, Marais BJ, Denholm JT. Preventive therapy for latent tuberculosis infection—the promise and the challenges. Int J Infect Dis 2017; 56: 68-76. [http://dx.doi.org/10.1016/j.ijid.2016.11.006] [PMID: 27872018]

[14] Liu BG, Xie M, Dong Y, *et al.* Antimicrobial mechanisms of traditional Chinese medicine and reversal of drug resistance: a narrative review. Eur Rev Med Pharmacol Sci 2022; 26(15): 5553-61. [PMID: 35993652]

[15] Caron WP, Mousa SA. Prevention strategies for antimicrobial resistance: a systematic review of the literature. Infect Drug Resist 2010; 3(May): 25-33. [PMID: 21694891]

[16] Sika-Paotonu D, Liligeto U. Group a streptococcal infection, acute rheumatic fever and rheumatic heart disease in the solomon islands. The Journal of Immunology 2(1_Supplement): 182.80-0. 2019 May 1.

[17] Hawkey PM, Warren RE, Livermore DM, *et al.* Treatment of infections caused by multidrug-resistant Gram-negative bacteria: report of the British Society for Antimicrobial Chemotherapy/Healthcare Infection Society/British Infection Association Joint Working Party. J Antimicrob Chemother 2018; 73 (Suppl. 3): iii2-iii78. [http://dx.doi.org/10.1093/jac/dky027] [PMID: 29514274]

[18] Laxminarayan R, Matsoso P, Pant S, *et al.* Access to effective antimicrobials: a worldwide challenge. Lancet 2016; 387(10014): 168-75. [http://dx.doi.org/10.1016/S0140-6736(15)00474-2] [PMID: 26603918]

[19] McCulloch TR, Wells TJ, Souza-Fonseca-Guimaraes F. Towards efficient immunotherapy for bacterial infection. Trends Microbiol 2022; 30(2): 158-69. [http://dx.doi.org/10.1016/j.tim.2021.05.005] [PMID: 34253452]

[20] Zhang L, Liang E, Cheng Y, *et al.* Is combined medication with natural medicine a promising therapy for bacterial biofilm infection? Biomed Pharmacother 2020; 128: 110184. [http://dx.doi.org/10.1016/j.biopha.2020.110184] [PMID: 32450528]

[21] Trastoy R, Manso T, Fernández-García L, *et al.* Mechanisms of bacterial tolerance and persistence in the gastrointestinal and respiratory environments. Clin Microbiol Rev 2018; 31(4): e00023-18. [http://dx.doi.org/10.1128/CMR.00023-18] [PMID: 30068737]

[22] Rosales-Castillo A, Jiménez-Guerra G, Ruiz-Gómez L, Expósito-Ruíz M, Navarro-Marí JM, Gutiérrez-Fernández J. Emerging Presence of Culturable Microorganisms in Clinical Samples of the Genitourinary System: Systematic Review and Experience in Specialized Care of a Regional Hospital. J Clin Med 2022; 11(5): 1348. [http://dx.doi.org/10.3390/jcm11051348] [PMID: 35268439]

[23] Leshem A, Liwinski T, Elinav E. Immune-Microbiota Interplay and Colonization Resistance in Infection. Mol Cell 2020; 78(4): 597-613. [http://dx.doi.org/10.1016/j.molcel.2020.03.001] [PMID: 32208169]

[24] Popoff MR. Bacterial Toxins, Current Perspectives. Toxins (Basel) 2020; 12(9): 570. [http://dx.doi.org/10.3390/toxins12090570] [PMID: 32899816]

[25] Reece ST, Kaufmann SHE. Host Defenses to Intracellular Bacteria. Clinical Immunology. Elsevier 2019; pp. 375-389.e1. Internet Available from: https://linkinghub.elsevier.com/retrieve/pii/B9780702068966000260 [http://dx.doi.org/10.1016/B978-0-7020-6896-6.00026-0]

[26] Bernard P. Management of common bacterial infections of the skin. Curr Opin Infect Dis 2008; 21(2): 122-8. [http://dx.doi.org/10.1097/QCO.0b013e3282f44c63] [PMID: 18317033]

[27] Gabillot-Carré M, Roujeau JC. Acute bacterial skin infections and cellulitis. Curr Opin Infect Dis 2007; 20(2): 118-23. [http://dx.doi.org/10.1097/QCO.0b013e32805dfb2d] [PMID: 17496568]

[28] Green RF, Selinger DS. Urinary tract infection and soft tissue abscess caused by Streptococcus pneumoniae. South Med J 1980; 73(11): 1550-1.

[http://dx.doi.org/10.1097/00007611-198011000-00046] [PMID: 7444538]

[29] Zhang H, Zhang G, Yang Y, *et al.* Antimicrobial resistance comparison of Klebsiella pneumoniae pathogens isolated from intra-abdominal and urinary tract infections in different organs, hospital departments and regions of China between 2014 and 2017. J Microbiol Immunol Infect 2021; 54(4): 639-48.
[http://dx.doi.org/10.1016/j.jmii.2020.03.009] [PMID: 32247662]

[30] Fakhraddin Raheem T. Ahmed Hasan Ali S, Prevalence and Multi-Drug Resistance Patterns of Uropathogenic E.coli isolated from Women Patients in Kirkuk city, Iraq. Iran J Med Microbiol 2022; 16(6): 609-14.

[31] LaPenna PA, Roos KL. Bacterial Infections of the Central Nervous System. Semin Neurol 2019; 39(3): 334-42.
[http://dx.doi.org/10.1055/s-0039-1693159] [PMID: 31378869]

[32] Palmu AAI, Herva E, Savolainen H, Karma P, Mäkelä PH, Kilpi TM. Association of clinical signs and symptoms with bacterial findings in acute otitis media. Clin Infect Dis 2004; 38(2): 234-42.
[http://dx.doi.org/10.1086/380642] [PMID: 14699456]

[33] Rosca A, Cerca N. Bacterial vaginosis. In: Singh SK, editor Diagnostics to pathogenomics of sexually transmitted infections [Internet] 1st ed Wiley; 2018 [cited 2024 Aug 3] 257-75. Available from: https://onlinelibrary.wiley.com/doi/10.1002/9781119380924.ch13
[http://dx.doi.org/10.1002/9781119380924.ch13]

[34] Fernando SM, Tran A, Cheng W, *et al.* Necrotizing Soft Tissue Infection: Diagnostic Accuracy of Physical Examination, Imaging, and LRINEC Score. Ann Surg 2019; 269(1): 58-65.
[http://dx.doi.org/10.1097/SLA.0000000000002774] [PMID: 29672405]

[35] Gemmel F, Dumarey N, Welling M. Future diagnostic agents. Semin Nucl Med 2009; 39(1): 11-26.
[http://dx.doi.org/10.1053/j.semnuclmed.2008.08.005] [PMID: 19038597]

[36] Martin JK II, Sheehan JP, Bratton BP, *et al.* A Dual-Mechanism Antibiotic Kills Gram-Negative Bacteria and Avoids Drug Resistance. Cell 2020; 181(7): 1518-1532.e14.
[http://dx.doi.org/10.1016/j.cell.2020.05.005] [PMID: 32497502]

[37] Magistro G, Stief CG. Vaccine Development for Urinary Tract Infections: Where Do We Stand? Eur Urol Focus 2019; 5(1): 39-41.
[http://dx.doi.org/10.1016/j.euf.2018.07.034] [PMID: 30093359]

[38] Zuckerman JM, Qamar F, Bono BR. Review of macrolides (azithromycin, clarithromycin), ketolids (telithromycin) and glycylcyclines (tigecycline). Med Clin North Am 2011; 95(4): 761-791, viii.
[http://dx.doi.org/10.1016/j.mcna.2011.03.012] [PMID: 21679791]

[39] Malabarba A. Section Review Anti-infectives: New approaches to the treatment of vancomycin-resistant bacterial infections. Expert Opin Ther Pat 1996; 6(7): 627-44.
[http://dx.doi.org/10.1517/13543776.6.7.627]

[40] Shahbaz K. Cephalosporins: pharmacology and chemistry. Pharmaceutical and Biological Evaluations 2017; 4(6): 234.
[http://dx.doi.org/10.26510/2394-0859.pbe.2017.36]

[41] Paladino JA. Linezolid: An oxazolidinone antimicrobial agent. Am J Health Syst Pharm 2002; 59(24): 2413-25.
[http://dx.doi.org/10.1093/ajhp/59.24.2413] [PMID: 12503340]

[42] Edson RS, Terrell CL. The aminoglycosides: streptomycin, kanamycin, gentamicin, tobramycin, amikacin, netilmicin, and sisomicin. Mayo Clin Proc 1987; 62(10): 916-20.
[http://dx.doi.org/10.1016/S0025-6196(12)65048-4] [PMID: 3657309]

[43] Grillon A, Schramm F, Kleinberg M, Jehl F. Comparative Activity of Ciprofloxacin, Levofloxacin and Moxifloxacin against *Klebsiella pneumoniae, Pseudomonas aeruginosa* and *Stenotrophomonas maltophilia* Assessed by Minimum Inhibitory Concentrations and Time-Kill Studies. Nguyen MH,

editor PLoS ONE 2016 Jun 3. (6)e0156690.

[44] Bernardino ALF, Kaushal D, Philipp MT. The antibiotics doxycycline and minocycline inhibit the inflammatory responses to the Lyme disease spirochete *Borrelia burgdorferi.* J Infect Dis 2009; 199(9): 1379-88.
[http://dx.doi.org/10.1086/597807] [PMID: 19301981]

[45] Foltzer MA, Reese RE. Trimethoprim-sulfamethoxazole and other sulfonamides. Med Clin North Am 1987; 71(6): 1177-94.
[http://dx.doi.org/10.1016/S0025-7125(16)30805-7] [PMID: 3320619]

[46] Nathwani D, Wood MJ. Penicillins. Drugs 1993; 45(6): 866-94.
[http://dx.doi.org/10.2165/00003495-199345060-00002] [PMID: 7691496]

[47] Dingsdag SA, Hunter N. Metronidazole: an update on metabolism, structure–cytotoxicity and resistance mechanisms. J Antimicrob Chemother 2018; 73(2): 265-79.
[http://dx.doi.org/10.1093/jac/dkx351] [PMID: 29077920]

[48] Hellinger WC, Brewer NS. Carbapenems and monobactams: imipenem, meropenem, and aztreonam. Mayo Clin Proc 1999; 74(4): 420-34.
[http://dx.doi.org/10.4065/74.4.420] [PMID: 10221472]

[49] Lee RA, Centor RM, Humphrey LL, *et al.* Appropriate use of short-course antibiotics in common infections: Best practice advice from the American college of physicians. Ann Intern Med 2021; 174(6): 822-7.
[http://dx.doi.org/10.7326/M20-7355] [PMID: 33819054]

[50] Spellberg B, Rice LB. Duration of Antibiotic Therapy: Shorter Is Better. Ann Intern Med 2019; 171(3): 210-1.
[http://dx.doi.org/10.7326/M19-1509] [PMID: 31284302]

[51] Boyles TH, Wasserman S. Diagnosis of bacterial infection. S Afr Med J 2015; 105(5): 419.
[http://dx.doi.org/10.7196/SAMJ.9647]

[52] Urban-Chmiel R, Marek A, Stępień-Pyśniak D, *et al.* Antibiotic Resistance in Bacteria—A Review. Antibiotics (Basel) 2022; 11(8): 1079.
[http://dx.doi.org/10.3390/antibiotics11081079] [PMID: 36009947]

[53] Chan KY, Chan TSY, Gill H, *et al.* Supportive care and symptom management in patients with advanced hematological malignancies: a literature review. Ann Palliat Med 2022; 11(10): 3273-91.
[http://dx.doi.org/10.21037/apm-22-691] [PMID: 36267009]

[54] Thwaites CL, Loan HT. Eradication of tetanus. Br Med Bull 2015; 116(1): 69-77.
[PMID: 26598719]

[55] Gould DJ, Moralejo D, Drey N, Chudleigh JH. Interventions to improve hand hygiene compliance in patient care. In: The Cochrane Collaboration, editor Cochrane Database of Systematic Reviews [Internet] 2010; p. CD005186.pub3. [cited 2024 Aug 3] Available from: https://doi.wiley.com/10.1002/14651858.CD005186.pub3
[http://dx.doi.org/10.1002/14651858.CD005186.pub3]

[56] Cunha CB, Opal SM. Antibiotic Stewardship. Med Clin North Am 2018; 102(5): 831-43.
[http://dx.doi.org/10.1016/j.mcna.2018.04.006] [PMID: 30126574]

[57] Stracy M, Snitser O, Yelin I, *et al.* Minimizing treatment-induced emergence of antibiotic resistance in bacterial infections. Science 2022; 375(6583): 889-94.
[http://dx.doi.org/10.1126/science.abg9868] [PMID: 35201862]

[58] Das DJ, Shankar A, Johnson JB, Thomas S. Critical insights into antibiotic resistance transferability in probiotic Lactobacillus. Nutrition 2020; 69: 110567.
[http://dx.doi.org/10.1016/j.nut.2019.110567] [PMID: 31733594]

[59] Friedman ND, Temkin E, Carmeli Y. The negative impact of antibiotic resistance. Clin Microbiol

Infect 2016; 22(5): 416-22.
[http://dx.doi.org/10.1016/j.cmi.2015.12.002] [PMID: 26706614]

[60] Tarín-Pelló A, Suay-García B, Pérez-Gracia MT. Antibiotic resistant bacteria: current situation and treatment options to accelerate the development of a new antimicrobial arsenal. Expert Rev Anti Infect Ther 2022; 20(8): 1095-108.
[http://dx.doi.org/10.1080/14787210.2022.2078308] [PMID: 35576494]

[61] Shariati A, Dadashi M, Chegini Z, *et al.* The global prevalence of Daptomycin, Tigecycline, Quinupristin/Dalfopristin, and Linezolid-resistant *Staphylococcus aureus* and coagulase–negative staphylococci strains: a systematic review and meta-analysis. Antimicrob Resist Infect Control 2020; 9(1): 56.
[http://dx.doi.org/10.1186/s13756-020-00714-9] [PMID: 32321574]

[62] Zurenko G, Gibson JK, Shinabarger DL, Aristoff PA, Ford CW, Tarpley WG. Oxazolidinones: a new class of antibacterials. Curr Opin Pharmacol 2001; 1(5): 470-6.
[http://dx.doi.org/10.1016/S1471-4892(01)00082-0] [PMID: 11764772]

[63] González-Bello C, Rodríguez D, Pernas M, Rodríguez Á, Colchón E. β-Lactamase Inhibitors To Restore the Efficacy of Antibiotics against Superbugs. J Med Chem 2020; 63(5): 1859-81.
[http://dx.doi.org/10.1021/acs.jmedchem.9b01279] [PMID: 31663735]

[64] Abram TJ, Cherukury H, Ou CY, *et al.* Rapid bacterial detection and antibiotic susceptibility testing in whole blood using one-step, high throughput blood digital PCR. Lab Chip 2020; 20(3): 477-89.
[http://dx.doi.org/10.1039/C9LC01212E] [PMID: 31872202]

[65] Dickmann LJ, Ware JA. Pharmacogenomics in the age of personalized medicine. Drug Discov Today Technol 2016; 21-22: 11-6.
[http://dx.doi.org/10.1016/j.ddtec.2016.11.003] [PMID: 27978982]

[66] Zhuo C, Wei X, Zhang Z, *et al.* An antibiotic stewardship programme to reduce inappropriate antibiotic prescribing for acute respiratory infections in rural Chinese primary care facilities: study protocol for a clustered randomised controlled trial. Trials 2020; 21(1): 394.
[http://dx.doi.org/10.1186/s13063-020-04303-4] [PMID: 32398065]

[67] Vallicelli C, Minghetti M, Sartelli M, *et al.* Antibiotic de-escalation in emergency general surgery. Antibiotics (Basel) 2022; 11(9): 1148.
[http://dx.doi.org/10.3390/antibiotics11091148] [PMID: 36139928]

[68] Goldenberg JZ, Yap C, Lytvyn L, *et al.* Probiotics for the prevention of Clostridium difficile-associated diarrhea in adults and children. Cochrane Database of Systematic Reviews [Internet] 2017 Dec 19 [cited 2024 Aug 3] 2017; 12. Available from: http://doi.wiley.com/10.1002/14651858.CD006095.pub4
[http://dx.doi.org/10.1002/14651858.CD006095.pub4]

[69] Pillai A, Nelson RL. Probiotics for treatment of Clostridium difficile-associated colitis in adults. Cochrane IBD Group, editor Cochrane Database of Systematic Reviews [Internet] 2008 Jan 23 [cited 2024 Aug 3] Available from: https://doi.wiley.com/10.1002/14651858.CD004611.pub2
[http://dx.doi.org/10.1002/14651858.CD004611.pub2]

[70] Masihi KN. Fighting infection using immunomodulatory agents. Expert Opin Biol Ther 2001; 1(4): 641-53.
[http://dx.doi.org/10.1517/14712598.1.4.641] [PMID: 11727500]

[71] Satlin MJ, Chen L, Gomez-Simmonds A, *et al.* Impact of a rapid molecular test for *Klebsiella pneumoniae* carbapenemase and ceftazidime-avibactam use on outcomes after bacteremia caused by carbapenem-resistant enterobacterales. Clin Infect Dis 2022; 75(12): 2066-75.
[http://dx.doi.org/10.1093/cid/ciac354] [PMID: 35522019]

[72] Boattini M, Bianco G, Charrier L, *et al.* Rapid diagnostics and ceftazidime/avibactam for KPC-producing Klebsiella pneumoniae bloodstream infections: impact on mortality and role of combination therapy. Eur J Clin Microbiol Infect Dis 2023; 42(4): 431-9.

[http://dx.doi.org/10.1007/s10096-023-04577-x] [PMID: 36806056]

[73] Petrak K. Nanotechnology and site-targeted drug delivery. J Biomater Sci Polym Ed 2006; 17(11): 1209-19.
[http://dx.doi.org/10.1163/156856206778667497] [PMID: 17176746]

[74] Liu Y, Li Y, Shi L. Controlled drug delivery systems in eradicating bacterial biofilm-associated infections. J Control Release 2021; 329: 1102-16.
[http://dx.doi.org/10.1016/j.jconrel.2020.10.038] [PMID: 33098913]

[75] Kakasis A, Panitsa G. Bacteriophage therapy as an alternative treatment for human infections. A comprehensive review. Int J Antimicrob Agents 2019; 53(1): 16-21.
[http://dx.doi.org/10.1016/j.ijantimicag.2018.09.004] [PMID: 30236954]

[76] Melero I, Martinez-Forero I, Dubrot J, Suarez N, Palazón A, Chen L. Palettes of vaccines and immunostimulatory monoclonal antibodies for combination. Clin Cancer Res 2009; 15(5): 1507-9.
[http://dx.doi.org/10.1158/1078-0432.CCR-08-2931] [PMID: 19240168]

[77] Lucero MG, Dulalia VE, Parreño RAN, Lim-Quianzon D, Nohynek H, Makela H, *et al.* Pneumococcal conjugate vaccines for preventing vaccine-type invasive pneumococcal disease and pneumonia with consolidation on x-ray in children under two years of age. In: The Cochrane Collaboration, editor Cochrane Database of Systematic Reviews [Internet] 2004; p. CD004977. [cited 2024 Aug 3] Available from: https://doi.wiley.com/10.1002/14651858.CD004977
[http://dx.doi.org/10.1002/14651858.CD004977]

[78] Tao S, Chen H, Li N, Liang W. The Application of the CRISPR-Cas System in Antibiotic Resistance. Infect Drug Resist 2022; 15: 4155-68.
[http://dx.doi.org/10.2147/IDR.S370869] [PMID: 35942309]

CHAPTER 5

Novel Strategies for Targeting Biofilm-Associated Bacterial Resistance

Archana Bagre[1,*], **Payal Saiju**[1] and **Amrendra Pratap Yadav**[2]

[1] *Department of Pharmaceutics, Lakshmi Narain College of Pharmacy, Bhopal, Madhya Pradesh, India*

[2] *Department of Pharmacy, Meerut Institute of Technology, Meerut, Uttar Pradesh, India*

Abstract: Biofilm is a 3D structure formed by surface-associated clusters of microbial cells, which are encased in an extracellular polymeric substance (EPS) called the matrix. Infections associated with biofilms can be irreversible and life-threatening. Understanding biofilm formation, its propagation, the mechanism of resistance development, and its identification/detection is crucial in today's context. We discuss in detail the reasons for the development of drug resistance mechanisms by highlighting the important structural and functional aspects of microbial biofilms. Exploring various biochemical factors, molecular mechanisms, and changes in host environments that contribute to the development of bacterial resistance within biofilms is essential for developing novel treatment strategies for biofilm eradication. The detailed revelation of multidisciplinary strategies for biofilm destruction necessitates the identification of target sites within the biofilm. Recent advancements in drug delivery systems have led to the use of numerous biofilm-fighting strategies. Therapeutic strategies include the use of nanotechnology, bioengineering, smart delivery systems that respond to stimuli, and modifications to particle surfaces, such as mixing with organic materials, among others. Therefore, this chapter is an effort to give an overview of current therapeutic strategies and future perspectives for the treatment of biofilm-associated infections.

Keywords: Biofilms, EPS Matrix, Novel drug delivery system, Resistance.

INTRODUCTION

Biofilm is a collection of microorganisms that adhere to the surface and nest within an extracellular polymeric matrix. It is primarily found in bacteria but may also be present in fungi, viruses, protozoa, or other microbes. It is a complicated arrangement of proteins, polysaccharides, and DNA in an extracellular polymeric matrix that protects bacteria [1]. Due to the complex structure of biofilms in comparison to the microbe, it can produce an unresponsive host immune system

* **Corresponding author Archana Bagre:** Department of Pharmaceutics, Lakshmi Narain College of Pharmacy, Bhopal, Madhya Pradesh, India; E-mail: pataskar.archana2609@gmail.com

Mukesh Kumar Singh, Gurdeep Singh, Amrendra Pratap Yadav & Papiya Bigoniya (Eds.)

that leads to the development of antibiotic resistance. Anton Van Leeuwenhoek defined biofilm as a cluster of bacteria that adheres to an inert or living surface in a hydrated polymeric matrix [2]. Recently, biofilms have gained significant attention due to their involvement in over 80% of chronic infections, particularly those associated with medical devices, chronic wounds, and respiratory illnesses. Within biofilms, bacteria exhibit enhanced resistance to antibiotics that is up to 1,000 times greater than that of their planktonic counterparts due to factors such as limited drug penetration, altered metabolic activity, activation of efflux pumps, and the presence of dormant persister cells. These properties make conventional antibiotic therapies largely ineffective, positioning biofilm research at the forefront of antimicrobial resistance (AMR) studies [3, 4].

Currently, biofilms are extensively used as models for antimicrobial drug screening and the development of anti-biofilm coatings, hydrogels, and vaccines. They more accurately mimic the *in vivo* conditions of chronic infections compared to traditional planktonic models. Moreover, biofilm studies have shed light on quorum sensing (QS) mechanisms that regulate virulence and resistance, offering new targets for non-lethal anti-virulence therapies. Understanding biofilm structure and behaviour is therefore essential for developing novel therapeutic strategies and medical materials aimed at overcoming biofilm-associated resistance [5, 6].

MICROBIAL BIOFILMS AND THEIR STRUCTURAL AND FUNCTIONAL ASPECTS

Biofilms are self-formed biopolymer matrices that contain exopolysaccharides (EPS), extracellular DNA (e-DNA), and extracellular proteins. The exopolysaccharides provide a strong and sticky structure for forming biofilms, which can be created inside or outside of cells; examples of important polysaccharides include alginate in *P. aeruginosa* and colonic acid in *E. coli.* Exopolysaccharides act as "molecular glue" and create specific changes in gene expression, such as the release of extracellular DNAs (eDNAs) through various mechanisms, including autolysis and lateral gene transfer. These e-proteins are building blocks of biofilm present on the outer surface of a bacterial cell. They are secretory in nature and not only help in the formation of biofilm but also in the aggregation, initial attachment, and the formation of bacterial cell clusters [4]. The formation of biofilms is possible in both Gram-positive and Gram-negative bacterial species. However, there are high chances of the development of biofilm-associated infection, particularly in patients receiving treatment in the ICU and those who have medical device assistance. The primary sites for biofilm formation are natural surfaces like heart valves, teeth, lungs, and ears, as well as catheters and other medical devices and stents that trigger extracellular signals

[7]. These biofilms differ in structure, location, and the type of organism involved.

1. Medical Device-Associated Biofilms
2. Chronic Wound Biofilms
3. Dental Biofilms (Oral Biofilms)
4. Lung Biofilms
5. Urinary Tract Biofilms
6. Gastrointestinal Biofilms
7. Polymicrobial Biofilms

STAGES OF BACTERIAL BIOFILM FORMATION

Specific genes regulate the dynamic and continuous process of film synthesis, which involves various stages. The following are the different stages of bacterial biofilm formation, as presented in Fig.(**1**).

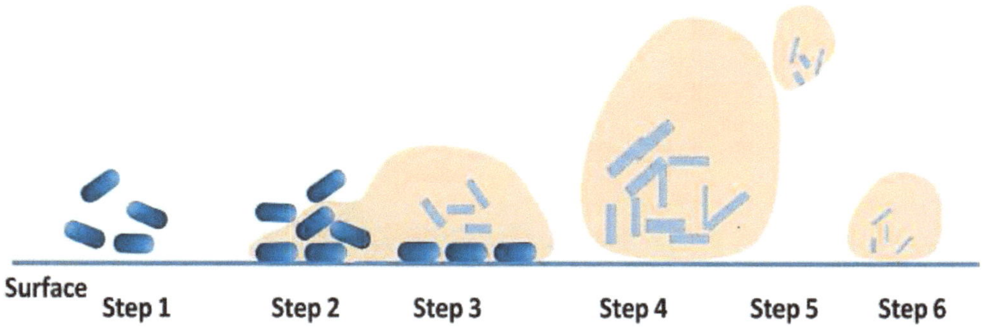

Fig. (1). Stages of bacterial biofilm formation (Step 1: Reversible Attachment; Step 2: Bacterial initial attachment and irreversible adhesion; Step 3: The extracellular matrix formation; Step 4: Microcolony formation; Step 5: Biofilm Maturation; Step 6: Biofilm Dispersal).

- Bacterial initial attachment and irreversible adhesion
- Extracellular matrix formation
- Microcolony formation
- Maturation of biofilm
- Dispersal of biofilm

Initial Attachment and Irreversible Adhesion

During an irreversible adhesion process, freely floating bacteria attach to a surface. Thereafter, bacterial cell proliferation occurs and other bacteria adhereto a site provided to them, leading to colonisation.

Matrix Formation

After the completion of colonisation, the formation of the extracellular matrix takes place. The matrix consists of exopolysaccharides (EPS), e-DNA, and extracellular proteins. The formation of an extracellular matrix is regulated by the quorum sensing mechanism (QS). The QS mechanism serves as a cell-to-cell communication channel that enables bacteria to detect, produce, and respond to extracellular signal molecules (autoinducers), thereby increasing cell population density through the regulation of genetic expression. This matrix is responsible for withstanding bacterial cells in highly stressful conditions (*i.e.*, reduced oxygen and nutrient availability), high osmotic pressure, or in the presence of antibiotics [8].

Microcolony Formation

The formation of microcolonies starts soon after a specific chemical signal. The microcolonies work together with others to share materials, distribute metabolic products, and get rid of waste.

Dispersion

This step involves the breakdown of mature biofilms and the formation of new biofilms. It is a complicated process, controlled by various environmental factors, *i.e.*, pH and nutrient levels, temperature, availability of glucose supply, and oxidative stress. Among these factors, signal transduction pathways like inhibition of c-di-GMP can promote the dispersal of biofilm [9].

QUORUM SENSING: ITS ROLE IN BACTERIAL BIOFILM DEVELOPMENT

Quorum sensing (QS) is a cell-to-cell communication process in which chemical signals activate genes that mediate an alteration in cell population density, followed by the further development of biofilm. It regulates all stages of biofilm development by activating genes and molecules for virulence [10]. In initial adhesion, it facilitates surface attachment and cell-to-cell communication to form microcolonies. The maturation of biofilm is regulated by QS through gene expression, which gives it shape. The thickness of biofilm and the dispersal of daughter cells are also regulated by QS [11].

DETECTION METHODS OF MICROBIAL BIOFILM

Biofilms can be detected by various methods, like Congo red agar, the tube method, the microtiter plate assay, CLSM (confocal laser scanning microscopy), the Congo red agar method, the crystal violet staining method, the tube method

(TM), the bioluminescent assay, piezoelectric sensors, fluorescent microscopic examination, etc [12]. As *in silico* image analysis advances, we can develop 3D biofilm images to enhance our understanding of the matrix [13].

The accurate detection and characterisation of bacterial biofilms are crucial for understanding their structure, development, and resistance mechanisms. Over the years, various qualitative and quantitative techniques have been developed for biofilm detection, each with distinct advantages and limitations.

Conventional methods include the Congo Red Agar (CRA) method, which detects slime production based on changes in colony colouration due to the interaction of bacterial exopolysaccharides with the Congo red dye. Another frequently used qualitative technique is the tube method (TM), where biofilm formation is visually assessed by staining the inner wall of test tubes with crystal violet following incubation with bacterial cultures.

The microtiter plate assay (MPA) is one of the most widely employed quantitative methods due to its reproducibility and scalability. This technique uses 96-well plates, where biofilms formed on the well surfaces are stained, typically with crystal violet, and quantified spectrophotometrically. Closely related is the crystal violet staining method, which can be applied to different surfaces and materials to evaluate biofilm mass.

Advanced techniques, like confocal laser scanning microscopy (CLSM), offer detailed structural insights by enabling high-resolution, three-dimensional visualisations of biofilms *in situ*. CLSM often uses fluorescent dyes or genetically encoded fluorophores to stain biofilm components, allowing researchers to analyse the architecture and viability of biofilm-associated cells.

Bioluminescent assays provide a dynamic and non-invasive means of monitoring biofilm growth and metabolic activity in real time, especially when using genetically modified bacteria that emit light in response to specific metabolic states. Similarly, fluorescent microscopy enables the visualisation of biofilms at the cellular level, particularly when combined with viability stains to differentiate between live and dead cells.

Piezoelectric sensors represent another innovative approach, where biofilm accumulation is detected based on changes in the resonant frequency of quartz crystal surfaces, offering a label-free and real-time monitoring option.

With the advent of computational tools and in silico image analysis, it has become possible to reconstruct three-dimensional models of biofilms based on imaging data, particularly from CLSM. These reconstructions facilitate a more comprehensive understanding of the biofilm matrix, cellular distribution, and potential diffusion barriers, which is helpful in the development of anti-biofilm strategies.

Collectively, the integration of classical and modern detection methods provides a robust framework for the study of biofilms, supporting both fundamental research and the development of therapeutics targeting biofilm-associated resistance [14].

MECHANISMS OF ANTIBIOTIC RESISTANCE THROUGH BIOFILMS

Antibiotic resistance is a state in which the drug/antibiotic loses its efficacy and increases the minimum inhibitory concentration (MIC) against microbes. The development of biofilm enables bacteria to withstand antibiotic pressure and exert resistance. It is theorised that resistance against antibiotics is due to their poor penetration inside the biofilm through neutralisation [4], the presence of enzymes like β-lactamases [15], a decrease in diffusion and adsorption mechanisms [16], a mutation in the target site, the formation of persister cells. Hence, the target for antibiotics is not active. Another reason for antibiotic resistance in biofilms is the presence of active antibiotic efflux pumps, as illustrated in Fig. (**2**). Efflux pumps are membrane proteins that localise near the cytoplasmic membranes of bacteria. The efflux pumps are responsible for maintaining bacterial homeostasis by expelling antibiotics, toxic substances, heavy metals, and metabolic products from bacterial cells.

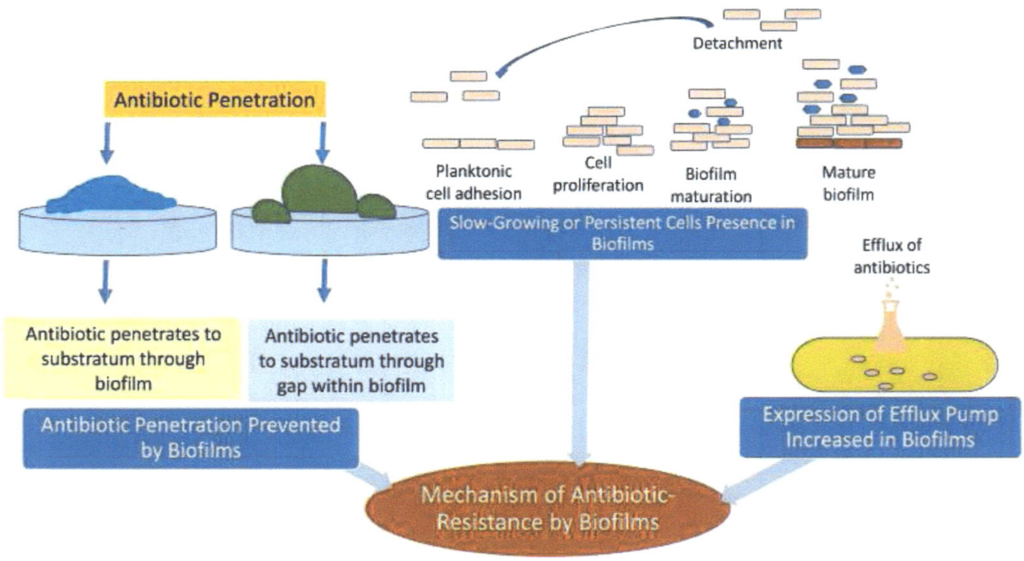

Fig. (2). Mechanism of antibiotic resistance by biofilms.

BASIC STRATEGIES FOR TARGETING BIOFILM-ASSOCIATED BACTERIAL RESISTANCE

A wide range of microbes, nearly 99%, can develop ms on both biotic and abiotic surfaces, significantly contributing to the development of antibiotic resistance. Biofilm is polymicrobial in nature, so there is competition for space and nutrients (due to horizontal gene transfer), which can increase the chances of survival and the development of antimicrobial resistance. Basic strategies for treating biofilm infections can include either prophylactic or therapeutic approaches. Prophylactic strategies involve inhibiting bacterial adhesion, preventing the formation of extracellular matrix, disrupting signalling between bacteria, or interfering with their metabolism [17]. Therapeutic strategies involve removing or destroying mature biofilms using physical, chemical, or biological methods. Physical approaches like scrubbing with jet sprays, brushes, UV rays, laser shocks, or ultrasounds are suggested, whereas chemical approaches involve the use of biofilm disruptors, antimicrobial disinfectants, and certain surfactants. In biological methods, approaches that use bacteriophage invasion are employed (Table **1**). Apart from conventional strategies, recently various novel targeted drug delivery systems (*i.e.*, active or passive targeting), controlled release systems for drug delivery, and smart drug delivery systems (having antibiotics) have been introduced for the eradication of bacterial biofilms and to avoid the development of resistance in bacteria through the delivery of antibiotics at optimum concentration. Recently, researchers have introduced smart drug delivery systems that respond to external or internal stimuli to combat biofilm-associated infections.

CONVENTIONAL APPROACHES FOR REMOVING BACTERIAL BIOFILMS

The effective way to control the biofilm includes some conventional approaches, *i.e.*, physical methods (removal by ultrasound, shock therapy, brushes, *etc.*), chemical methods (use of bio-disruptors or antimicrobial disinfectants such as surfactants, quaternary ammonium compounds, Povidone-Iodine, *etc.*), and biological methods (bacteriophage invasion and probiotics, *etc.*). Both physical and chemical methods for removing biofilms are challenging, especially when bacteria are present within those biofilms. These methods are tactical, time-consuming, and expensive. These methods create a synergistic effect that enhances biofilm disruption. Other than these methods, application of environmental factors is also useful, which includes inadequate supply of nutrients and dysfunctioning of the QS system.

Table 1. Basic strategies for targeting biofilm-associated bacterial resistance.

Basic Strategies for Targeting Biofilm-associated Bacterial Resistance	
Prevention of Biofilm Maturation	**Destroying Mature Biofilm**
▪ Inhibiting bacterial adhesion ▪ Inhibiting ECM formation ▪ Interfering with signaling between bacteria ▪ Interfering with metabolism	1. Physical Method Scrubbing by jet sprays, Brushes UV rays laser shock Ultrasound 2. Chemical Method Biofilm disruptors Antimicrobial disinfectants Surfactants Povidone-iodine 3. Biological Methods Phage Invasion Role of Probiotics

Limitations of Conventional Approaches for Removing Bacterial Biofilms

Conventional antimicrobial therapies, which primarily include systemic or topical administration of antibiotics and antiseptics, have long been the mainstay for treating bacterial infections. However, their effectiveness against biofilm-associated infections is markedly limited due to several intrinsic and extrinsic factors related to biofilm biology.

Limited Antibiotic Penetration

Biofilms are structured microbial communities embedded within a self-produced extracellular polymeric substance matrix (EPS) composed of polysaccharides, proteins, lipids, and extracellular DNA. This matrix acts as a physical and chemical barrier, impeding the diffusion of antibiotics into the deeper layers of the biofilm. As a result, bacteria located in the core of the biofilm are exposed to sub-inhibitory concentrations of antibiotics, which not only promote survival but may also induce resistance mechanisms [18].

Altered Microenvironment

Within biofilms, there are significant gradients in oxygen, pH, and nutrients. These gradients result in heterogeneous bacterial populations, including slow-growing or dormant cells known as "persister cells." . These cells are metabolically inactive and thus highly tolerant to antibiotics, especially those targeting active cellular processes such as cell wall synthesis or protein translation [19].

Phenotypic Resistance and Tolerance

Unlike genetic resistance, which involves mutations or the acquisition of resistance genes, phenotypic tolerance in biofilms is transient and reversible. Bacteria in biofilms can exhibit up to a 1,000-fold increase in minimum inhibitory concentration (MIC) compared to their planktonic counterparts. This tolerance is primarily due to the biofilm lifestyle rather than the presence of resistance genes, rendering conventional antibiotics significantly less effective [20].

Inadequate Host Immune Clearance

Biofilms also hinder effective immune responses. The EPS matrix protects embedded bacteria from phagocytosis and limits the access of immune effectors like antibodies and complement proteins. Consequently, even when the immune system is activated, it may fail to eradicate bacteria residing in biofilms, leading to chronic infections [21].

Recurrence and Chronicity of Infections

The resilience of biofilms often leads to the recurrence of infections following antibiotic treatment. Once treatment stops, persister cells can repopulate the biofilm, leading to chronic and relapsing infections, particularly in cases such as chronic wounds, cystic fibrosis lung infections, and indwelling medical devices [22].

Biofilm-Associated Resistance to Medical Devices

The colonisation of medical implants and catheters with bacteria that form biofilm presents a unique challenge. Conventional antibiotic prophylaxis or systemic treatment often fails to clear these infections, frequently necessitating the surgical removal of the infected device, a costly and invasive intervention [23].

Development of Multidrug Resistance (MDR)

Sub-inhibitory concentrations of antibiotics within biofilms can act as a selective pressure, promoting the emergence and horizontal transfer of resistance genes. This phenomenon exacerbates the global problem of antimicrobial resistance [23].

NOVEL APPROACHES FOR REMOVING BACTERIAL BIOFILMS

Researchers have applied recent advancements in nanotechnology, bioengineering, surface modification in particulate systems, and the integration of organic materials with particulate systems to eradicate biofilm-associated infections [13]. The developments in liposome and nanoparticle-based drug delivery systems serve as either intrinsic treatments or carriers for antimicrobial compounds. Specific targeting within the biofilm can be achieved by a drug delivery system using particles (nanoparticles, liposomes, *etc.*) with targeting ligands, whereas non-specific targeting is based on charge interactions and environmental factors.

The interaction of the carrier system with biofilms depends not only on its physicochemical properties but also on the heterogeneous nature of bacterial exopolysaccharides. Physicochemical properties include particle size and shape, charge on its surface, hydrophilicity/hydrophobicity, and the functional group associated with it. Exopolysaccharide is structurally a critical matrix component composed of plentiful polymer molecules having an electrical charge. The interaction of the carrier system with the bacterial surface and EPS is a systematic process that occurs in three steps:

1. Transfer of nanoparticles to the vicinity of bacterial biofilm.
2. Adhesion of nanoparticles to the biofilm surface.
3. The biofilm facilitates the movement of nanoparticles.

Each step of the interaction is influenced by biochemical and physicochemical factors like zeta potential, local environmental factors, the charges on the biofilm matrix, EPS viscosity, cell density, resistance during external mass transfer, etc [4, 14]. Nanoparticles can interact with components of the biofilm, which are basically proteins, carbohydrates, lipids, or nucleic acids. Interaction can be electrostatic, van der Waals, or ionic [15]. Some nanoparticles show antibacterial activity via different mechanisms, *i.e.*, disruption of cell wall interactions with proteins or nucleic acids, inhibition of biofilm development process, buildup of reactive oxygen species (ROS), *etc* [24]. Metal nanoparticles (Ag, Au, Zn, Cu) have the ability to release metal cations (ROS products), which can produce devastating effects on cells and SH groups on enzymes [24, 25].

In addition to nanoparticles, liposomes, which serve as a carrier system, also have the ability to interact with both the bacterial biopolymer matrix and bacterial cell membranes. The interaction of liposomes with biofilms is due to their specificity towards the target, high drug payload, low immunogenicity, and ability to reduce drug toxicity. Moreover, this process leads to the fusion of vesicles with drug-carrying liposomes, which disrupts the bacterial membrane and releases the loaded drug or bioactive molecule, allowing it to be absorbed internally. Consequently, after internal use, the antibiotic is able to eradicate the infection [26].

SMART DELIVERY SYSTEM FOR BIOFILM-ASSOCIATED BACTERIAL INFECTION

Over the past few decades, the unprecedented development in the biomedical nanotechnology field and the conversion of conventional drug delivery systems into smart drug delivery systems with stimuli-responsive characteristics have been introduced for the treatment of biofilm-associated bacterial infections. Smart (intelligent) drug delivery systems are the carrier systems that release the drug at the proper rates at the site of action [27]. The design of a smart drug delivery system, which modifies the physiochemical characteristics of the carrier system based on the environmental conditions within biofilms, has tremendous potential for treating these infections and overcoming associated resistance. The optimum level of the drug/antibiotic to produce the desired therapeutic action at the site can be activated mainly by two types: internally responsive smart carrier systems and externally responsive smart carrier systems. Recently, researchers have designed some approaches that combine both internally and externally responsive carrier systems [28].

Internal Stimuli-responsive Smart Drug Delivery System

Inside the microorganism, some internally regulated systems can target the release of antimicrobial agents. Internally regulated or self-regulated systems may include pH, the presence of enzymes, or an oxygen gradient. The change in these systems at the diseased site can trigger physical or chemical changes in the carrier system, which can further activate the release of the antimicrobial agent inside the bacteria.

pH-responsive System

The inside environment of the biofilm in the bacteria is acidic. Variations in pH can provide a potential method for treating bacterial biofilm-associated infections by creating a pH-responsive carrier system. This system can be introduced by two methods: either by introducing a protonated group in nanoparticles that undergo alteration in their physicochemical properties when the environmental pH changes or by the formation of an acid-sensitive chemical bond, which can have acid-sensitive linkages in the structure. Many researchers have used this charge-shifting approach to formulate pH-responsive carriers for biofilm. Researchers recently formulated and investigated a novel vancomycin-loaded nanovesicle against biofilms [13]. Chlorhexidine-loaded silica nanoparticles work better when their surface is changed with poly(4-vinylpyridine) because the modification makes them more responsive to pH changes.

Enzyme-responsive System

At the site of bacterial infection, there is a presence of overexpressed endogenous enzymes. A design of a carrier system for particular overexpressed enzymes, controlling the release of drugs/antibiotics, can be beneficial for biofilm-associated infection. Enzyme-responsive nanocarriers release the drug through an enzyme-degradable moiety that commonly uses bacteria-secreted enzymes as a stimulus, *i.e.*, HAS, hyaluronan synthases, membrane-bound enzymes, lipases, gelatinases, phospholipases, phosphatases, matrix metalloproteinases, glutamyl endonucleases, *etc*. The hyaluronidase-responsive system is the most commonly used approach for targeting biofilms. Hyaluronidase-responsive nanocarriers and graphene-mesoporous silica nanocarrier systems act as capping agents to protect the drug, which is contained inside [29]. Similarly, mesoporous ruthenium nanoparticles were designed for the delivery of ascorbic acid (as a prodrug) coated with hyaluronic acid and then bound to molybdenum disulfide to the outer surface, which was precoated with ciprofloxacin (a catalyst) [30]. Bacteria widely distribute lipases, which have the ability to hydrolyse carboxyl ester bonds and initiate the release of antibiotics within the biofilm. Some researchers have investigated combining an enzyme and pH-responsive approach with micellar nanocarriers for biofilm-associated infection. These polymeric micelles contain hydrophilic polyethylene glycol, which acts as an enzyme-responsive system, and poly β-amino ester, which acts as a pH-responsive system. This carrier system is positively charged at pH 5.0, while it is negatively charged at physiological pH 7.8. These mixed shell-type polymeric micelles bind to the bacterial cell surface; later, they are degraded by bacterial enzymes to release the antibiotic moiety and kill bacteria inside the biofilm [31]. We designed gelatinase-responsive gelatin nanoparticles, encapsulated with bioactives and loaded into patches, to treat Vibrio vulnificus biofilms. Glutamyl endonuclease (V8) enzyme, which is present in *S. aureus*, has the ability to break amide linkages. The enzyme-responsive metal nanocarrier is formulated by assembling poly-l-glutamic acid (PG) and polyallylamine hydrochloride (PAH) onto silver nanoparticles combined with mesoporous silica (Ag-MSN). In this context, poly-l-glutamic acid (PG) serves as a degradable motif [32].

Hypoxia-responsive System

Recently, hypoxia-responsive drug delivery systems have utilised drug molecules that are sensitive to oxygen-deficient levels inside bacteria. However, this approach had been previously utilised by researchers for targeting tumours. These systems are designed to enhance drug delivery and therapeutic efficacy by releasing antimicrobial drugs selectively in oxygen-deficient areas and maximising the desired concentration at the site of action while minimising systemic toxicity. Li and his research group formulated a hypoxia-responsive supramolecular smart drug delivery system, the lactose-modified azocalix [4] arene carrier system loaded with antibiotics. This customised carrier system shows increased antimicrobial efficacy due to drug accumulation inside the biofilm and controlled release at the infection site [33].

External Stimuli-responsive Smart Drug Delivery Systems

These are specially designed stimuli-responsive systems that externally regulate the release of an antibacterial agent from a carrier system at a desired strength during a desired time duration for the treatment of biofilm-associated bacterial infection. To date, numerous carrier systems have been designed to detect changes in external stimuli, such as light, temperature, and magnetic fields.

Light-responsive System

Light-responsive carrier systems commonly use external stimuli for biofilm-associated bacterial infections due to their non-invasive nature, high spatiotemporal response, ease of use, and convenience. This type of carrier system can either cleave a covalent bond using light to release an antimicrobial agent (*i.e.*, photochemically triggered) or absorb photon energy and convert it into heat, which may induce local hyperthermia within the biofilm (*i.e.*, photothermally triggered). Many biomedical applications implement the light-responsive approach. Photochemically triggered carrier systems are synthesised by adding light-responsive groups, such as azobenzene, Diazonaphthoquinone (DNQ), Indocyanine green (ICG), and O-nitrobenzyl, to the carrier systems. Various researchers have implemented this approach for the treatment of biofilm-associated infections. Yuan and his research group formulated a nanoplatform consisting of l-arginine, indocyanine green, and mesoporous polydopamine to eradicate biofilm. The surface of mesoporous polydopamine was modified by l-arginine, followed by the further addition of the light-responsive group indocyanine green. Under exposure to near-infrared radiation, the carrier system produces reactive oxygen species, which initiate a cascade of enzymes to release nitric oxide and trigger the destruction of biofilm [34]. In another study, Li and his group formulated protease-conjugated gold nanorods, which illuminated under NIR radiation and caused hyperthermia locally. Due to the photothermal properties of this carrier system, biofilm destruction and the removal of residual endotoxins, including the inhibition of the quorum-sensing system, occur to stop further synthesis of new bacterial biofilm [35].

Temperature-responsive System

A temperature-responsive drug delivery system is designed with the use of temperature-sensitive polymers with a lower critical solution temperature, which can release antibiotics when the temperature rises inside the bacteria. These carriers, designed to accumulate inside the microorganism and physically disrupt the biofilm, respond to temperature fluctuations [36]. The temperature-responsive hydrogel, which provides high and sustained antimicrobial action on surgical sites, is composed of poly (N-isopropylacrylamide-co-dimethylbutyrolactone acrylate-co-Jeffamine M-1000 acrylamide) and is loaded with tobramycin and vancomycin, as formulated by Overstreet [37]. On the other hand, Choi and his colleagues developed a novel coating method that utilises multilayered temperature-responsive polymer brushes, which prevent bacterial adhesion and the formation of biofilm on titanium surfaces during orthopaedic surgery [38].

Magnetic Field-responsive System

Magnetic field-responsive carrier systems find widespread use in imaging, controlled drug release, and therapeutic applications across various diseases. They release the drug under the influence of an external magnetic field by two types of mechanisms: inducing magnetic hyperthermia for drug release or providing direction for drug targeting. Recently, the combination of an external magnetic field with magnetic carriers has been explored in the field of targeted biofilm eradication. Abenojar and his group designed glycol chitin-based D-amino acid-loaded magnetic hydrogel nanoparticles for the disruption and eradication of biofilm in *S. aureus* [39]. Nickel and his group designed shape-selected magnetic nanoparticles as penetration enhancers for the biocide cetyltrimethylammonium bromide (CTAB) by increasing transport inside the biofilm, which exerts its action after magnetic stimulation and is harmful to bacteria [40]. In another study, Ji and his team designed and introduced enzyme glucose oxidase-coated magnetic nanoparticles that penetrated biofilms under the influence of a magnetic field. After penetration, nanoparticles lead to the generation of ROS and the depletion of nutrients through the action of enzymes [41].

CONCLUSION

The biofilm produced by bacteria hinders the treatment of infections, and various environmental factors influence its growth. The structure of biofilm offers physical protection to bacteria even at extreme levels of antibiotics. The bacterial biofilms can survive not only the harsh conditions and high levels of antibiotics but also offer physical protection to the bacteria from other varied and distinct microorganisms. Various approaches have been developed to overcome the risks associated with biofilms, including methods to prevent biofilm formation and technologies that can penetrate existing biofilms to ensure drug release at the appropriate site. The developments in liposome- and nanoparticle-based drug delivery systems serve as either intrinsic treatment or as carriers for antimicrobial compounds. Specific targeting inside the biofilm can be achieved by a particulate drug delivery system (nanoparticles, liposomes, *etc.*) with the development of the technology. Smart delivery systems for biofilm-associated bacterial infections offer more effective ways to treat biofilms through various approaches, like pH-responsive ones.

REFERENCES

[1] Jabber Al-Saady MAA, Aldujaili NH, Rabeea Banoon S, Al-Abboodi A. Antimicrobial properties of nanoparticles in biofilms. Bionatura 2022; 7(4): 1-9.
[http://dx.doi.org/10.21931/RB/2022.07.04.71]

[2] Sahoo K, Meshram S. Biofilm formation in chronic infections: a comprehensive review of pathogenesis, clinical implications and novel therapeutic approaches. Cureus 2024; 16(10): e70629-9.

[3] Hall CW, Mah TF. Molecular mechanisms of biofilm-based antibiotic resistance and tolerance in pathogenic bacteria. FEMS Microbiol Rev 2017; 41(3): 276-301.
[http://dx.doi.org/10.1093/femsre/fux010] [PMID: 28369412]

[4] Sharma D, Misba L, Khan AU. Antibiotics *versus* biofilm: an emerging battleground in microbial communities. Antimicrob Resist Infect Control 2019; 8(1): 76.
[http://dx.doi.org/10.1186/s13756-019-0533-3] [PMID: 31131107]

[5] Høiby N, Bjarnsholt T, Givskov M, Molin S, Ciofu O. Antibiotic resistance of bacterial biofilms. Int J Antimicrob Agents 2010; 35(4): 322-32.
[http://dx.doi.org/10.1016/j.ijantimicag.2009.12.011] [PMID: 20149602]

[6] Donlan RM. Biofilm formation: a clinically relevant microbiological process. Clin Infect Dis 2001; 33(8): 1387-92.
[http://dx.doi.org/10.1086/322972] [PMID: 11565080]

[7] Mishra A, Aggarwal A, Khan F. Medical device-associated infections caused by biofilm-forming microbial pathogens and controlling strategies. Antibiotics (Basel) 2024; 13(7): 623.
[http://dx.doi.org/10.3390/antibiotics13070623] [PMID: 39061305]

[8] Afrasiabi S, Partoazar A. Targeting bacterial biofilm-related genes with nanoparticle-based strategies. Front Microbiol 2024; 15: 1387114.
[http://dx.doi.org/10.3389/fmicb.2024.1387114] [PMID: 38841057]

[9] Toyofuku M, Inaba T, Kiyokawa T, Obana N, Yawata Y, Nomura N. Environmental factors that shape biofilm formation. Biosci Biotechnol Biochem 2016; 80(1): 7-12.
[http://dx.doi.org/10.1080/09168451.2015.1058701] [PMID: 26103134]

[10] Raina S, Vizio DD, Odell M, Clements M, Vanhulle S, Keshavarz T. Microbial quorum sensing: a tool or a target for antimicrobial therapy? Biotechnol Appl Biochem 2009; 54(2): 65-84.
[http://dx.doi.org/10.1042/BA20090072] [PMID: 19594442]

[11] Kang X, Yang X, He Y, *et al.* Strategies and materials for the prevention and treatment of biofilms. Mater Today Bio 2023; 23: 100827.
[http://dx.doi.org/10.1016/j.mtbio.2023.100827] [PMID: 37859998]

[12] Hassan A, Usman J, Kaleem F, Omair M, Khalid A, Iqbal M. Evaluation of different detection methods of biofilm formation in the clinical isolates. Braz J Infect Dis 2011; 15(4): 305-11. [http://dx.doi.org/10.1016/S1413-8670(11)70197-0] [PMID: 21860999]

[13] Hassan D, Omolo CA, Fasiku VO, Mocktar C, Govender T. Novel chitosan-based pH-responsive lipid-polymer hybrid nanovesicles (OLA-LPHVs) for delivery of vancomycin against methicillin-resistant *Staphylococcus aureus* infections. Int J Biol Macromol 2020; 147: 385-98. [http://dx.doi.org/10.1016/j.ijbiomac.2020.01.019] [PMID: 31926237]

[14] Fulaz S, Vitale S, Quinn L, Casey E. Nanoparticle–Biofilm Interactions: The Role of the EPS Matrix. Trends Microbiol 2019; 27(11): 915-26. [http://dx.doi.org/10.1016/j.tim.2019.07.004] [PMID: 31420126]

[15] Panda SK, Buroni S, Tiwari V, Nascimento da Silva LC. Editorial: Insights Into New Strategies to Combat Biofilms. Front Microbiol 2021; 12: 742647. [http://dx.doi.org/10.3389/fmicb.2021.742647] [PMID: 34630368]

[16] Sheng Y, Chen Z, Wu W, Lu Y. Engineered organic nanoparticles to combat biofilms. Drug Discov Today 2023; 28(2): 103455. [http://dx.doi.org/10.1016/j.drudis.2022.103455] [PMID: 36403883]

[17] Ciofu O, Rojo-Molinero E, Macià MD, Oliver A. Antibiotic treatment of biofilm infections. Acta Pathol Microbiol Scand Suppl 2017; 125(4): 304-19. [http://dx.doi.org/10.1111/apm.12673] [PMID: 28407419]

[18] Donlan RM, Costerton JW. Biofilms: survival mechanisms of clinically relevant microorganisms. Clin Microbiol Rev 2002; 15(2): 167-93. [http://dx.doi.org/10.1128/CMR.15.2.167-193.2002] [PMID: 11932229]

[19] Bergsbaken T, Fink SL, Cookson BT. Pyroptosis: host cell death and inflammation. Nat Rev Microbiol 2009; 7(2): 99-109. [http://dx.doi.org/10.1038/nrmicro2070] [PMID: 19148178]

[20] Mah TFC, O'Toole GA. Mechanisms of biofilm resistance to antimicrobial agents. Trends Microbiol 2001; 9(1): 34-9. [http://dx.doi.org/10.1016/S0966-842X(00)01913-2] [PMID: 11166241]

[21] Costerton JW, Stewart PS, Greenberg EP. Bacterial Biofilms: A Common Cause of Persistent Infections. Science (1979) 284(5418): 1318-22. 1999 May 21.

[22] Bjarnsholt T. The role of bacterial biofilms in chronic infections. Acta Pathol Microbiol Scand Suppl 2013; 121(s136): 1-58. [http://dx.doi.org/10.1111/apm.12099] [PMID: 23635385]

[23] Donlan RM. Biofilms and device-associated infections. Emerg Infect Dis 2001; 7(2): 277-81. [http://dx.doi.org/10.3201/eid0702.010226] [PMID: 11294723]

[24] Joshi AS, Singh P, Mijakovic I. Interactions of gold and silver nanoparticles with bacterial biofilms: Molecular interactions behind inhibition and resistance. Int J Mol Sci 2020; 21(20): 7658. [http://dx.doi.org/10.3390/ijms21207658] [PMID: 33081366]

[25] Moradi F, Ghaedi A, Fooladfar Z, Bazrgar A. Recent advance on nanoparticles or nanomaterials with anti-multidrug resistant bacteria and anti-bacterial biofilm properties: A systematic review. Heliyon 2023; 9(11): e22105. [http://dx.doi.org/10.1016/j.heliyon.2023.e22105] [PMID: 38034786]

[26] Wang DY, van der Mei HC, Ren Y, Busscher HJ, Shi L. Lipid-Based Antimicrobial Delivery-Systems for the Treatment of Bacterial Infections. Front Chem 2020; 7: 872. [http://dx.doi.org/10.3389/fchem.2019.00872] [PMID: 31998680]

[27] Sousa A, Phung AN, Škalko-Basnet N, Obuobi S. Smart delivery systems for microbial biofilm therapy: Dissecting design, drug release and toxicological features. J Control Release 2023; 354: 394-

416.
[http://dx.doi.org/10.1016/j.jconrel.2023.01.003] [PMID: 36638844]

[28] Liu Y, Busscher HJ, Zhao B, *et al.* Surface-Adaptive, Antimicrobially Loaded, Micellar Nanocarriers with Enhanced Penetration and Killing Efficiency in Staphylococcal Biofilms. ACS Nano 2016; 10(4): 4779-89.
[http://dx.doi.org/10.1021/acsnano.6b01370] [PMID: 26998731]

[29] Ding M, Zhao W, Song LJ, Luan SF. Stimuli-responsive nanocarriers for bacterial biofilm treatment. Rare Met 2022; 41(2): 482-98.
[http://dx.doi.org/10.1007/s12598-021-01802-4] [PMID: 34366603]

[30] Ji H, Dong K, Yan Z, *et al.* Bacterial Hyaluronidase Self-Triggered Prodrug Release for Chemo-Photothermal Synergistic Treatment of Bacterial Infection. Small 2016; 12(45): 6200-6.
[http://dx.doi.org/10.1002/smll.201601729] [PMID: 27690183]

[31] Liu Y, Lin A, Liu J, *et al.* Enzyme-responsive mesoporous ruthenium for combined chemo-photothermal therapy of drug-resistant bacteria. ACS Appl Mater Interfaces 2019; 11(30): 26590-606.
[http://dx.doi.org/10.1021/acsami.9b07866] [PMID: 31264823]

[32] Xu J, Danehy R, Cai H, *et al.* Microneedle Patch-Mediated Treatment of Bacterial Biofilms. ACS Appl Mater Interfaces 2019; 11(16): 14640-6.
[http://dx.doi.org/10.1021/acsami.9b02578] [PMID: 30933463]

[33] Li JJ, Hu Y, Hu B, *et al.* Lactose azocalixarene drug delivery system for the treatment of multidrug-resistant pseudomonas aeruginosa infected diabetic ulcer. Nat Commun 2022; 13(1): 6279.
[http://dx.doi.org/10.1038/s41467-022-33920-7] [PMID: 36270992]

[34] Yuan Z, Lin C, He Y, *et al.* Near-Infrared Light-Triggered Nitric-Oxide-Enhanced Photodynamic Therapy and Low-Temperature Photothermal Therapy for Biofilm Elimination. ACS Nano 2020; 14(3): 3546-62.
[http://dx.doi.org/10.1021/acsnano.9b09871] [PMID: 32069025]

[35] Li W, Geng X, Liu D, Li Z. Near-Infrared Light-Enhanced Protease-Conjugated Gold Nanorods As A Photothermal Antimicrobial Agent For Elimination Of Exotoxin And Biofilms. Int J Nanomedicine 2019; 14: 8047-58.
[http://dx.doi.org/10.2147/IJN.S212750] [PMID: 31632017]

[36] Hu Y, Ruan X, Lv X, *et al.* Biofilm microenvironment-responsive nanoparticles for the treatment of bacterial infection. Nano Today 2022; 46: 101602.
[http://dx.doi.org/10.1016/j.nantod.2022.101602]

[37] Overstreet DJ, Badha VS, Heffernan JM, *et al.* Temperature-responsive PNDJ hydrogels provide high and sustained antimicrobial concentrations in surgical sites. Drug Deliv Transl Res 2019; 9(4): 802-15.
[http://dx.doi.org/10.1007/s13346-019-00630-5] [PMID: 30891707]

[38] Lee JW, Dai Z, Lee C, *et al.* Tuning Molecular Interactions for Highly Reproducible and Efficient Formamidinium Perovskite Solar Cells *via* Adduct Approach. J Am Chem Soc 2018; 140(20): 6317-24.
[http://dx.doi.org/10.1021/jacs.8b01037] [PMID: 29723475]

[39] Abenojar EC, Wickramasinghe S, Ju M, *et al.* Magnetic Glycol Chitin-Based Hydrogel Nanocomposite for Combined Thermal and D -Amino-Acid-Assisted Biofilm Disruption. ACS Infect Dis 2018; 4(8): 1246-56.
[http://dx.doi.org/10.1021/acsinfecdis.8b00076] [PMID: 29775283]

[40] Nickel R, Kazemian MR, Wroczynskyj Y, Liu S, van Lierop J. Exploiting shape-selected iron oxide nanoparticles for the destruction of robust bacterial biofilms – active transport of biocides *via* surface charge and magnetic field control. Nanoscale 2020; 12(7): 4328-33.
[http://dx.doi.org/10.1039/C9NR09484A] [PMID: 32043517]

[41] Ji Y, Han Z, Ding H, *et al.* Enhanced eradication of bacterial/fungi biofilms by glucose oxidase-

modified magnetic nanoparticles as a potential treatment for persistent endodontic infections. ACS Appl Mater Interfaces 2021; 13(15): 17289-99.
[http://dx.doi.org/10.1021/acsami.1c01748] [PMID: 33827209]

CHAPTER 6

Co-Infections and Opportunistic Pathogens in Ameliorating Disease Outcomes

Rakesh Kumar[1,*], **Vivek Raj**[2], **Vandana**[3], **Biplab Pal**[1] and **Vikas Sharma**[1]

[1] *School of Pharmaceutical Sciences, Lovely Professional University, Phagwara- 144411, Punjab, India*

[2] *Department of Biotechnology, Patna Women's College, Patna, Bihar, India*

[3] *Indus Institute of Management, Indus University, Rancharda via Thaltej, Ahmedabad, Gujarat. 382114, India*

Abstract: The clinical course of primary infections is frequently complicated by co-infections and opportunistic pathogens, which have a substantial impact on disease outcomes. Multiple pathogens can worsen illness severity, make identification more difficult, and reduce the effectiveness of treatment. Advanced molecular methods, such as polymerase chain reaction (PCR) and next-generation sequencing (NGS), are necessary for accurate diagnosis of co-infections because they can identify many pathogens at once and offer detailed insights into the microbial ecology. Treatment plans must be customized to target the particular infections after they have been discovered, taking into account the patient's immunological condition as well as any possible drug-drug interactions. Opportunistic infections, caused by pathogens that exploit weakened immune defenses, further complicate treatment. These infections often require a combination of antimicrobial therapies and immunomodulatory treatments to restore immune function and control pathogen proliferation. The interplay between co-infections and opportunistic pathogens necessitates a multidisciplinary approach, involving infectious disease specialists, microbiologists, and immunologists, to optimize patient outcomes. Advances in personalized medicine, including the use of biomarker-driven therapies and immune profiling, are showing promise in improving the management of co-infections. Early detection and targeted treatment are critical in preventing the progression of disease and reducing mortality rates. Future research should focus on understanding the mechanisms of pathogen interaction within the host and developing novel therapeutic strategies to mitigate the impact of co-infections and opportunistic pathogens on disease outcomes.

Keywords: Antimicrobial therapy, Co-infections, Disease outcomes, Diagnosis, Molecular techniques, Opportunistic pathogens.

* **Corresponding author Rakesh Kumar:** School of Pharmaceutical Sciences, Lovely Professional University, Phagwara- 144411, Punjab, India; E-mail:csrakeshk@gmail.com

Mukesh Kumar Singh, Gurdeep Singh, Amrendra Pratap Yadav & Papiya Bigoniya (Eds.)

INTRODUCTION

Co-infections

Co-infections occur when a host is simultaneously infected by two or more distinct pathogens. These infections can be caused by a combination of viruses, bacteria, fungi, or parasites. Co-infections are of particular concern because they can complicate diagnosis, exacerbate symptoms, and affect treatment outcomes. The interaction between pathogens in co-infections can lead to either antagonistic or synergistic effects. In an antagonistic interaction, one pathogen may suppress the growth of another, potentially resulting in milder symptoms. Conversely, in a synergistic interaction, the pathogens may enhance each other's virulence, leading to more severe disease progression. Co-infections are common in conditions where the immune system is compromised or already weakened by a primary infection. For instance, individuals with HIV are often susceptible to co-infections such as tuberculosis (TB), as HIV weakens the immune system, increasing susceptibility to other pathogens [1]. Another common example is the co-occurrence of hepatitis B and C viruses in patients, which complicates liver disease management [2].

Co-infections can also occur in the context of viral epidemics and pandemics. For example, during the COVID-19 pandemic, co-infections with influenza and other respiratory pathogens were frequently observed, often worsening the clinical outcomes in affected patients [3]. In such cases, the presence of more than one pathogen can make treatment more complex, as the therapeutic strategies must account for multiple causative agents.

Opportunistic Pathogens

Opportunistic pathogens are microorganisms that usually do not cause disease in a healthy host but can lead to infections in individuals with weakened immune systems. These pathogens take advantage of certain conditions, such as a compromised immune system, disruptions in the normal microbial flora, or breaches in the body's physical barriers, like skin or mucosal membranes. Opportunistic infections are especially prevalent in immunocompromised individuals, such as those undergoing chemotherapy, organ transplant recipients on immunosuppressive drugs, or people living with chronic diseases like HIV/AIDS [4]. In such individuals, pathogens that are usually harmless or kept in check by a healthy immune system can cause serious infections. Common opportunistic pathogens include *Candida albicans*, which can cause fungal infections, and *Pseudomonas aeruginosa*, a bacterium responsible for respiratory and urinary tract infections. HIV/AIDS is a prime example of a condition where opportunistic pathogens become a significant concern. As the HIV attacks and destroys CD4+ T cells, the immune system becomes progressively weaker, allowing various opportunistic pathogens, such as *Pneumocystis jirovecii* (which causes pneumonia) and Cytomegalovirus (which can lead to blindness or gastrointestinal diseases), to proliferate and cause severe infections [4].

Opportunistic pathogens can also arise in hospital settings, where patients are often vulnerable due to invasive procedures, immunosuppressive treatments, or prolonged antibiotic use. Hospital-acquired infections (HAIs), caused by opportunistic bacteria like *Staphylococcus aureus* and *Clostridioides difficile*, pose serious risks to patient health and can lead to outbreaks in healthcare settings [5].

The Epidemiological Significance

Co-infections and opportunistic pathogens play a crucial role in the epidemiology of human diseases, often complicating diagnosis, treatment, and outcomes. Co-infections occur when a host is simultaneously infected by two or more pathogens, which can interact in ways that exacerbate disease severity. Opportunistic pathogens, on the other hand, typically cause illness only when the host's immune system is weakened, such as in cases of immunodeficiency or chronic disease. The epidemiological significance of co-infections is particularly evident in diseases like HIV/AIDS, tuberculosis, and malaria. For instance, HIV-positive individuals are at an increased risk of contracting tuberculosis, a leading cause of death among those with HIV. Approximately one-sixth of the global population is affected by coinfections, involving over 270 pathogen taxa. These coinfections can alter infection dynamics and influence both individual and population-level disease outcomes [1, 47]. These co-infections can lead to more severe disease progression and complications due to immune system compromise. Similarly, malaria patients are often more susceptible to bacterial and viral infections, increasing morbidity and mortality rates [6]. Opportunistic pathogens, such as *Pneumocystis jirovecii* and *Candida albicans*, are another concern in immunocompromised populations, including those undergoing chemotherapy or organ transplantation. These pathogens take advantage of weakened immune defenses to cause life-threatening infections that would not typically occur in healthy individuals. For example, *Pneumocystis pneumonia* is a common cause of death in patients with AIDS, particularly in regions with limited access to antiretroviral therapy. In 2023, an estimated 8.2 million people were newly diagnosed with TB worldwide, up from 7.5 million in 2022. Co-infections with HIV, SARS-CoV-2, influenza, and various bacterial and fungal pathogens complicate TB management, especially in low- and middle-income countries (LMICs) [7, 48].

Paradox of Co-infections in Disease Amelioration

The paradox of co-infections in disease amelioration highlights how the presence of certain secondary infections can modulate immune responses, potentially altering the severity, progression, and outcomes of a primary disease. While co-infections are often assumed to exacerbate disease severity, research has shown that in some cases, they may ameliorate disease progression. This counterintuitive phenomenon has gained attention as scientists explore how pathogens interact with one another and the host immune system.

Modulation of Immune Responses by Co-infections

Co-infections can modulate immune responses through several mechanisms, including immune competition, immune suppression, and immune redirection. For example, during a co-infection, pathogens may compete for host immune resources, leading to a dampened immune response to one or both infections. This "immune trade-off" may result in reduced inflammation or tissue damage, alleviating the clinical severity of the primary infection. One notable example of this phenomenon is the interaction between helminth infections and viral or bacterial pathogens. Helminths, which are parasitic worms, have evolved mechanisms to evade the host's immune system, often inducing a regulatory or anti-inflammatory immune response. This can reduce the hyperinflammatory response that may be associated with viral or bacterial infections, as observed in conditions like tuberculosis or certain viral diseases. In such cases, helminth co-infections may paradoxically protect against severe outcomes by tempering the host's immune activation [8].

Impact on Disease Progression and Outcomes

The impact of co-infections on disease progression and outcomes depends on several factors, including the type of pathogens involved, the timing of infection, and the host's immune status. In some instances, co-infections may lead to immune suppression, allowing one pathogen to dominate and cause a more severe disease. For example, HIV co-infection with tuberculosis can severely impair immune responses, leading to worsened outcomes due to the unchecked progression of tuberculosis [9]. However, in other cases, the presence of a co-infection can limit the progression of the primary infection. For instance, some studies have suggested that helminth infections may reduce the severity of autoimmune diseases like multiple sclerosis by modulating immune responses toward a more anti-inflammatory state [10].

MECHANISMS OF INTERACTION BETWEEN CO-INFECTIONS AND HOST IMMUNITY

Co-infections occur when multiple pathogens infect a host simultaneously, complicating the immune response, as shown in Fig. (**1**). The interaction between these pathogens and host immunity can modulate the immune system in various ways, with potential consequences for disease progression, immune evasion, and overall health outcomes. Understanding these mechanisms is crucial in managing diseases with high rates of co-infection, such as HIV, tuberculosis (TB), and malaria.

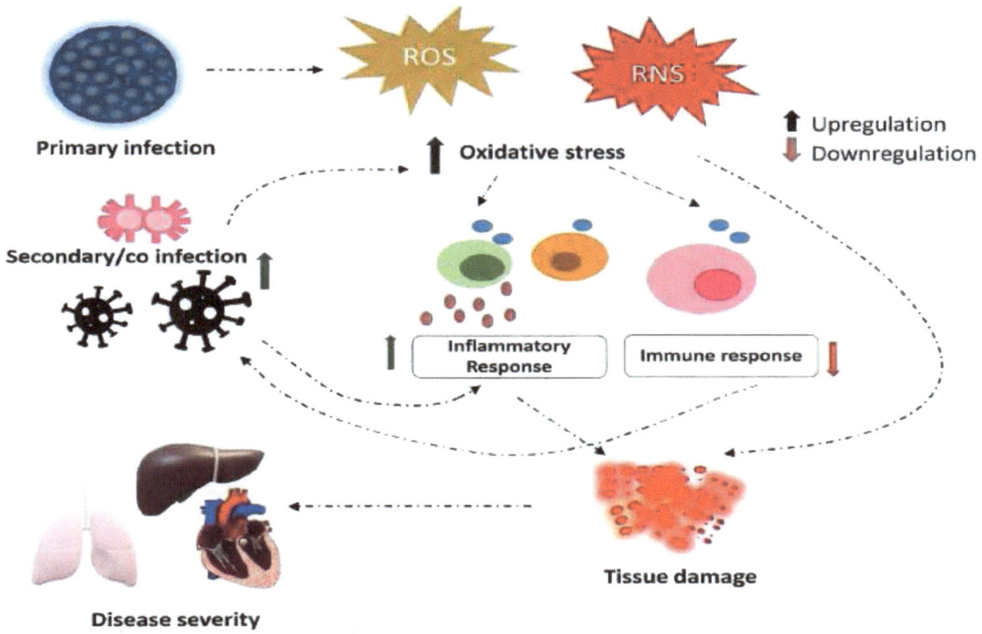

Fig. (1). Co-infection affects immunological severity and oxidative stress. Primary infections cause oxidative stress, which is then exacerbated by secondary/co-infections and ultimately results in immune response dysregulation. Together, these resulted in tissue damage and disease severity.

Immunological Modulation by Co-infections

When the immune system encounters a co-infection, it responds to each pathogen through distinct but overlapping mechanisms. Pathogens stimulate different immune pathways, including the innate and adaptive immune responses. Co-infections can induce competitive or cooperative interactions between these immune pathways, altering their normal functions. Competitive interactions arise when immune responses to one pathogen inhibit the response to another. For example, HIV co-infection with TB impairs the host's ability to mount an effective immune response to TB by depleting CD4+ T-cells, essential for controlling *Mycobacterium tuberculosis* infection. This results in an increased risk of TB reactivation and progression in HIV-infected individuals [11]. Cooperative interactions occur when the immune response to one pathogen facilitates the immune response to another. For instance, malaria and helminth co-infections can amplify immune activation by promoting a generalized immune response that targets both pathogens. However, this enhanced response may also lead to immune dysregulation and increased tissue damage [12]. Co-infections can also manipulate immune evasion strategies, where one pathogen alters immune signaling to benefit both itself and the secondary pathogen. For example, cytomegalovirus (CMV) infection during HIV co-infection can increase immune exhaustion by overactivating T-cells, thus weakening the immune system further [13].

Pathogen-pathogen Interactions

Pathogen-pathogen interactions during co-infections can significantly influence disease progression, immune responses, and overall host health. These interactions are often complex, involving competition or cooperation between pathogens, as well as their modulation of host immunity. Understanding these mechanisms can help improve strategies for managing co-infections and their associated risks. One prominent mechanism of pathogen-pathogen interaction is competition for resources. When two pathogens infect the same host, they may compete for nutrients, such as iron or glucose, which are essential for their survival and replication. For example, *Mycobacterium tuberculosis* and HIV can coinfect individuals, where tuberculosis limits the availability of key nutrients, impairing HIV replication, and also compromises host immunity, facilitating HIV persistence [14].

Another mechanism is immune modulation. Some pathogens can alter host immune responses in ways that favor the survival of other pathogens. For instance, in co-infections with *Helicobacter pylori* and Hepatitis C virus (HCV), H. pylori can skew the immune response toward a Th2 phenotype, suppressing antiviral Th1 responses and potentially enhancing HCV persistence. Such immune modulation can lead to chronic infections and increased disease severity [15].

Cytokine crosstalk is another critical factor, where the immune response to one pathogen can affect the outcome of a second infection. In co-infections with influenza and bacterial pneumonia, influenza infection induces type I interferons that suppress neutrophil recruitment, facilitating bacterial superinfections [16].

Examples of Co-infections that Ameliorate Disease Outcomes

Co-infections, where a host is infected by two or more pathogens at the same time, can sometimes lead to unexpected outcomes in terms of disease severity. While many co-infections exacerbate disease, there are instances where one infection can actually ameliorate the outcome of another. These examples often involve complex interactions between pathogens, the host immune system, and other biological factors.

Helminth Infections and Autoimmune Diseases

Helminths, or parasitic worms, are known to modulate the immune system in ways that can have both positive and negative effects on other diseases. One of the most well-documented instances where helminth infections ameliorate disease outcomes is in autoimmune diseases, such as multiple sclerosis (MS) and inflammatory bowel disease (IBD). Helminths induce a regulatory immune response by increasing the production of anti-inflammatory cytokines, such as interleukin-10 (IL-10) and transforming growth factor-beta (TGF-β), and by promoting the development of regulatory T cells (Tregs). This immune modulation can reduce the severity of autoimmune diseases, where the immune system mistakenly attacks the body's own tissues. In fact, experimental infection with helminths, or treatment with helminth-derived products, has been shown to reduce the severity of MS in both animal models and clinical studies [17 - 19].

Measles Virus and Asthma

Another example of co-infection improving disease outcomes is seen with the measles virus and its potential protective effect against asthma. Epidemiological data have suggested that individuals who experience measles in childhood have a lower risk of developing asthma later in life. Measles virus infections may suppress immune hyperreactivity that is often responsible for allergic diseases like asthma [20]. This observation is supported by the hygiene hypothesis, which proposes that reduced exposure to infections in childhood may increase the risk of allergic diseases due to insufficient immune system training. Measles infection can promote a shift from a Th2-dominated immune response, which is associated with allergies, to a Th1-dominated response, reducing the likelihood of developing asthma [21].

HIV and HTLV-1 Co-infection

Human T-lymphotropic virus type 1 (HTLV-1) and human immunodeficiency virus (HIV) are retroviruses that often co-infect individuals, particularly in areas where both viruses are endemic, such as certain regions of Africa, South America, and Japan. Interestingly, HIV-HTLV-1 co-infections can sometimes result in slower HIV progression. HTLV-1 stimulates the immune system, leading to increased T-cell activation and proliferation. This immune activation is paradoxically beneficial for individuals co-infected with HIV, as it helps maintain a more functional immune response against HIV in the early stages of infection. Some studies have reported that individuals co-infected with HTLV-1 and HIV have a delayed progression to AIDS compared to those infected with HIV alone. However, it is important to note that not all studies have confirmed this effect, and the long-term consequences of HIV-HTLV-1 co-infection can vary depending on other factors, such as viral load and immune system health [22, 23].

GB Virus C and HIV

GB virus C (GBV-C), also known as hepatitis G virus, is a flavivirus that infects humans but does not cause any known disease. Interestingly, studies have shown that GBV-C infection can have a beneficial effect on individuals with HIV. People co-infected with GBV-C and HIV tend to have slower disease progression, higher CD4+ T cell counts, and better survival outcomes compared to those infected with HIV alone. The protective effect of GBV-C is thought to be due to its interference with HIV replication. GBV-C can inhibit the expression of HIV co-receptors on T cells, such as CCR5 and CXCR4, thereby reducing HIV's ability to infect these cells. Additionally, GBV-C infection has been shown to increase the production of antiviral cytokines like interferon gamma (IFN-γ), which helps control HIV replication [22, 23].

Plasmodium falciparum and Hepatitis B Virus

In malaria-endemic regions, co-infection with *Plasmodium falciparum* (the parasite responsible for malaria) and hepatitis B virus (HBV) is common. Some studies suggest that co-infection with HBV may protect against severe malaria outcomes. The proposed mechanism involves the immune system's altered response to co-infection, where chronic HBV infection dampens the inflammatory response to malaria [24, 25].

CASE STUDIES: HOW OPPORTUNISTIC PATHOGENS INFLUENCE DISEASE OUTCOMES

Opportunistic pathogens are microbes that do not typically cause disease in a healthy host but can cause infections when the host's immune system is weakened or compromised. These pathogens take advantage of weakened immune responses due to conditions such as immunodeficiency, chronic diseases, or medical interventions like chemotherapy, organ transplants, or prolonged antibiotic use. While they are often part of the normal microbiota, opportunistic pathogens can lead to significant morbidity and mortality in vulnerable populations. A few case studies illustrate how opportunistic pathogens influence disease outcomes.

Case Study 1: *Pseudomonas aeruginosa* in Cystic Fibrosis

Cystic fibrosis (CF) is a genetic disorder that severely affects the respiratory and digestive systems, leading to the production of thick, sticky mucus that traps bacteria in the lungs. One of the most notable opportunistic pathogens in CF patients is *Pseudomonas aeruginosa*, a gram-negative bacterium that thrives in moist environments. Normally, *P. aeruginosa* poses little threat to healthy individuals. However, in CF patients, the pathogen can establish chronic lung infections due to the impaired clearance of mucus and weakened local immunity. Over time, this bacterium undergoes genetic changes that allow it to persist and evade the host's immune responses. Chronic infections with *P. aeruginosa* are associated with progressive lung damage, increased inflammation, and, ultimately, respiratory failure in CF patients. Studies have shown that chronic infection with *P. aeruginosa* correlates with decreased lung function and higher mortality rates in CF patients. Early detection and aggressive treatment, including antibiotics and airway clearance techniques, are critical in managing these infections and improving long-term outcomes [26].

Case Study 2: *Candida albicans* in HIV/AIDS

Human Immunodeficiency Virus (HIV) infection leads to the progressive weakening of the immune system, particularly affecting CD4+ T-cells. As HIV progresses to Acquired Immunodeficiency Syndrome (AIDS), patients become increasingly susceptible to opportunistic infections. *Candida albicans*, a fungus commonly found on the skin and mucosal surfaces, is a notable opportunistic pathogen in this population. In healthy individuals, *C. albicans* causes mild, self-limiting infections. However, in HIV-positive individuals with low CD4+ counts, the pathogen can cause persistent and invasive infections, particularly in the oral cavity and esophagus (thrush). *C. albicans* infections in HIV/AIDS patients can be painful, impair nutrition, and significantly reduce quality of life. Invasive candidiasis, where the pathogen enters the bloodstream and spreads to other organs, can occur in severely immunocompromised patients and is life-threatening. Prophylactic antifungal treatments and antiretroviral therapy (ART) have been shown to reduce the incidence of these infections and improve disease outcomes [27].

Case Study 3: *Aspergillus fumigatus* in Transplant Recipients

Solid organ transplant recipients are at high risk for opportunistic infections due to the immunosuppressive therapies necessary to prevent organ rejection. One of the most feared pathogens in this population is *Aspergillus fumigatus*, a ubiquitous mold that can cause invasive aspergillosis. In healthy individuals, inhaled *A. fumigatus* spores are typically cleared by the immune system. However, in immunocompromised transplant recipients, particularly those who have undergone lung or bone marrow transplants, *A. fumigatus* can cause severe lung infections that can spread to other organs, including the brain and kidneys. Invasive aspergillosis is associated with high morbidity and mortality, especially if diagnosis and treatment are delayed. Early antifungal therapy, combined with careful monitoring of immunosuppressive drug levels, is essential in improving the prognosis for transplant recipients [28].

Case Study 4: *Clostridioides difficile* in Antibiotic-Associated Diarrhea

Clostridioides difficile (formerly *Clostridium difficile*) is a bacterium that causes severe diarrhea and colitis, particularly in individuals who have recently received antibiotics. Antibiotics can disrupt the normal gut microbiota, allowing *C. difficile* to proliferate and produce toxins that damage the intestinal lining. *Clostridioides difficile* infections (CDI) are most common in hospitalized patients, especially those undergoing prolonged antibiotic treatment. The infection can range from mild diarrhea to life-threatening inflammation of the colon, known as pseudomembranous colitis. CDI is a major cause of morbidity and mortality in healthcare settings, particularly among elderly patients. Treatment typically involves the cessation of the inciting antibiotic and administration of targeted antibiotics like vancomycin or fidaxomicin. Fecal microbiota transplantation (FMT) has also emerged as an effective therapy for recurrent CDI, helping to restore a healthy gut microbiome [29].

ROLE OF CYTOKINES AND CHEMOKINES

Cytokines and chemokines are pivotal in orchestrating the immune response during infections. Cytokines are small proteins secreted by cells that affect the behavior of other cells, while chemokines are a subset of cytokines that specifically induce chemotaxis in nearby cells. During co-infections, the interplay of these signaling molecules can lead to altered immune responses. The presence of multiple pathogens can lead to an exaggerated or dysregulated cytokine response, commonly referred to as a "cytokine storm." For instance, in viral-bacterial co-infections, such as the influenza virus and *Streptococcus pneumoniae*, the host may experience a surge in pro-inflammatory cytokines like IL-6, TNF-α, and IL-1β, which can result in severe lung inflammation and tissue damage [30].

This hyper-inflammatory state not only exacerbates disease severity but also compromises the immune system's ability to effectively clear both infections. Moreover, chemokine profiles can change significantly during co-infections. Different pathogens can induce specific chemokines that attract distinct immune cell populations, leading to a skewed immune response. For example, during HIV and tuberculosis (TB) co-infection, the altered production of chemokines such as CXCL10 can influence the recruitment and activation of T cells, leading to impaired control of TB [31]. The resultant imbalance in immune cell distribution can further compromise the host's ability to combat either infection.

IMMUNE EVASION AND PATHOGEN PERSISTENCE

Pathogens have evolved various mechanisms to evade the host immune response, particularly in the context of co-infections. One common strategy is the modulation of cytokine and chemokine signaling pathways. For example, certain viruses, such as HIV and influenza, can inhibit the production of type I interferons (IFNs) and other cytokines critical for antiviral immunity, thereby prolonging their survival in the host [32]. This not only allows the primary pathogen to persist but also creates an immunosuppressive environment that can enable secondary infections to flourish. Furthermore, pathogens can exploit immune cell exhaustion. During chronic infections, such as HIV, the continuous stimulation of T cells can lead to a state of exhaustion characterized by the upregulation of inhibitory receptors such as PD-1 and CTLA-4. This exhausted state can impair the ability of T cells to respond to co-infecting pathogens [33]. In this scenario, the host becomes susceptible to secondary infections as the immune system's capacity to mount effective responses is significantly diminished. Co-infections can also lead to the phenomenon of "antigenic competition." When two pathogens share similar antigens, they can compete for immune recognition, potentially leading to suboptimal immune responses. For example, in malaria and HIV co-infections, the presence of malaria antigens can distract the immune system from effectively targeting HIV-infected cells, thereby enhancing HIV replication and persistence [34].

THERAPEUTIC IMPLICATIONS

Co-infections, where an individual is infected with two or more pathogens simultaneously, pose significant challenges to public health and therapeutic management. Understanding the interplay between co-infecting organisms can lead to enhanced therapeutic strategies, yet it also presents complex clinical challenges. This discussion explores the potential benefits of exploiting co-infections for therapeutic gain and the challenges inherent in managing these complex clinical scenarios.

Potential Benefits of Exploiting Co-infections

Enhanced Immunological Response

One of the most promising aspects of co-infections is the potential for a synergistic immunological response. Research has indicated that exposure to certain pathogens can cause the immune system to respond more effectively to subsequent infections. For instance, studies have shown that individuals with a history of viral infections, such as influenza, may have heightened immune responses to subsequent bacterial infections [35]. This phenomenon can be exploited therapeutically; for example, vaccines that leverage prior immune responses may enhance protection against specific pathogens, particularly in high-risk populations.

Targeting Multiple Pathogens

Another potential benefit of exploiting co-infections lies in the ability to develop treatments that target multiple pathogens simultaneously. Combination therapies are already a staple in managing diseases like HIV, where antiretroviral therapy is used to suppress the virus while also addressing opportunistic infections [36]. By developing multidrug regimens that address various coinfecting organisms, healthcare providers can enhance treatment efficacy, reduce morbidity, and improve patient outcomes.

Epidemiological Insights

Studying co-infections also provides valuable epidemiological insights that can inform public health strategies. Understanding the dynamics of co-infections can lead to improved surveillance and management strategies. For example, the co-occurrence of malaria and HIV in sub-Saharan Africa has led to targeted interventions that address both diseases concurrently, optimizing resource allocation and improving health outcomes [37]. By integrating approaches for managing multiple infections, health systems can become more efficient and effective.

Challenges in Managing Co-infections

Diagnostic Complexity

Despite the potential benefits, managing co-infections presents significant diagnostic challenges. Many co-infections share overlapping symptoms, making it difficult for healthcare providers to accurately diagnose the primary infection. For instance, the symptoms of viral respiratory infections can mimic those of bacterial pneumonia, complicating treatment decisions [38]. Misdiagnosis can lead to inappropriate treatments, exacerbating patient conditions, and contributing to the development of antimicrobial resistance.

Treatment Interactions

Another challenge is the potential for drug interactions when managing multiple infections. Many patients with co-infections are treated with multiple medications, which can lead to adverse drug reactions and reduced treatment efficacy. For instance, the use of certain antiretrovirals can complicate the management of tuberculosis, as some antiretrovirals may inhibit the metabolism of anti-TB medications, leading to suboptimal treatment outcomes [39]. Therefore, healthcare providers must carefully consider the pharmacokinetics and pharmacodynamics of each drug to avoid harmful interactions.

Increased Morbidity and Mortality

Co-infections are associated with increased morbidity and mortality rates, complicating management strategies. The presence of one infection can exacerbate the severity of another, leading to a vicious cycle of declining health. For example, patients with HIV are more susceptible to opportunistic infections, which can significantly reduce their lifespan [40]. This necessitates a holistic approach to treatment that addresses not just the infections but also the underlying health issues and immune status of the patient.

FUTURE DIRECTIONS AND RESEARCH GAPS IN PATHOGEN INTERACTIONS

Emerging Research on Pathogen Interactions

Recent advances in technologies such as genomics and microbiome studies are transforming our understanding of pathogen interactions. Historically, most research focused on single pathogens in isolation. However, the complex dynamics of co-infections and multi-pathogen interactions are gaining attention, revealing significant implications for disease outcomes and public health strategies.

Microbiome Studies

The human microbiome plays a critical role in modulating immune responses and pathogen behavior. Research indicates that microbial communities can influence susceptibility to infections and disease severity. For example, the gut microbiome has been shown to affect the course of viral infections like influenza [41].

Emerging studies are exploring how alterations in the microbiome due to diet, antibiotics, and environmental factors can affect pathogen interactions. The interplay between bacterial and viral pathogens within the microbiome can lead to synergistic or antagonistic effects, influencing the severity and transmission dynamics of infectious diseases [42].

Genomics and Metagenomics

Genomic technologies enable researchers to study multiple pathogens simultaneously and to understand their interactions at the molecular level. Metagenomic sequencing allows for the identification of viral, bacterial, and fungal communities in a single sample, providing insights into how these organisms interact. For instance, the discovery of viral entities in the microbiome that can inhibit bacterial growth, such as bacteriophages targeting pathogenic bacteria, opens new avenues for therapeutic strategies [43].

Pathogen-Pathogen Interactions

Understanding the interactions between different pathogens can elucidate mechanisms of disease progression and resistance. For instance, co-infections of HIV and tuberculosis are well-documented, with evidence suggesting that HIV can enhance the susceptibility to tuberculosis infection through immune system modulation [44]. However, many other potential interactions remain unexplored. The identification of such interactions can help in developing more effective treatment and prevention strategies. Depending on the pathogen's virulence factors, the host's susceptibility, the pathogen's mode of entrance, the pathogen's mode of transmission, and several environmental conditions, the host-pathogen interaction can result in either infection or immunity. It will be easier to create more effective control strategies against EIDs if the study comprehends the mechanisms of the molecular elements involved in host-pathogen interactions during infection, as shown in Fig. (**2**).

Implications for Global Health and Disease Management

The recognition of pathogen interactions has profound implications for global health and disease management. Traditional approaches focusing on single-pathogen interventions may need to be reevaluated in light of these findings.

Public Health Strategies

Current public health strategies often overlook the complexities of co-infections. By integrating knowledge of pathogen interactions into surveillance and intervention strategies, health authorities can better predict outbreaks and manage resources. For instance, vaccination campaigns may need to consider the presence of co-infecting pathogens that could diminish vaccine efficacy [45].

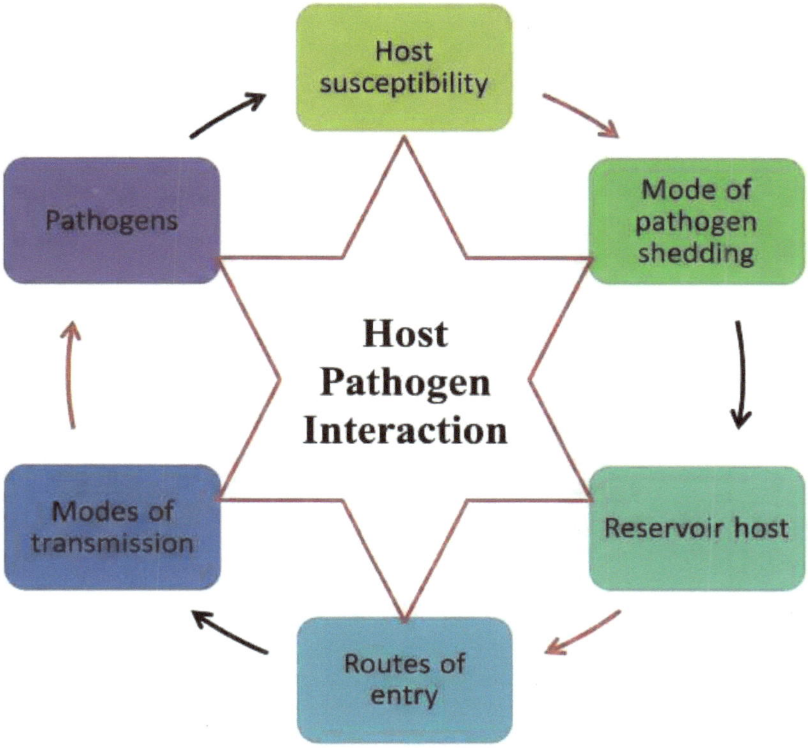

Fig. (2). Host-pathogen interaction.

Therapeutic Approaches

The development of combination therapies targeting multiple pathogens may be necessary to address co-infections effectively. For example, understanding how bacteria can enhance or inhibit viral infections could lead to innovative therapeutic strategies that leverage these interactions to enhance patient outcomes [46].

Global Health Policies

As global travel and trade increase, the risk of multi-pathogen outbreaks rises. Policies must adapt to these challenges by promoting collaborative international research that focuses on pathogen interactions. This will require interdisciplinary approaches that bridge microbiology, epidemiology, and public health.

EXPERIMENTAL MODELS TO STUDY CO-INFECTION

According to various research studies, there are some experimental models for studying co-infection, including *in vitro, in vivo, ex vivo*, and *in silico* systems. *In vitro* cell cultures allow controlled analysis of pathogen interactions, while organoids provide a more realistic tissue architecture [50]. *In vivo* models, like mice and humanized mice, enable exploration of systemic immune responses [53]. *Ex vivo* tissue cultures maintain native microenvironments [54]. *In silico* models simulate interactions computationally [55]. These models collectively provide insights into co-infection model types, description, advantages, and limitations, as shown in Table **1**.

Table 1. Various experimental models to study co-infection.

Model Type	Description	Advantages	Limitations	References
***In vitro* Cell Culture**	Co-culture of host cells (*e.g*., epithelial, macrophages) with multiple pathogens	Controlled environment, high reproducibility, cost-effective	Lacks systemic immune responses; limited tissue complexity	[49]
Organoids	3D mini-organs derived from stem cells to mimic tissue microenvironments	Physiologically relevant; better tissue architecture than 2D culture	Expensive, technical complexity, and limited immune components	[50]
Animal Models (Mice, Ferrets, Zebrafish)	Whole-organism infection models to simulate co-infection scenarios	Full immune response; suitable for *in vivo* pathogenesis studies	Ethical issues, interspecies differences, and higher cost	[51]
Humanized Mice	Mice engrafted with human immune cells or tissues to mimic the human immune response.	Allows human-specific pathogen study; models chronic infection	Complex, expensive, partial immune function	[52, 53]
***Ex vivo* Tissue Culture**	Human or animal tissues cultured and infected with pathogens	Preserves tissue architecture; useful for lung or gut co-infection models	Limited viability; variable results from donor tissue	[54]
Computational Models (*In silico*)	Simulations of host-pathogen interactions using machine learning models	No ethical constraints; rapid hypothesis generation	Requires experimental validation; limited by data quality	[55]

CONCLUSION

The relationship between co-infections and opportunistic pathogens significantly influences disease outcomes. Co-infections, the simultaneous presence of two or more infectious agents in a host, can lead to more severe disease manifestations, as seen in conditions like HIV/AIDS, where the presence of opportunistic pathogens like *Pneumocystis jirovecii* increases morbidity and mortality. These pathogens thrive in immunocompromised individuals, further undermining the host's immune response and complicating treatment regimens. However, the relationship is not solely detrimental. In some cases, opportunistic pathogens can modulate immune responses beneficially. For instance, certain viral infections may stimulate an adaptive immune response that enhances protection against other pathogens. This dual role underscores the necessity of understanding how these interactions influence overall disease progression and patient outcomes. The effects of co-infections can vary greatly depending on the pathogen involved, the host's immune status, and the timing of infections, illustrating the need for a nuanced approach to treatment. Moreover, understanding the dynamics of co-infections can guide the development of targeted therapies that address not only the primary infection but also the effects of secondary pathogens. This approach may involve tailored vaccination strategies, combination therapies, and personalized medicine that consider the unique pathogen interactions present in each patient. The integration of co-infection knowledge into treatment paradigms is not merely an academic exercise but a necessary evolution in healthcare that can lead to more effective and holistic patient care.

REFERENCES

[1] Pawlowski A, Jansson M, Sköld M, Rottenberg ME, Källenius G. Tuberculosis and HIV Co-Infection. PLoS Pathog 2012; 8(2): e1002464. [http://dx.doi.org/10.1371/journal.ppat.1002464] [PMID: 22363214]

[2] Martins AN, Perez RM, Moreira RC. Hepatitis B and C co-infection in a Brazilian population: viral genotype distribution and clinical characteristics. Rev Soc Bras Med Trop 2019; 52.

[3] Lansbury L, Lim B, Baskaran V, Lim WS. Co-infections in people with COVID-19: a systematic review and meta-analysis. J Infect 2020; 81(2): 266-75. [http://dx.doi.org/10.1016/j.jinf.2020.05.046] [PMID: 32473235]

[4] Kaplan JE, Hanson D, Dworkin MS, *et al.* Epidemiology of human immunodeficiency virus-associated opportunistic infections in the United States in the era of highly active antiretroviral therapy. Clin Infect Dis 2000; 30(s1) (Suppl. 1): S5-S14. [http://dx.doi.org/10.1086/313843] [PMID: 10770911]

[5] Weiner-Lastinger LM, Pattabiraman V, Konnor RY, *et al.* The impact of coronavirus disease 2019 (COVID-19) on healthcare-associated infections in 2020: A summary of data reported to the National Healthcare Safety Network – ADDENDUM. Infect Control Hosp Epidemiol 2022; 43(1): 137. [http://dx.doi.org/10.1017/ice.2022.10] [PMID: 35043780]

[6] Roberds A, Ferraro E, Luckhart S, Stewart VA. HIV-1 impact on malaria transmission: A complex and relevant global health concern. Front Cell Infect Microbiol 2021; 11: 656938.

[http://dx.doi.org/10.3389/fcimb.2021.656938] [PMID: 33912477]

[7] Riccardi N, Rotulo GA, Castagnola E. Definition of opportunistic infections in immunocompromised children on the basis of etiologies and clinical features: A summary for practical purposes. Curr Pediatr Rev 2019; 15(4): 197-206.
[http://dx.doi.org/10.2174/1573396315666190617151745] [PMID: 31242834]

[8] Maizels RM, McSorley HJ, Smyth DJ. Helminths in the hygiene hypothesis: sooner or later? Clin Exp Immunol 2018; 175(1): 44-54.
[PMID: 24749722]

[9] Kwan CK, Ernst JD. HIV and tuberculosis: a deadly human syndemic. Clin Microbiol Rev 2011; 24(2): 351-76.
[http://dx.doi.org/10.1128/CMR.00042-10] [PMID: 21482729]

[10] Correale J, Farez MF. The impact of parasite infections on the course of multiple sclerosis. J Neuroimmunol 2011; 233(1-2): 6-11.
[http://dx.doi.org/10.1016/j.jneuroim.2011.01.002] [PMID: 21277637]

[11] Lawn SD, Wilkinson RJ. Immune reconstitution disease associated with parasitic infections following antiretroviral treatment. Parasite Immunol 2006; 28(11): 625-33.
[http://dx.doi.org/10.1111/j.1365-3024.2006.00900.x] [PMID: 17042934]

[12] Hartgers FC, Yazdanbakhsh M. Co-infection of helminths and malaria: modulation of the immune responses to malaria. Parasite Immunol 2006; 28(10): 497-506.
[http://dx.doi.org/10.1111/j.1365-3024.2006.00901.x] [PMID: 16965285]

[13] Smith C, Khanna R, Gamadia L. Role of cytomegalovirus-specific CD8+ T cells in immune modulation and viral persistence. Nat Rev Immunol 2013; 13(6): 494-507.

[14] Bell LC, Noursadeghi M, Boyton RJ. Tuberculosis and HIV co-infection. Front Immunol 2019; 10: 206.

[15] Kamdar ZN, Rutkowski MR, Denduluri SK. Pathogen-pathogen interactions in coinfected hosts. J Immunol 2019; 202(7): 1925-33.

[16] Shahangian A, Chow EK, Tian X, Iwasaki A, Type I. IFNs suppress bacterial infection. Nat Immunol 2009; 10(5): 512-8.

[17] Maizels RM, Yazdanbakhsh M. Immune Regulation by helminth parasites: cellular and molecular mechanisms. Nat Rev Immunol 2003; 3(9): 733-44.
[http://dx.doi.org/10.1038/nri1183] [PMID: 12949497]

[18] Weinstock JV, Elliott DE. Helminth infections decrease pathogenesis in T-cell-mediated autoimmunity. J Immunol 2009; 182(12): 6668-73.

[19] Correale J, Farez M. Association between parasite infection and immune responses in multiple sclerosis. Ann Neurol 2007; 61(2): 97-108.
[http://dx.doi.org/10.1002/ana.21067] [PMID: 17230481]

[20] Shaheen SO, Barker DJP, Heyes CB, *et al.* Measles and atopy in Guinea-Bissau. Lancet 1996; 347(9018): 1792-6.
[http://dx.doi.org/10.1016/S0140-6736(96)91617-7] [PMID: 8667923]

[21] Strachan DP. Family size, infection and atopy: the first decade of the "hygiene hypothesis". Thorax 2000; 55(Suppl 1).

[22] Xiang J, Wünschmann S, Diekema DJ, *et al.* Effect of coinfection with GB virus C on survival among patients with HIV infection. N Engl J Med 2001; 345(10): 707-14.
[http://dx.doi.org/10.1056/NEJMoa003364] [PMID: 11547739]

[23] Tillmann HL, Heiken H, Knapik-Botor A, *et al.* Infection with GB virus C and reduced mortality among HIV-infected patients. N Engl J Med 2001; 345(10): 715-24.
[http://dx.doi.org/10.1056/NEJMoa010398] [PMID: 11547740]

[24] Murray MJ, Murray AB, Murray MB, *et al.* Viral hepatitis and malaria in Nigerians. Lancet 1977; 310(8040): 1316-8.

[25] Hoffmann CJ, Thio CL. Clinical implications of HIV and hepatitis B co-infection in Asia and Africa. Lancet Infect Dis 2007; 7(6): 402-9.
[http://dx.doi.org/10.1016/S1473-3099(07)70135-4] [PMID: 17521593]

[26] Høiby N. Recent advances in the treatment of *Pseudomonas aeruginosa* infections in cystic fibrosis. BMC Med 2011; 9(1): 32.
[http://dx.doi.org/10.1186/1741-7015-9-32] [PMID: 21463524]

[27] Pappas PG, Kauffman CA, Andes DR, *et al.* Clinical practice guideline for the management of candidiasis: 2016 update by the Infectious Diseases Society of America. Clin Infect Dis 2016; 62(4): 409-17.
[http://dx.doi.org/10.1093/cid/civ1194]

[28] Kosmidis C, Denning DW. The clinical spectrum of pulmonary aspergillosis. Thorax 2015; 70(3): 270-7.
[http://dx.doi.org/10.1136/thoraxjnl-2014-206291] [PMID: 25354514]

[29] Kelly CR, Kahn S, Kashyap P, Laine L, Rubin D, Atreja A, *et al.* Update on fecal microbiota transplantation 2015: Indications, methodologies, outcomes, and future directions. Gastroenterology 2015; 149(1): 223-37.
[http://dx.doi.org/10.1053/j.gastro.2015.05.008] [PMID: 25982290]

[30] McAuley DF, *et al.* Influenza and secondary bacterial pneumonia: A cytokine storm. Lancet Respir Med 2020; 8(5): 485-6.

[31] Hernández R, *et al.* Chemokine profiles in HIV and tuberculosis co-infection. J Infect Dis 2019; 220(1): 97-106.

[32] Schoggins JW, *et al.* Pan-viral specificity of IFN-induced genes reveals new roles for cGAS in viral infections. Cell Host Microbe 2011; 10(5): 513-25.

[33] Wherry EJ, *et al.* T cell exhaustion. Nat Immunol 2007; 8(3): 277-85.
[PMID: 17220892]

[34] Kantor JJ, *et al.* Co-infection with malaria and HIV: effects on HIV replication and immune activation. Curr Opin HIV AIDS 2015; 10(1): 55-61.
[PMID: 25389805]

[35] Meyer KC, Goss M, Hurst R. Viral and bacterial interactions in respiratory infections: A review. J Infect Dis 2018; 217(7): 1085-91.
[PMID: 29762690]

[36] Hernández AV, Negrón RM, González FA. Antiretroviral therapy and opportunistic infections in HIV patients: A review. Curr HIV Res 2019; 17(2): 122-30.

[37] Baal MK, Koudstaal J, De Groot E. The epidemiology of malaria and HIV co-infection in sub-Saharan Africa: A systematic review. Malar J 2020; 19(1): 1-13.
[PMID: 31898492]

[38] López-Cedrón R, de Dios L, Cuadrado C. Diagnostic challenges in co-infections: Implications for treatment. Infect Dis (Lond) 2022; 54(4): 252-9.

[39] Gupta A, Muliya VS, Thakur R. Drug interactions in HIV and tuberculosis co-infected patients: A review. J Antimicrob Chemother 2021; 76(5): 1030-41.

[40] Nachega JB, Hislop M, Dowdy D. The impact of co-infections on HIV management in sub-Saharan Africa: A review. AIDS Res Hum Retroviruses 2018; 34(1): 1-9.
[PMID: 29161879]

[41] Zhu L, Wang X, Yang H. Gut microbiome and influenza infection: A new area of research. Nat Rev

Gastroenterol Hepatol 2020; 17(12): 773-86.
[PMID: 33067592]

[42] Lloyd-Price J, Abu-Ali G, Huttenhower C. The healthy human microbiome. Genome Med 2016; 8(1): 51.
[http://dx.doi.org/10.1186/s13073-016-0307-y] [PMID: 27122046]

[43] Wang J, Zhang Y, Liu L. Microbiome–pathogen interactions: Implications for human health and disease. Nat Rev Microbiol 2019; 17(9): 585-94.

[44] Corbett EL, Watt CJ, Walker N, *et al.* The growing burden of tuberculosis: global trends and interactions with the HIV epidemic. Arch Intern Med 2003; 163(9): 1009-21.
[http://dx.doi.org/10.1001/archinte.163.9.1009] [PMID: 12742798]

[45] Mann SM, Wykes MN, O'Connor J. Co-infection and its impact on vaccine efficacy: A review of the literature. Front Microbiol 2020; 11: 564857.

[46] Reddy SK, Trivedi NA, Wang L. Exploiting pathogen interactions for therapeutic advances. Nat Rev Microbiol 2020; 18(10): 695-711.

[47] Gorsich EE, Etienne RS, Medlock J, *et al.* Opposite outcomes of coinfection at individual and population scales. Proc Natl Acad Sci USA 2018; 115(29): 7545-50.
[http://dx.doi.org/10.1073/pnas.1801095115] [PMID: 29967175]

[48] Cioboata R, Balteanu MA, Osman A, *et al.* Coinfections in tuberculosis in low- and middle-income countries: Epidemiology, clinical implications, diagnostic challenges, and management strategies—a narrative review. J Clin Med 2025; 14(7): 2154.
[http://dx.doi.org/10.3390/jcm14072154] [PMID: 40217604]

[49] Johnson RM, *et al.* Cellular models of viral co-infection. Virol J 2015; 12: 45.

[50] Bartfeld S, *et al.* Modeling infectious diseases and host-pathogen interactions in human organoids. Cell Host Microbe 2015; 17(6): 706-20.

[51] Wu X, *et al.* A mouse model of co-infection with influenza virus and *Streptococcus pneumoniae*. Nat Protoc 2018; 13(4): 705-21.
[PMID: 29543794]

[52] Billerbeck E, *et al.* Humanized mouse models for hepatitis C and human immune system studies. J Clin Invest 2013; 123(3): 1034-42.

[53] Shultz LD, *et al.* Humanized mice in translational biomedical research. Nat Rev Immunol 2012; 12(11): 786-98.
[http://dx.doi.org/10.1038/nri3311] [PMID: 23059428]

[54] Sajti E, *et al.* Transcriptomic differences in *ex vivo* human tissue infections. Nat Commun 2020; 11: 1-14.

[55] Marino S, Hogue IB, Ray CJ, Kirschner DE. A methodology for performing global uncertainty and sensitivity analysis in systems biology. J Theor Biol 2008; 254(1): 178-96.
[http://dx.doi.org/10.1016/j.jtbi.2008.04.011] [PMID: 18572196]

CHAPTER 7

Unraveling the Complexities of Coinfection Diagnosis and Treatment

Monika Singh[1,*], **Nitin Kumar**[2], **Sadish Kumar Shanmugam**[3] and **Moumita Barman**[4]

[1] *Department of Pharmacology, I.T.S College of Pharmacy, Ghaziabad, India*

[2] *Department of Pharmacognosy, Meerut Institute of Technology, Meerut, India*

[3] *Department of Pharmaceutical Chemistry, I.T.S College of Pharmacy, Ghaziabad, India*

[4] *Department of Pharmaceutics, I.T.S College of Pharmacy, Ghaziabad, India*

Abstract: Coinfections, characterized by the simultaneous presence of multiple pathogenic agents in a single host, pose significant challenges to accurate diagnosis and effective treatment. This chapter focuses on cases with overlapping clinical symptoms that obscure the identification of individual infections, emphasizing the need for a comprehensive diagnostic strategy. A multi-tiered approach integrating advanced imaging, biofluid analysis, and molecular techniques, particularly multiplex PCR assays, is discussed for detecting multiple pathogens in animal models. The complexity of coinfections is further highlighted by difficulties in treatment, including potential drug interactions and distinct resistance patterns. The chapter concludes by outlining essential steps for implementing advanced diagnostics and personalized therapeutic strategies to improve patient outcomes in cases of coinfection.

KEYWORDS: Coinfection, Diagnosis, Disease, Host response, Pathogenic agents, Treatment.

INTRODUCTION

When an individual has simultaneous infection with more than one pathogenic microorganism, it is known as coinfection. A typical scenario is for an individual to be infected with a virus (such as HIV) along with a bacterium like *Mycobacterium tuberculosis* or two different viral infections concurrently, such as HIV and hepatitis C [1].

* **Corresponding author Monika Singh:** Department of Pharmacology, I.T.S College of Pharmacy, Ghaziabad, India; E-mail: monikas@its.edu.in

Mukesh Kumar Singh, Gurdeep Singh, Amrendra Pratap Yadav & Papiya Bigoniya (Eds.)

However, in medicine, it is the trickiest of all because you are not talking about one but many infecting agents, interacting amongst themselves and with the host response. Coinfections can dramatically change the progression, virulence, and remediate response of the involved diseases, making them a vital area in all clinical and research fields [2].

Coinfections frequently manifest with overlapping symptoms, so identifying all of the associated pathogens can be difficult. For example, an individual with a viral respiratory infection and a bacterial respiratory infection can sometimes have fever, cough, and fatigue, making the clinical assessment of these symptoms challenging. The combined effects of multiple pathogens may lead to a greater viral or bacterial disease burden. For example, a patient with influenza and bacterial pneumonia may experience greater respiratory distress than a patient with influenza or another type of pneumonia [3, 4].

One pathogen involved in a coinfection may modulate the immune response of the host in ways that may facilitate or impair the establishment of the second pathogen. For example, some viruses can suppress immune responses, which may allow for easier bacterial infection. Pathogens can compete for the same resources of the host, such as nutrients [5], or utilize host cells that share cellular receptors. This competition can determine which pathogen is most likely to become dominant or how severe the infectious stage will be. Some pathogens may make changes to the host physiology or the surrounding environment, which may influence other pathogens' survival or multiplication. For instance, a bacterial infection may lead to tissue destruction, which will provide access to another pathogen. In treating diseases, there are a number of complexities, including drug interactions. Some drugs for one infection may interact with those for the other and may hence reduce their effectiveness or increase the chances of side effects. The identified comorbid bacterial infections also amplify the extent of antibiotic resistance, especially if broad-spectrum antibiotics are used without necessarily testing for all the bacteria. It may cause the infections to be trickier to control, treat, and contain [6]. The transmission of coinfections is not limited to single infections, as they appear more complicated. For instance, one pathogen may enhance the effects of another, as observed with HIV, which makes one more vulnerable to the rest of the STIs. Completing the coinfected patients' history and clearly identifying all pathogens in patients are complicated tasks in public health systems, especially in regions with the presence of multiple infectious diseases [7]. In many cases, control measures take time because the different pathogens require concerted efforts, which can cost a lot of money. Consequently, coinfections are highly applicable in global health since they infect persons who have little or no access to health facilities. Managing coinfections is critical in enhancing the health status of those regions [8].

It can be concluded that coinfection is a very complicated process that interrelates several pathogens in one host. Such interactions can profoundly change the development of diseases, the difficulty of their diagnosis and treatment, and the hindrances experienced in the field of public health. The knowledge of and approaches to coinfections are a focal research aspect that has significant implications for single-patient care on global fitness [9].

EPIDEMIOLOGY OF COINFECTIONS

- **Prevalence of Coinfections**

Compromised Immune Systems: Immunocompromised persons are at high risk of developing other infections. Their immune system is not as strong, and thus, they find it difficult to combat several diseases. For instance, people living with HIV are more prone to infections, including TB, fungal infections, and viral infections such as hepatitis [10].

Endemic Regions: Another factor is that coinfections also occur in areas where some infectious diseases are comparatively more prevalent. For instance, in Sub-Saharan Africa, malaria, TB, and HIV are communicable diseases; the diseases frequently occur at the same time. It should, however, be noted that these regions have environmental, socio-economic, and healthcare conditions that allow for the proliferation of multiple pathological agents [11].

- **Patterns of Coinfections**
    - ***HIV and Tuberculosis (TB):*** HIV weakens the immune system, allowing latent TB infections to become active, making this coinfection particularly dangerous [12].
    - ***HIV and Malaria***: Malaria can worsen HIV infection by increasing viral replication, and HIV weakens the immune response to malaria, leading to more severe illness [13].
    - ***Helminth Infections and Malaria***: In tropical regions, helminth (parasitic worm) infections are common and can coexist with malaria. These interactions can lead to more severe anaemia and immune dysregulation [14].
    - ***COVID-19 and Respiratory Infections***: During the COVID-19 pandemic, many patients experienced coinfections with other respiratory pathogens like influenza or bacterial pneumonia, which compounded the severity of the illness [15].

- **Impact of Coinfections**
    - ***Increased Disease Severity***: Coinfections can make diseases more severe. For example, people suffering from both malaria and HIV experience severe malaria symptoms [16].

- ***Complicated Treatment***: Treating coinfections can be more challenging as the drugs used to treat one infection may interact with or affect the treatment of the other [17].
- ***Impact on Public Health***: The prevalence of coinfections requires careful public health management, especially in areas where resources are limited. Integrated disease management strategies are crucial to address overlapping diseases in affected regions [18].
  - **Pathogen-Pathogen Interactions:** Pathogen-pathogen interactions in coinfections occur when one pathogen influences the behaviour, entry, or virulence of another. These interactions can significantly affect the course of diseases, leading to more severe outcomes [19]. Here is a closer look at how certain pathogens can facilitate or enhance the virulence of others:
- ***Facilitation of Entry***: Some pathogens can damage tissues, suppress the immune system, or create conditions that make it easier for secondary infections to occur [20].
- ***Influenza and Bacterial Pneumonia:*** Influenza weakens the respiratory tract's defences, particularly the epithelial cells that form a barrier against bacteria. This makes it easier for bacteria, such as *Streptococcus pneumoniae* or *Staphylococcus aureus*, to enter the lungs and cause secondary bacterial pneumonia. Influenza also impairs the immune system's ability to clear bacteria from the lungs, allowing bacterial infections to thrive after the viral infection [21].
- ***HIV and Opportunistic Infections***: HIV primarily targets and destroys CD^{4+} cells, gradually weakening the immune system. Once the immune system deteriorates, the person becomes more susceptible to opportunistic infections like tuberculosis, as well as fungal and viral infections. These pathogens might not cause severe disease in individuals with healthy immune systems, but become life-threatening in those with HIV [22].
- ***Enhanced Virulence:*** Certain pathogens not only allow other infections to occur but can also increase the virulence or severity of these secondary pathogens [23].
- ***HIV and Tuberculosis (TB):*** TB is often latent in people with healthy immune systems. HIV accelerates TB progression and complicates treatment, as the two diseases require complex and prolonged treatment regimens [24].
- ***Malaria and HIV:*** HIV positive persons are more susceptible to suffering severe malaria because their immune system cannot control the parasite. At the same time, malaria exacerbates HIV by increasing the replication of the virus and the activation of the immune system, further weakening the body's defences [25].

- ***Hepatitis C Virus (HCV) and HIV:*** HIV speeds up the progression of liver damage caused by HCV, causing liver diseases like cirrhosis and liver cancer, in a shorter period [26].
- ***Immune Modulation*:** Some pathogens actively modulate the immune system, creating an atmosphere that is more conducive to other infections [27].
- ***Helminths (Parasitic Worms) and Tuberculosis (TB)*:** In some areas where helminth infections are endemic, coinfections with TB are common. This immunomodulation can make it more difficult for the body to control TB, leading to increased susceptibility or worsening of the disease [28].
- ***HIV and Cytomegalovirus (CMV):*** CMV, a herpesvirus, is usually asymptomatic in healthy individuals but becomes a significant problem in those with HIV [29].
- ***Synergistic Effects on Disease Severity*:** Coinfections can cause a combined impact, where two pathogens have an impact greater than their individual effects [30].
- ***Methicillin-Resistant Staphylococcus Aureus (MRSA) and Influenza:*** Coinfection with MRSA and influenza in the lungs can lead to severe necrotizing pneumonia. The immune response to influenza creates an environment in the lungs that allows MRSA to proliferate, causing more severe tissue damage than either pathogen alone would cause [31].
- ***COVID-19 and Bacterial Contagions*:** Throughout the COVID-19 pandemic, secondary bacterial infections were common in critically ill patients. The immune suppression caused by severe COVID-19, coupled with prolonged hospitalization, allowed bacteria like *Pseudomonas aeruginosa* or *Acinetobacter baumannii* to infect the lungs, thereby increasing mortality Fig. (**1**) [32].

CHALLENGES IN DIAGNOSIS

Diagnosing coinfections presents significant challenges due to the complex interplay of pathogens, overlapping symptoms, host factors, and the limitations of available diagnostic tools [33]. Here is a deeper exploration of these challenges:

• Overlapping Symptoms

Coinfections often present with non-specific or similar symptoms, making it difficult to distinguish between different infections based solely on clinical presentation.

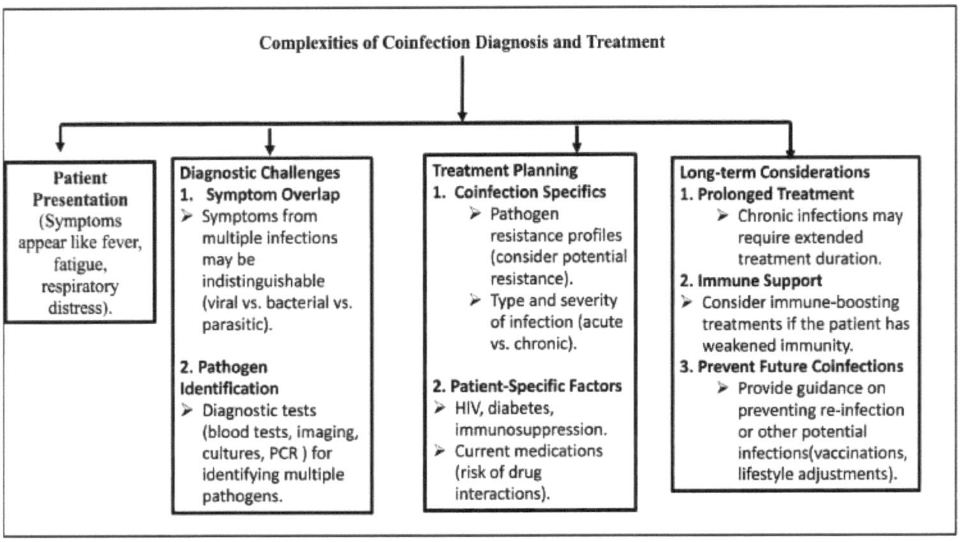

Fig. (1). This flowchart illustrates the step-by-step process of diagnosing and treating coinfections. It begins with the patient's presentation, diagnostic challenges, and treatment planning.

- ***Malaria and Dengue*:** Both diseases are prevalent in tropical regions and often present with symptoms like fever, headache, muscle pain, and fatigue. Since these symptoms are common to many infectious diseases, including influenza and COVID-19, differentiating between them based on clinical signs alone is challenging. Misdiagnosis can lead to inappropriate treatment, which may worsen patient outcomes [34].
- ***HIV and Tuberculosis*:** In individuals with HIV, TB may present with atypical symptoms or resemble other opportunistic infections, further complicating diagnosis. Indications like chronic cough, night sweats and weight loss overlap with other respiratory infections or conditions like fungal infections [35].

Diagnostic Tools and Techniques

Several diagnostic techniques are used to identify coinfections, but each has limitations that can affect their reliability.

- ***Molecular Techniques (PCR, Multiplex Assays):*** Polymerase Chain Reaction (PCR) is highly precise and sensitive for the detection of the genetic material of pathogens. It can simultaneously detect multiple pathogens in a single sample (*e.g.*, multiplex PCR). However, PCR may detect low levels of pathogens that do not causing active disease but merely colonize the body. This makes it challenging to distinguish between a true infection and non-pathogenic colonization [36].

- ***Serological Tests*:** Serological tests detect antibodies or antigens related to specific pathogens. They are useful in diagnosing infections like HIV, hepatitis, and some bacterial infections. However, serological tests often cannot distinguish between active and past infections, especially in individuals with chronic infections where antibody levels may remain elevated long after the infection is cleared [37].
- ***Imaging Techniques*:** Imaging tools like chest X-rays and CT scans are supportive in diagnosing respiratory infections like TB or pneumonia. However, they may show non-specific patterns of inflammation or infection that can be triggered by various pathogens [38].

○ Host Factors

Host factors, particularly immune status, significantly impact how coinfections present and how they can be diagnosed.

- ***Immunosuppression:*** Conditions like HIV/AIDS, chemotherapy, or organ transplantation weaken the immune system, masking typical symptoms of infections. For example, a person with advanced HIV may not exhibit the classic signs of TB (*e.g.*, fever, cough), making diagnosis more difficult. Immunocompromised individuals may also develop infections from normally non-pathogenic organisms, further complicating diagnosis [39].
- ***Comorbidities:*** Chronic diseases like diabetes or chronic kidney disease can alter the course of infections, making it harder to identify coinfections. These underlying conditions can also exacerbate the severity of infections [40].

○ Immune Evasion and Modulation

Many pathogens have evolved mechanisms to manipulate the individual's immune response, complicating diagnosis and treatment.

- ***HIV:*** HIV weakens the immune system's ability to detect and fight other infections. This immune suppression allows opportunistic infections like TB, *Pneumocystis jirovecii* pneumonia (PCP), or fungal infections to flourish undetected until they become severe [41].
- ***Epstein-Barr Virus (EBV):*** EBV can evade the immune system by infecting B-cells and remaining latent for long periods. It can later reactivate and cause coinfections with other pathogens such as HIV or *cytomegalovirus* (CMV), often without immediate symptoms [42].

○ Cytokine Storms and Immune Dysregulation

In some cases, coinfections can trigger excessive immune responses, leading to cytokine storms or severe immune dysregulation.

- ***Cytokine Storms:*** A cytokine storm is an extreme production of pro-inflammatory cytokines through the immune system due to infection. Coinfections, especially with viral and bacterial pathogens (*e.g*., COVID-19 and secondary bacterial infections), can trigger these overwhelming immune responses [43].
- ***Hemophagocytic Lymphohistiocytosis (HLH):*** HLH is a life-threatening condition due to unrestrained immune activation. It can be triggered by infections, including coinfections like EBV and leishmaniasis. The overactive immune system destroys its own cells and tissues, causing organ damage [44].

○ Immune Exhaustion

Chronic infections can lead to immune exhaustion, where the immune system becomes less effective at fighting infections over time, increasing susceptibility to additional infections [45].

- ***Chronic Viral Infections and HIV*:** HIV is a prime example of a chronic infection that causes immune exhaustion. HIV leads to the depletion of immune cells, making it easier for other infections to take hold [46].
- ***Hepatitis B Virus (HBV) and HIV*:** Chronicity of the two infections in coinfected HIV/ HBV patients results in immune exhaustion. This leads to a diminished ability to mount an immune response to new infecting agents and an inability to eliminate the prevailing infection, creating a vicious cycle of increased disease severity [47].

○ Implications for Clinical Management

- ***Early Detection*:** There are fundamental enhancements todiagnostic techniques in an attempt to identify coinfections at the beginning, especially in immunocompromised patients or in regions with a high prevalence of several pathogens [48].
- ***Comprehensive Testing*:** Diagnosing patients with coinfections requires clinicians to complement molecular diagnostics and serology with imaging. This may require multiplex testing, whereby a sample from a patient is tested for a number of pathogens at once [49].

- ***Tailored Treatment*:** Dealing with infections usually necessitates treatment plans that consider possible interactions between medications and the requirement to combat various pathogens [50].

Diagnosis is further confounded by overlapping symptoms, immune subversion by burrowing parasites, and the risk of severe immune dysregulation (*e.g.*, cytokine storms). Further improvements in molecular diagnostics, along with a more holistic approach to human case management, can improve outcomes in the coinfected population Table **1** [51].

Table 1. Vigorous complications in identifying and treating coinfections.

S.No.	Complexity	Diagnosis Challenges	Treatment Challenges
1.	Overlay of Symptoms	Coinfections often cause similar symptoms, making differentiation difficult.	The risk of mistreatment due to misdiagnosis or symptom masking.
2.	Several Pathogens	Need for advanced diagnostics to identify all pathogens involved.	Treatment must be comprehensive, addressing all pathogens simultaneously.
3.	Diagnostic Sensitivity	Standard tests may not detect all infections, especially chronic or low-level infections.	The risk of missing one pathogen, leading to incomplete treatment.
4.	Host Features	Host genetics, immunity, and co-morbidities influence diagnostic accuracy.	Individualized treatments may be necessary, increasing complexity in clinical decision-making.
5.	Pathogen Interaction	Pathogens may enhance each other's virulence, complicating diagnosis.	Interaction between pathogens can increase disease severity, requiring more aggressive treatment.
6.	Coinfection with Resistant Strains	Some pathogens may be resistant to first-line treatments, delaying effective diagnosis.	May require broad-spectrum or combination therapies, increasing toxicity risks.
7.	Treatment Duration	Length of treatment may need adjustment due to the chronic nature of some infections.	Long-term treatment risks include toxicity, side effects, and patient non-compliance.
8.	Coexisting Conditions	Underlying diseases (*e.g.*, HIV, diabetes) complicate the detection and interpretation of results.	Treatments may interact with medications for underlying conditions.
9.	Antimicrobial Resistance	Pathogens may exhibit resistance, especially in coexisting bacterial and viral infections.	Multiple pathogens may require different treatments, increasing the risk of drug interactions and resistance.
10.	Immune System Modulation	Coinfections can alter immune response, making it harder to detect specific pathogens.	Immune-modulating treatments (*e.g.*, steroids) may worsen one infection while treating another.

TREATMENT STRATEGIES

Coinfections present a special challenge, not only because of the varied microbes involved, but also because of the complexities in tailoring antimicrobial pharmacotherapies for individual patients, integrating multisite care, and coordinating multiple drug therapies across different sectors of a healthcare system [52]. Detailed guidelines on how to treat coinfections are provided:

- **Antimicrobial Stewardship**

Antimicrobial stewardship entails selecting the most appropriate antimicrobial therapy to treat infections while minimising the likelihood of inducing antimicrobial resistance. As a result, coinfections complicate optimal patient care.

- ***Challenge of Multi-Pathogen Treatment*:** Often, coinfections are a combination of multiple pathogens with varied sensitivities to antimicrobial agents, necessitating the selection of drugs that are efficacious against both infections, while also posing the threat of promoting drug resistance [53].
- ***Antibiotic Resistance*:** The inappropriate or excessive use of antibiotics might thereby confer selection for the development of drug-resistant strains, especially those involved in coinfections with bacteria. For example, a broad-spectrum antibiotic regimen is recommended for a flu patient witha secondary bacterial pneumonia (such as *Staphylococcus aureus*) [54].
- ***Targeted Therapy:*** Antimicrobial stewardship is crucial, using narrow-spectrum antibiotics whenever possible in order to reduce collateral damage to the microbiome and selection for resistance. This is particularly challenging in those who are coinfected, requiring specific pathogen identification (*e.g.,* through PCR and culture) to guide direct and narrow therapeutic treatments [55].

    - **Drug-Drug Interactions**

Treating coinfections often involves polypharmacy, or the practice of numerous drugs, which increases the likelihood of drug-drug interactions that can affect treatment efficacy or lead to adverse effects.

- ***HIV and Tuberculosis (TB):*** HIV and TB coinfection have become model diseases for the significance of addressing drug-drug interactions. For example, TB treatment often includes the drug Rifampin, which can make many antiretroviral drugs less effective by speeding up their metabolism in the liver.

Consequently, the dosing may be different, and in extreme cases of drug-drug interactions, alternative drugs to rifampicin, such as rifabutin, are prescribed [56].

- ***Antifungals and Antiretrovirals:*** In cases where fungal infections (such as cryptococcal meningitis) occur alongside HIV, it is often necessary to administer antifungal medications (like fluconazole) in addition to antiretroviral therapy (ART). However, it is important to note that antifungal drugs can have interactions with antiretroviral medications, which may result in heightened toxicity or decreased levels of the drugs in the body. This can make the treatment process more complex [57, 58].

○ Tailoring Treatment to the Individual

Effective treatment of coinfections must be personalized, taking into account the patient's immune status, comorbidities, and potential for drug resistance.

- ***Immune Status:*** In immunocompromised patients (*e.g.*, those with HIV or undergoing chemotherapy), certain infections like pneumocystis pneumonia (PCP) or cytomegalovirus (CMV) may require aggressive treatment and preventive measures. Immunocompromised patients may also have difficulty tolerating certain drugs, so treatment plans need to be modified accordingly [59].
- ***Comorbidities:*** In patients with weakened immune systems (such as those with HIV or undergoing chemotherapy), specific infections like pneumocystis pneumonia (PCP) or cytomegalovirus (CMV) may need intensive treatment and preventive actions. These patients may also have difficulty tolerating certain medications, so treatment plans must be modified as needed [60].
- ***Drug Resistance:*** This is especially important in areas where antimicrobial resistance is common, such as multidrug-resistant TB or drug-resistant malaria. Diagnostic tests for drug resistance, like genotypic testing for HIV or TB, are crucial for choosing effective treatments [61].

○ Innovative Approaches

Emerging therapies offer new strategies for managing coinfections, especially in cases where conventional antimicrobials may not be effective or are associated with significant side effects.

- ***Host-Directed Therapies (HDTs):*** Rather than directly targeting the pathogen, HDTs aim to improve the host's immune response to infections. HDTs can be particularly beneficial in coinfections where the immune system is compromised, such as in HIV or cancer patients [62].

- ***Immunomodulatory Drugs:*** These drugs can be useful in treating coinfections where immune dysregulation is a concern, such as in COVID-19 and secondary bacterial infections [63].
- ***Phage Therapy:*** Bacteriophages (viruses that contaminate bacteria) are being explored as alternatives to antibiotics, particularly in treating drug-resistant bacterial infections. Phage therapy can be an effective approach in coinfections where bacterial pathogens have developed resistance to traditional antibiotics, such as MRSA coinfections in influenza or COVID-19 patients [64].
- ***Phage Therapy for Sepsis:*** In cases of sepsis caused by multidrug-resistant bacteria, phage therapy can be used to specifically target the bacterial pathogen without affecting the normal microbiome [65].
- ***Probiotics:*** The use of probiotics (beneficial bacteria) has shown promise in restoring the gut microbiome, which can be disrupted by antibiotics or infections. Probiotics may help prevent secondary infections, especially in patients receiving prolonged antibiotic therapy for coinfections [66].
- ***Combination Therapies:*** Combining dissimilar types of therapies (*e.g.,* antibiotics with HDTs or phage therapy) can offer synergistic benefits in treating coinfections. Combination therapies are particularly important in cases where pathogens interact to enhance each other's virulence or resistance [67].

CASE STUDIES

- **HIV and Tuberculosis:** The immunosuppressive effects of HIV increase susceptibility to TB, particularly in regions where TB is endemic. TB is the main cause of death among people living with HIV due to the way these infections interact [68].
- **COVID-19 and Secondary Bacterial Infections:** During the COVID-19 pandemic, secondary bacterial infections significantly worsened the prognosis of patients, especially those with severe viral infections [69].
- **Malaria and Helminth Infections:** Malaria and helminth (parasitic worm) coinfections are common in many tropical and subtropical regions. These coinfections can alter immune responses and complicate treatment, leading to unique challenges in endemic areas [70].

FUTURE DIRECTIONS

- **Research Needs:** Identifying gaps in our understanding of coinfection biology and pathogenesis, particularly in the context of emerging pathogens, is crucial. More research is needed to fully understand how different pathogens interact within the host. For example, in HIV and TB coinfections, while much is known about how HIV weakens the immune system, the precise molecular mechanisms that allow TB to exploit this weakness remain unclear. Understanding these interactions at a deeper level can lead to better treatment options [71].

- **Diagnostic Advances:** This technology can be especially useful in identifying coinfections with rare or difficult-to-culture organisms [72].
- **Personalized Medicine:** Future treatment strategies may involve using algorithms that account for a patient's immune status, microbiome composition, genetic factors, and the types of coinfecting pathogens present. These personalized regimens can minimize drug interactions and resistance, while maximizing therapeutic outcomes [73].
- **Global Health Implications:** Global health policies should prioritize coinfection research and funding, especially in endemic regions. Educational programs for healthcare providers are also essential, ensuring that clinicians can recognize and effectively manage coinfections [74].

CONCLUSION

Coinfections pose a complex challenge that demands comprehensive strategies for both diagnosis and treatment. As research into the interactions between pathogens and the host progresses, our approach to managing these cases must also evolve. Effective coinfection management will increasingly depend on integrating advanced diagnostic technologies, such as next-generation sequencing and multiplex assays, which can identify multiple pathogens simultaneously. Personalized treatment plans, tailored to each patient's specific immune status and infection profile, will become crucial in improving patient outcomes. By focusing on these areas, this chapter can enhance patient care and alleviate the global burden of coinfections, particularly in regions where such diseases are endemic.

ACKNOWLEDGEMENT

The authors express their gratitude to the ITS College of Pharmacy and Meerut Institute of Technology for their assistance throughout the study.

REFERENCES

[1] Ali S, Ur-Rehman T, Lougher E, Mutimer D, Ali M, Paudyal V. Impact of HIV and chronic kidney disease comorbidities on hepatitis C treatment choices, drug-drug interactions and hepatitis C cure. Int J Clin Pharm 2020; 42: 515-26.

[2] Singer M. Pathogen-pathogen interaction. Virulence 2010; 1(1): 10-8. [http://dx.doi.org/10.4161/viru.1.1.9933] [PMID: 21178409]

[3] Aghbash PS, Eslami N, Shirvaliloo M, Baghi HB. Viral coinfections in COVID-19. J Med Virol 2021; 93(9): 5310-22. [http://dx.doi.org/10.1002/jmv.27102] [PMID: 34032294]

[4] Manohar P, Loh B, Nachimuthu R, Hua X, Welburn SC, Leptihn S. Secondary Bacterial Infections in Patients With Viral Pneumonia. Front Med (Lausanne) 2020; 7: 420. [http://dx.doi.org/10.3389/fmed.2020.00420] [PMID: 32850912]

[5] Fuster D, Sanvisens A, Bolao F, Rivas I, Tor J, Muga R. Alcohol use disorder and its impact on chronic hepatitis C virus and human immunodeficiency virus infections. World J Hepatol 2016; 8:

1295-308.

[6] Mancuso G, Midiri A, Gerace E, Biondo C. Bacterial Antibiotic Resistance: The Most Critical Pathogens. Pathogens 2021; 10(10): 1310. [http://dx.doi.org/10.3390/pathogens10101310] [PMID: 34684258]

[7] Jal S, Chhotaray S, Pattnaik G, *et al.* Dengue fever coinfection in COVID-19 era: A public health concern. Health Sci Rep 2024; 7(5): e2089. [http://dx.doi.org/10.1002/hsr2.2089] [PMID: 38784250]

[8] Osakunor DNM, Sengeh DM, Mutapi F. Coinfections and comorbidities in African health systems: At the interface of infectious and noninfectious diseases. PLoS Negl Trop Dis 2018; 12(9): e0006711. [http://dx.doi.org/10.1371/journal.pntd.0006711] [PMID: 30235205]

[9] McArdle AJ, Turkova A, Cunnington AJ. When do co-infections matter? Curr Opin Infect Dis 2018; 31(3): 209-15. [http://dx.doi.org/10.1097/QCO.0000000000000447] [PMID: 29698255]

[10] Kc R, Adhikari S, Bastola A, *et al.* Opportunistic Respiratory Infections in HIV Patients Attending Sukraraj Tropical and Infectious Diseases Hospital in Kathmandu, Nepal. HIV AIDS (Auckl) 2019; 11: 357-67. [http://dx.doi.org/10.2147/HIV.S229531] [PMID: 31920403]

[11] Tay S, Badu K, Mensah AA, Gbedema SY. The prevalence of malaria among HIV seropositive individuals and the impact of the co- infection on their hemoglobin levels. Ann Clin Microbiol Antimicrob 2015; 14(1): 10. [http://dx.doi.org/10.1186/s12941-015-0064-6] [PMID: 25857950]

[12] Afkhami S, Lai R, D'agostino MR, Vaseghi-Shanjani M, Zganiacz A, Yao Y, Jeyanathan M, Xing Z. Single-dose mucosal immunotherapy with chimpanzee adenovirus-based vaccine accelerates tuberculosis disease control and limits its rebound after antibiotic cessation. J Infect Dis. 2019; 220: 1355-1366.

[13] Berger O, Gan X, Gujuluva C, Burns AR, Sulur G, Stins M, *et al.* CXC and CC chemokine receptors on coronary and brain endothelia. Mol Med. 1999; 5: 795–805.

[14] Allen JE, Maizels RM.Diversity and dialogue in immunity to helminths. Nat. Rev. Immunol 2011; 11:375–388.

[15] Losier A, Gupta G, Caldararo M, Dela Cruz CS. The Impact of Coronavirus Disease 2019 on Viral, Bacterial, and Fungal Respiratory Infections. Clin Chest Med 2023; 44(2): 407-23. [http://dx.doi.org/10.1016/j.ccm.2022.11.018] [PMID: 37085229]

[16] Baeten J, Chohan B, Lavreys L, Chohan V, McClelland R, Certain L, *et al.* HIV-1 subtype D infection is associated with faster disease progression than subtype A in spite of similar plasma HIV-1 loads. J Infect Dis. 2007; 195: 1177–1180.

[17] Mohsen S, Dickinson JA, Somayaji R. Update on the adverse effects of antimicrobial therapies in community practice. Can Fam Physician 2020; 66(9): 651-9. [PMID: 32933978]

[18] Assah F, Mbanya JC, Dagogo-Jack S. Diabetes mellitus in developing countries and underserved communities. Adv Exp Med Biol. 2017; 498.

[19] Abdullah AS, Moffat CS, Lopez-Ruiz FJ, Gibberd MR, Hamblin J, Zerihun A. Host–Multi-Pathogen Warfare: Pathogen Interactions in Co-infected Plants. Front Plant Sci 2017; 8: 1806. [http://dx.doi.org/10.3389/fpls.2017.01806] [PMID: 29118773]

[20] Balloux F, van Dorp L. Q&A: What are pathogens, and what have they done to and for us? BMC Biol 2017; 15(1): 91. [http://dx.doi.org/10.1186/s12915-017-0433-z] [PMID: 29052511]

[21] Prasso JE, Deng JC. Postviral Complications. Clin Chest Med 2017; 38(1): 127-38.

[http://dx.doi.org/10.1016/j.ccm.2016.11.006] [PMID: 28159155]

[22] Abdoli A, Falahi S, Kenarkoohi A. COVID-19-associated opportunistic infections: a snapshot on the current reports. Clin Exp Med 2021; 22(3): 327-46.
[http://dx.doi.org/10.1007/s10238-021-00751-7] [PMID: 34424451]

[23] Beceiro A, Tomás M, Bou G. Antimicrobial resistance and virulence: a successful or deleterious association in the bacterial world? Clin Microbiol Rev 2013; 26(2): 185-230.
[http://dx.doi.org/10.1128/CMR.00059-12] [PMID: 23554414]

[24] Bruchfeld J, Correia-Neves M, Källenius G. Tuberculosis and HIV Coinfection. Cold Spring Harb Perspect Med 2015; 5(7): a017871.
[http://dx.doi.org/10.1101/cshperspect.a017871] [PMID: 25722472]

[25] Hochman S, Kim K. The Impact of HIV Coinfection on Cerebral Malaria Pathogenesis. J Neuroparasitology 2012; 3: 1-18.
[http://dx.doi.org/10.4303/jnp/235547] [PMID: 22545215]

[26] Chen JY, Feeney ER, Chung RT. HCV and HIV co-infection: mechanisms and management. Nat Rev Gastroenterol Hepatol 2014; 11(6): 362-71.
[http://dx.doi.org/10.1038/nrgastro.2014.17] [PMID: 24535328]

[27] Acosta IC, Alonzo F III. The Intersection between Bacterial Metabolism and Innate Immunity. J Innate Immun 2023; 15(1): 782-803.
[http://dx.doi.org/10.1159/000534872] [PMID: 37899025]

[28] McSorley HJ, Maizels RM. Helminth infections and host immune regulation. Clin Microbiol Rev 2012; 25(4): 585-608.
[http://dx.doi.org/10.1128/CMR.05040-11] [PMID: 23034321]

[29] Yu Q, Ding X, Wang W, Lou Y. Pneumocystis jiroveci pneumonia with cytomegalovirus infection diagnosed by metagenomic next-generation sequencing in a patient with nephrotic syndrome. Medicine (Baltimore) 2021; 100(31): e26842.
[http://dx.doi.org/10.1097/MD.0000000000026842] [PMID: 34397856]

[30] Hébert-Dufresne L, Althouse BM. Complex dynamics of synergistic coinfections on realistically clustered networks. Proc Natl Acad Sci USA 2015; 112(33): 10551-6.
[http://dx.doi.org/10.1073/pnas.1507820112] [PMID: 26195773]

[31] Jia L, Zhao J, Yang C, *et al.* Severe pneumonia caused by coinfection with influenza virus followed by methicillin-resistant *Staphylococcus aureus* induces higher mortality in mice. Front Immunol 2019; 9: 3189.
[http://dx.doi.org/10.3389/fimmu.2018.03189] [PMID: 30761162]

[32] Bongiovanni M, Barda B. *Pseudomonas aeruginosa* Bloodstream Infections in SARS-CoV-2 Infected Patients: A Systematic Review. J Clin Med 2023; 12(6): 2252.
[http://dx.doi.org/10.3390/jcm12062252] [PMID: 36983256]

[33] Wu H, Zhou HY, Zheng H, Wu A. Towards Understanding and Identification of Human Viral Co-Infections. Viruses 2024; 16(5): 673.
[http://dx.doi.org/10.3390/v16050673] [PMID: 38793555]

[34] Bai Y, Tao X. Comparison of COVID-19 and influenza characteristics. J Zhejiang Univ Sci B 2021; 22(2): 87-98.
[http://dx.doi.org/10.1631/jzus.B2000479] [PMID: 33615750]

[35] Huang L, Crothers K. HIV-associated opportunistic pneumonias. Respirology 2009; 14(4): 474-85.
[http://dx.doi.org/10.1111/j.1440-1843.2009.01534.x] [PMID: 19645867]

[36] Yang S, Rothman RE. PCR-based diagnostics for infectious diseases: uses, limitations, and future applications in acute-care settings. Lancet Infect Dis 2004; 4(6): 337-48.
[http://dx.doi.org/10.1016/S1473-3099(04)01044-8] [PMID: 15172342]

[37] Vainionpaa R, Leinikki P. . Diagnostic techniques: Serological and molecular approaches. Encyclopedia of virology 2008; 29-37.

[38] Beigelman-Aubry C, Schmidt S. Pulmonary Infections: Imaging with CT. Med Radiol (Berl) 2016; 27: 131-61.
[http://dx.doi.org/10.1007/978-3-319-30355-0_8]

[39] Bhatt A, Quazi Syed Z, Singh H. Converging Epidemics: A Narrative Review of Tuberculosis (TB) and Human Immunodeficiency Virus (HIV) Coinfection. Cureus 2023; 15(10): e47624.
[http://dx.doi.org/10.7759/cureus.47624] [PMID: 38021882]

[40] Prasad N, Patel MR. Infection-Induced Kidney Diseases. Front Med (Lausanne) 2018; 5: 327.
[http://dx.doi.org/10.3389/fmed.2018.00327] [PMID: 30555828]

[41] Vidya Vijayan KK, Karthigeyan KP, Tripathi SP, Hanna LE. Pathophysiology of CD4+ T-Cell Depletion in HIV-1 and HIV-2 Infections. Front Immunol 2017; 8: 580.
[http://dx.doi.org/10.3389/fimmu.2017.00580] [PMID: 28588579]

[42] de Melo Silva J, Pinheiro-Silva R, Dhyani A, Pontes GS. Cytomegalovirus and Epstein-Barr Infections: Prevalence and Impact on Patients with Hematological Diseases. BioMed Res Int 2020; 2020(1): 1627824.
[http://dx.doi.org/10.1155/2020/1627824] [PMID: 33163531]

[43] Costa Silva RCM, Bandeira-Melo C, Paula Neto HA, Vale AM, Travassos LH. COVID-19 diverse outcomes: Aggravated reinfection, type I interferons and antibodies. Med Hypotheses2022; 167: 110943.

[44] Koumadoraki E, Madouros N, Sharif S, Saleem A, Jarvis S, Khan S. Hemophagocytic Lymphohistiocytosis and Infection: A Literature Review. Cureus 2022; 14(2): e22411.
[http://dx.doi.org/10.7759/cureus.22411] [PMID: 35345677]

[45] Segerstrom SC, Miller GE. Psychological stress and the human immune system: a meta-analytic study of 30 years of inquiry. Psychol Bull 2004; 130(4): 601-30.
[http://dx.doi.org/10.1037/0033-2909.130.4.601] [PMID: 15250815]

[46] Paiardini M, Müller-Trutwin M. HIV -associated chronic immune activation. Immunol Rev 2013; 254(1): 78-101.
[http://dx.doi.org/10.1111/imr.12079] [PMID: 23772616]

[47] Cheng Z, Lin P, Cheng N. HBV/HIV coinfection: Impact on the development and clinical treatment of liver diseases. Front Med (Lausanne) 2021; 8: 713981.
[http://dx.doi.org/10.3389/fmed.2021.713981] [PMID: 34676223]

[48] Arvanitis M, Anagnostou T, Fuchs BB, Caliendo AM, Mylonakis E. Molecular and nonmolecular diagnostic methods for invasive fungal infections. Clin Microbiol Rev 2014; 27(3): 490-526.
[http://dx.doi.org/10.1128/CMR.00091-13] [PMID: 24982319]

[49] Hanson KE, Couturier MR. Multiplexed molecular diagnostics for respiratory, gastrointestinal, and central nervous system infections. Clin Infect Dis 2016; 63(10): 1361-7.
[http://dx.doi.org/10.1093/cid/ciw494] [PMID: 27444411]

[50] Birger RB, Kouyos RD, Cohen T, *et al.* The potential impact of coinfection on antimicrobial chemotherapy and drug resistance. Trends Microbiol 2015; 23(9): 537-44.
[http://dx.doi.org/10.1016/j.tim.2015.05.002] [PMID: 26028590]

[51] Yong YK, Wong WF, Vignesh R, *et al.* Dengue Infection - Recent Advances in Disease Pathogenesis in the Era of COVID-19. Front Immunol 2022; 13: 889196.
[http://dx.doi.org/10.3389/fimmu.2022.889196] [PMID: 35874775]

[52] Navasardyan I, Miwalian R, Petrosyan A, Yeganyan S, Venketaraman V. HIV–TB Coinfection: Current Therapeutic Approaches and Drug Interactions. Viruses 2024; 16(3): 321.
[http://dx.doi.org/10.3390/v16030321] [PMID: 38543687]

[53] Nikjeh O, Rejali S, Sasaninia K, Venketaraman V. Overcoming Treatment Challenges in HIV-Associated Mycobacterial Diseases: New Therapeutic Frontiers. Int J Mol Sci. 2025; 26: 10325.

[54] Llor C, Bjerrum L. Antimicrobial resistance: risk associated with antibiotic overuse and initiatives to reduce the problem. Ther Adv Drug Saf 2014; 5(6): 229-41.
[http://dx.doi.org/10.1177/2042098614554919] [PMID: 25436105]

[55] Khadse SN, Ugemuge S, Singh C. Impact of antimicrobial stewardship on reducing antimicrobial resistance. Cureus 2023; 15(12): e49935.
[http://dx.doi.org/10.7759/cureus.49935] [PMID: 38179391]

[56] Navasardyan I, Miwalian R, Petrosyan A, Yeganyan S, Venketaraman V. HIV–TB Coinfection: Current Therapeutic Approaches and Drug Interactions. Viruses 2024; 16(3): 321.
[http://dx.doi.org/10.3390/v16030321] [PMID: 38543687]

[57] Hurt WJ, Harrison TS, Molloy SF, Bicanic TA. Combination Therapy for HIV-Associated Cryptococcal Meningitis—A Success Story. J Fungi (Basel) 2021; 7(12): 1098.
[http://dx.doi.org/10.3390/jof7121098] [PMID: 34947080]

[58] Rice DP Jr, Faragon JJ, Banks S, Chirch LM. HIV/HCV antiviral drug interactions in the era of direct-acting antivirals. J Clin Transl Hepatol 2016; 4(3): 234-40.
[http://dx.doi.org/10.14218/JCTH.2016.00026] [PMID: 27777891]

[59] Dropulic LK, Lederman HM. Overview of Infections in the Immunocompromised Host. Microbiol Spectr 2016; 4(4): 4.4.43.
[http://dx.doi.org/10.1128/microbiolspec.DMIH2-0026-2016] [PMID: 27726779]

[60] Betônico CCR, Titan SMO, Correa-Giannella MLC, Nery M, Queiroz M. Management of diabetes mellitus in individuals with chronic kidney disease: therapeutic perspectives and glycemic control. Clinics (São Paulo) 2016; 71(1): 47-53.
[http://dx.doi.org/10.6061/clinics/2016(01)08] [PMID: 26872083]

[61] Seung KJ, Keshavjee S, Rich ML. Multidrug-resistant tuberculosis and extensively drug-resistant tuberculosis. Cold Spring Harb Perspect Med 2015; 5(9): a017863.
[http://dx.doi.org/10.1101/cshperspect.a017863] [PMID: 25918181]

[62] Hawn TR, Matheson AI, Maley SN, Vandal O. Host-directed therapeutics for tuberculosis: can we harness the host? Microbiol Mol Biol Rev 2013; 77(4): 608-27.
[http://dx.doi.org/10.1128/MMBR.00032-13] [PMID: 24296574]

[63] Fajgenbaum DC, June CH. Cytokine Storm. N Engl J Med 2020; 383(23): 2255-73.
[http://dx.doi.org/10.1056/NEJMra2026131] [PMID: 33264547]

[64] Lin DM, Koskella B, Lin HC. Phage therapy: An alternative to antibiotics in the age of multi-drug resistance. World J Gastrointest Pharmacol Ther 2017; 8(3): 162-73.
[http://dx.doi.org/10.4292/wjgpt.v8.i3.162] [PMID: 28828194]

[65] Aranaga C, Pantoja LD, Martínez EA, Falco A. Phage therapy in the era of multidrug resistance in bacteria: A systematic review. Int J Mol Sci 2022; 23(9): 4577.
[http://dx.doi.org/10.3390/ijms23094577] [PMID: 35562968]

[66] Hemarajata P, Versalovic J. Effects of probiotics on gut microbiota: mechanisms of intestinal immunomodulation and neuromodulation. Therap Adv Gastroenterol 2013; 6(1): 39-51.
[http://dx.doi.org/10.1177/1756283X12459294] [PMID: 23320049]

[67] Diallo K, Dublanchet A. Benefits of combined phage–antibiotic therapy for the control of antibiotic-resistant bacteria: A literature review. Antibiotics (Basel) 2022; 11(7): 839.
[http://dx.doi.org/10.3390/antibiotics11070839] [PMID: 35884092]

[68] Hamada Y, Getahun H, Tadesse BT, Ford N. HIV-associated tuberculosis. Int J STD AIDS 2021; 32(9): 780-90.
[http://dx.doi.org/10.1177/0956462421992257] [PMID: 33612015]

[69] Fazel P, Sedighian H, Behzadi E, Kachuei R, Imani Fooladi AA. Interaction Between SARS-CoV-2 and Pathogenic Bacteria. Curr Microbiol 2023; 80(7): 223.
[http://dx.doi.org/10.1007/s00284-023-03315-y] [PMID: 37222840]

[70] Hotez PJ, Brindley PJ, Bethony JM, King CH, Pearce EJ, Jacobson J. Helminth infections: the great neglected tropical diseases. J Clin Invest 2008; 118(4): 1311-21.
[http://dx.doi.org/10.1172/JCI34261] [PMID: 18382743]

[71] Devi P, Khan A, Chattopadhyay P, *et al.* Co-infections as modulators of disease outcome: Minor players or major players? Front Microbiol 2021; 12: 664386.
[http://dx.doi.org/10.3389/fmicb.2021.664386] [PMID: 34295314]

[72] Nafea AM, Wang Y, Wang D, *et al.* Application of next-generation sequencing to identify different pathogens. Front Microbiol 2024; 14: 1329330.
[http://dx.doi.org/10.3389/fmicb.2023.1329330] [PMID: 38348304]

[73] Goetz LH, Schork NJ. Personalized medicine: motivation, challenges, and progress. Fertil Steril 2018; 109(6): 952-63.
[http://dx.doi.org/10.1016/j.fertnstert.2018.05.006] [PMID: 29935653]

[74] Obeagu EI, Obeagu GU, Ubosi NI, Uzoma IC, Tayrab EMA. Concurrent management of HIV and malaria: A comprehensive review of strategies to enhance quality of life. Medicine (Baltimore) 2024; 103(14): e37649.
[http://dx.doi.org/10.1097/MD.0000000000037649] [PMID: 38579091]

CHAPTER 8

Novel Drug Delivery Systems to Combat Antimicrobial Resistance

Sanjay Kumar Gupta[1,*], Astha Verma[2], Akash Gupta[1], Sumit Sahu[1], Nousheen Khatoon[1], Anjila Firdous[1] and Mohammad Adnan Raza[1]

[1] *Department of Pharmacology, Rungta College of Pharmaceutical Sciences and Research, Chhattisgarh– 490024, India*

[2] *Department of Pharmaceutics, Shri Rawatpura Sarkar Institute of Pharmacy, Chhattisgarh, – 490024, India*

Abstract: Antimicrobial resistance (AMR) poses a major threat to global health, as infections remain a leading cause of death worldwide. With few new antibiotics being developed, researchers are turning to innovative delivery methods for existing drugs to combat AMR. The novel carriers contribute several advantages over conventional antibiotic administration methods, including enhanced solubility, improved stability, increased permeability through cellular barriers and into bacterial biofilms, higher bioavailability, extended drug half-life, targeted delivery to specific tissues, and even the ability to bypass bacterial efflux pumps that contribute to resistance. Novel carriers such as liposomes, polymeric nanoparticles (PNPs), nanoemulsions, dendrimers, carbon nanotubes, and metal nanoparticles have emerged as promising solutions, offering the potential to create sophisticated drug delivery systems in the form of antibiotic-carrying nanoparticles. Other promising approaches, including the development of stimuli-responsive drug delivery systems, combination therapies within a single delivery system, advanced surface modification techniques, and biological delivery vehicles like bacteriophages and extracellular vesicles, are being engineered to deliver antibiotics directly to specific bacterial species. Additionally, 3D-printed drug delivery devices, smart hydrogels, and implantable devices are also being developed to treat biofilm-associated infections. While many are still in developmental stages, these novel approaches offer significant potential to revitalize existing antibiotics, overcome resistance mechanisms, and provide more effective treatments for bacterial infections in the face of growing AMR.

Keywords: 3D printed drug delivery, Antimicrobial resistance, Multidrug-resistant, Novel carriers, Resistance mechanisms, Smart hydrogels.

* **Corresponding author Sanjay Kumar Gupta:** Department of Pharmacology, Rungta College of Pharmaceutical Sciences and Research, Chhattisgarh– 490024, India; E-mail: sanjay.gupta0311@gmail.com

Mukesh Kumar Singh, Gurdeep Singh, Amrendra Pratap Yadav & Papiya Bigoniya (Eds.)

INTRODUCTION

Overview of Antimicrobial Resistance (AMR)

Increased mortality and long-standing infections related to antimicrobial resistance have become a global health crisis by killing the effectiveness of conventional antibiotics. In this regard, the challenge posed by AMR needs some innovative solutions. Some new drug delivery systems have been developed, which hold promise for antimicrobial drugs. The present paper focuses on recent developments in the field of novel drug delivery systems (NDDSs) to improve the delivery and efficacy of antimicrobial agents [1]. The current review has discussed several approaches that include nanotechnology-based carriers, liposomes, polymeric nanoparticles (PNPs), and dendrimers. Some of these particles are considered very promising in infectious disease treatment due to their ability to cross biological barriers and target the pathogen with minimized mechanisms of drug resistance [2]. The critical areas addressed in this respect include enhancement of drug solubility, stability, and bioavailability, as well as controlled release and targeted delivery to infection sites. The strategies have also been elaborated in detail relating to the combination of NDDS with antimicrobial peptides and smart systems responsive to environmental stimuli [3]. Considering the synergistic potential in conjunction with current antimicrobial therapy, which may mitigate AMR, NDDS has the potential to transform the future treatment landscape of infectious diseases. Accordingly, future research directions and clinical translation of these technologies are critically examined to address the multifaceted challenges posed by AMR [4].

Antibiotics, also called "*antimicrobial agents*", are chemical substances made by a microorganism that kill or slow the growth of another microorganism. The development of resistant microorganisms and their resistance mechanisms, since the discovery of antimicrobial drugs in 1937, has given rise to the idea of AMR [5]. Another characteristic of infection-causing bacteria that contributes to the explanation of AMR is their resistance to the effects of antimicrobial drugs, which either stop their growth or eliminate them. There are additional aspects to this ailment as well, like substantial medical costs, frequent examinations, and subsequent visits. Due to the innate capacity of resistant bacteria to survive, mutate, and adapt to resistance to stress and increased exposure to antimicrobial chemicals, antibiotic-resistant bacteria are an inevitable part of the evolutionary process [6]. In 2001, the World Health Organization (WHO) established the Global Strategy for Containment of AMR and defined the appropriate use of antimicrobials as "cost-effective use of antimicrobials which maximizes clinical therapeutic effect while minimizing drug-related toxicity and the development of antimicrobial resistance" [7]. Antibiotic-resistant bacteria and ARGs can be found in the environment, which can also act as an incubator for resistance. Consequently, it is the predominant means of dispersing resistant bacteria associated with fecal matter in water, sewage systems, and organic fertilizers(8).

AMR refers to the ability of microorganisms, which include bacteria, viruses, fungi, and parasites, to resist the therapeutic effects of medications that were previously effective in fighting them. This phenomenon reduces the effectiveness of drugs such as antibiotics and antivirals, which raises morbidity, mortality, and healthcare costs [9]. Combating AMR has become a critical global health priority that demands immediate and coordinated action from legislators, medical professionals, academics, and the general public. When bacteria, viruses, fungi, and parasites resist antimicrobial drugs, traditional treatments become ineffective, and the risk of infection rises. Although AMR is a naturally occurring phenomenon, in recent decades, human influences have greatly accelerated and aggravated its advancement [10].

Current Challenges in Treating Resistant Infections

Antibiotic resistance in multidrug-resistant (MDR) pathogens, such as Methicillin-Resistant *Staphylococcus aureus* (MRSA), *Vancomycin-resistant Enterococci* (VRE), and Carbapenem-resistant Enterobacteriaceae (CRE), has reduced treatment choices and raised death rates. The creation of biofilms increases treatment complexity by conferring up to 1,000-fold resistance on microorganisms. Additionally, bacteria lessen the efficiency of antibiotics by using β-lactamases and efflux pumps [11]. The paucity of novel antibiotics and inadequate medication penetration into hard-to-reach regions hampers the treatment of resistant diseases. Inadequate dosage and prolonged antibiotic exposure also contribute to the development of resistance during therapy, favouring resistant bacteria [12].

Limitations of Current Systems

Such limitations add to the more general difficulties in managing resistant infections, such as the rise of microorganisms that are MDR, the development of biofilms that impede therapy, and a notable decrease in the discovery of novel medicines. These elements work together to highlight the critical need for creative solutions, such as new drug delivery methods, to increase the effectiveness of antibiotics, target resistant bacteria, and boost treatment results [13].

- **Non-specific drug distribution:** Medications used in conjunction with conventional antibiotic therapy are distributed non-specifically throughout the body, which may have negative consequences and cause systemic toxicity, including disturbance of the gut microbiota [14].
- Sub-therapeutic dosing: Sub-therapeutic exposure promotes the development of resistance, as current medication delivery methods often fall short of sustaining the best possible drug concentrations at infection sites over time [15].
- Insufficient biofilm penetration: In general, biofilm matrices shield bacteria from exposure to high drug concentrations, making conventional antibiotics ineffective in breaking through them and leading to chronic infections [16].
- Fast drug degradation: Bacterial enzymes, such as *β-lactamases*, rapidly break down antibiotics, drastically shortening their effective half-lives and requiring larger dosages that raise the possibility of adverse effects [17].
- Poor solubility and chemical stability: Many antibiotics, especially those that are hydrophobic, have poor solubility and chemical stability, which makes it difficult for them to reach therapeutic concentrations at the site of infection [18].
- Lack of targeting: Current medication delivery strategies are unable to successfully target certain bacterial cells or tissues, which increases the risk of side effects to beneficial microbial populations and renders the therapy ineffective [12].
- Treatment difficulties for chronic infections: Due to their low penetration, which leaves them with persistent and difficult-to-eradicate infections, antibiotics are especially difficult to treat for chronic and intracellular infections [19].

Importance of NDDS

An increasing worldwide health concern, AMR jeopardizes the effectiveness of existing medications and raises morbidity and death rates. The use of NDDS has become a critical tactic in overcoming the drawbacks of traditional therapy, increasing the efficacy of antimicrobial medicines, and delaying the onset of resistance [20]. The importance of NDDS in battling AMR (Table **1**) is the main focus of this chapter, which also emphasizes how it may improve treatment results, lower resistance mechanisms, and increase medication targeting [21].

Table 1. Significance of NDDS in the management and prevention of AMR.

Characteristic	Description	Importance of AMR	Reference
Enhanced Drug Targeting	Antibiotics are better delivered to infection sites using NDDS, increasing drug availability at the site of action.	Minimizes adverse effects, improves effectiveness, and lowers systemic exposure.	[30, 31]

(Table 1) cont.....

Characteristic	Description	Importance of AMR	Reference
Improved Bioavailability	Poorly soluble antibiotics are made more soluble and stable using liposomes, NPs, and other carriers.	High drug concentrations at the site of infection enhance the effectiveness of treatment, particularly for hydrophobic drugs.	[32]
Reduced Systemic Toxicity	NDDS reduces the amount of antibiotics that reach healthy tissues.	Reduces the need for higher doses, lowers the risk of toxicity and side effects.	[22]
Preservation of Microbiota	Targeted delivery minimizes exposure to non-target regions, such as the gut microbiome, and helps maintain useful microorganisms.	Maintains the general microbial balance by assisting in the prevention of commensal bacteria from developing resistance.	[33]
Efflux Pump Evasion	By avoiding bacterial efflux pumps, nanocarriers help raise medication concentrations within cells.	Increases the effectiveness of antibiotics by overcoming one of the main resistance mechanisms.	[34]
Biofilm Penetration	The distribution of drugs to bacteria encased in biofilms, which are often resistant to therapy, is improved by NDDS.	Enhances the management of biofilm-associated infections, including infections brought on by catheter use and persistent wounds.	[26]
Enzyme Protection	Antibiotics are shielded by NDDS from being broken down by bacterial enzymes, such as β-lactamases.	Makes antibiotics more durable and potent, increasing their ability to combat resistant bacteria.	[17]
Controlled and Sustained Release	With the use of NDDS, therapeutic medication levels may be maintained throughout time with delayed and sustained drug release.	Prevents sub-therapeutic amounts from occurring, which lowers the likelihood that resistance will develop.	[3]
Co-Delivery of Therapeutics	Adjuvants (such as immune modulators and resistance inhibitors) and antibiotics may be administered together thanks to NDDS.	Targets many resistance routes and strategies to improve therapy.	[35]
Combination Therapy	NDDS makes it possible to target MDR illnesses by delivering numerous antibiotics or antibiotic combinations together with adjuvants.	Enhances the effectiveness of therapy by preventing the development of resistance by targeting germs from many directions.	[28]
Prevention of Resistance Development	The amount of time that bacteria may be exposed to therapeutic doses of antibiotics reduces their ability to mutate.	Reduces the development of resistant bacterial strains.	[36]

- ***Enhanced Drug Targeting and Bioavailability:*** Delivering effective medication concentrations to infection sites is a significant difficulty in antimicrobial treatment. NPs and liposomes are examples of NDDS that improve bioavailability and allow for tailored distribution [22]. By using passive (like improved permeability) or active (like ligand-receptor interactions) techniques to enable site-specific targeting, they may ensure higher medication concentrations at the infection site while lowering systemic exposure. Moreover, NDDS increases the stability and solubility of poorly soluble antibiotics, particularly those that are hydrophobic, thereby boosting their therapeutic effectiveness [23].

- ***Reduction of Systemic Toxicity and Side Effects:*** The non-specific distribution of conventional antibiotics often results in adverse effects. By directing medicines towards the infection site and minimising their exposure to healthy tissues, NDDS lessens toxicity. This makes it possible to use smaller dosages, which reduce side effects and protect the microbiota by limiting the exposure of antibiotics to non-target areas, a crucial step in halting the development of resistance in beneficial bacteria [24].
- ***Overcoming Bacterial Resistance Mechanisms:*** To avoid antibiotics, bacteria develop resistance mechanisms such as biofilm development, efflux pumps, and enzyme degradation. With the provision of other drug delivery channels, NDDS assists in overcoming these obstacles. Drug accumulation within resistant bacteria is increased *via* efflux pump evasion using nanocarriers [25]. By directly administering high antibiotic concentrations to the microorganisms inside biofilms, NDDS also improves biofilm penetration. It also provides enzyme protection, preventing the breakdown of antibiotics (by β-lactamases, for example) and preserving their effectiveness [26].
- ***Sustained and Controlled Release***: The secret to avoiding resistance is to keep therapeutic medication levels constant. Antibiotics are released gradually and under control with the help of NDDS, maintaining long-term optimum concentrations. By exposing bacteria to effective medication concentrations over time, this protracted drug release lowers the risk of resistant mutations and avoids sub-therapeutic levels that may foster resistance [3].
- ***Combination Therapy and Co-Delivery:*** NDDS makes it possible to co-deliver antibiotics with adjuvants, immune modulators, or resistance inhibitors to increase the effectiveness of the antibiotic. This makes it possible to combine antibiotics with β-lactamase inhibitors or efflux pumps to overcome resistance and achieve synergistic effects [27, 28]. NDDS provides combination medicines that target various bacterial pathways to reduce the development of resistance in cases of MDR infections. For example, liposomal carriers enhance bacterial elimination by concurrently delivering antibiotics and anti-biofilm chemicals [29].

Impact of NDDS

NDDS enhances the precision and efficiency of antimicrobial therapies. It reduces drug misuse and overexposure, which are key contributors to AMR. By enabling targeted and controlled release, NDDS minimizes side effects and improves therapeutic outcomes. Thus, NDDS represents a promising strategy for combating the global threat of AMR, as cited in Table **1**.

Biological Barriers to Drug Delivery

Biological barriers such as mucus layers, cellular membranes, and efflux pumps limit antimicrobial drug penetration. These barriers reduce drug bioavailability, contributing to subtherapeutic levels and treatment failure [37]. Limited drug access can promote microbial survival and the emergence of resistance. Overcoming these barriers is crucial to enhancing antimicrobial efficacy and combating resistance.

Three primary biological barriers in bacterial infections are as follows:

- ***Bacterial Biofilms***: These structures, formed by communities of bacteria, secrete an extracellular matrix that hinders drug penetration, significantly reducing the bioavailability of antimicrobials. Strategies designed for mucosal delivery may be adapted to enhance drug delivery to biofilm sites.
- ***Bacterial Cellular Envelope***: Particularly in Gram-negative bacteria, the outer membrane can limit drug diffusion. Enhancing penetration through this barrier is essential for reaching intracellular bacterial targets. Lehr suggests reevaluating approaches to avoid promoting antimicrobial resistance.
- ***Host Cell Membrane***: Intracellular pathogens, such as Mycobacteria, can hide within host cells, thereby complicating treatment. Effective antimicrobials must be able to cross these membranes, necessitating a better understanding of drug delivery methods [26].

Current approaches, primarily systemic administration, often fall short, as they do not effectively target infection sites. Localized delivery methods, such as topical or inhalation therapies, can enhance drug concentrations at infection sites while minimizing systemic exposure [38]. The limited efficacy of existing antimicrobials and the emergence of resistance are largely due to inadequate drug delivery, which results in sub-therapeutic exposure of pathogens. Collaborations among pharmaceutical scientists, microbiologists, and pathologists are essential for overcoming these barriers [39].

Mechanisms of AMR

Antibiotics have been used for many years to cure or prevent disease in animals raised for food. Antibiotics from the majority of antimicrobial groups used in humans are frequently found in animal feed in quantities ranging from lower therapeutic levels to higher therapeutic levels [40]. There is evidence to support the hypothesis that giving antibiotics to animals may cause the growth of organisms resistant to antibiotics and that humans who eat those animals may contract these infections. Antibiotic types and dosages are reflected in the patterns of AMR observed in animals [41]. AMR can spread from animals to people in several ways, but the most frequent one is by the direct oral route, which includes eating meat and consuming excrement in tainted food or water. Direct interaction with the animals is an additional common path [42]. The various sources of antimicrobial agents in the human body are illustrated in Fig. (**1**).

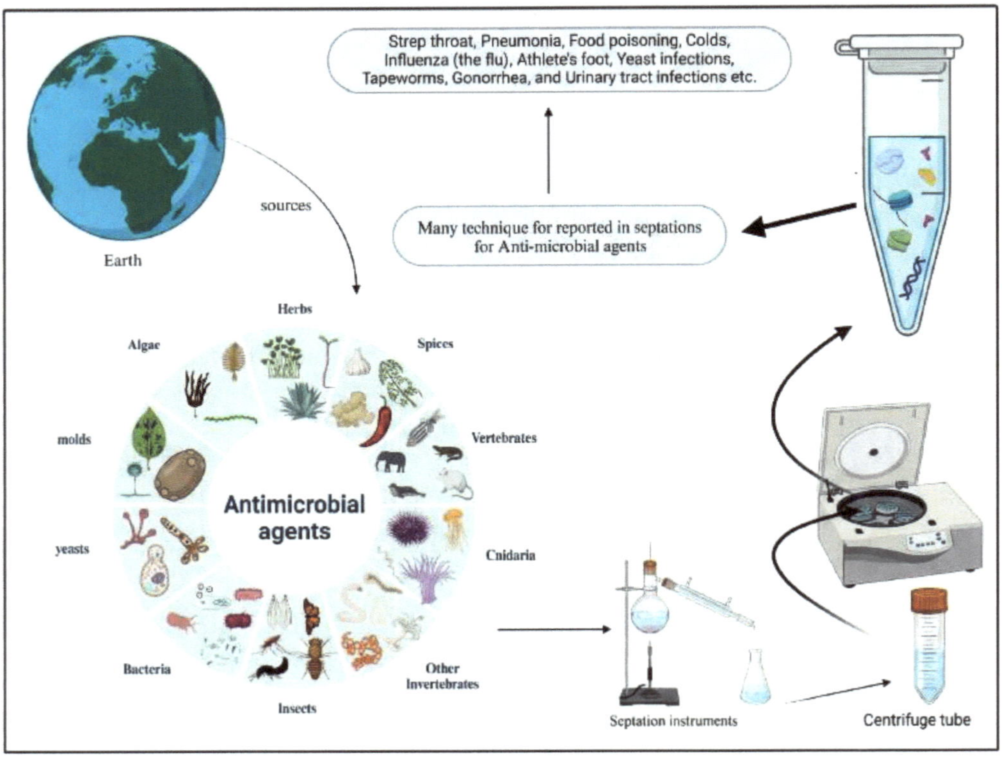

Fig. (1). Sources of antimicrobial agents to the human body.

There are four primary types of processes underlying AMR:

- **Reducing Drug Intake**

Antibacterial drugs cannot enter gram-negative bacteria because of their outer lipopolysaccharide barrier. It reduces the porin channel or mutation that changes the selectivity of the porin channel, leading to resistance [43].

- **Modification of Drug Targets**

Bacteria can alter targets of antimicrobial agents, such as PBPs (penicillin-binding proteins) in Gram-positive bacteria, which leads to reduced drug binding. Resistance to glycopeptides and lipopeptides is also common in Gram-positive bacteria [44]. Mechanisms for ribosomal target modification include mutations, methylation, or ribosomal protection, affecting various drug classes. Mutations in Deoxyribonucleic acid (DNA) gyrase or topoisomerase can confer resistance to drugs targeting nucleic acid synthesis. Enzymatic mutations affecting metabolic pathway inhibitors (like sulfonamides) also play a role [25].

- **Drug Inactivation**

Bacteria can degrade drugs or modify them through chemical group transfers. β-lactamases are prominent in the hydrolysis of β-lactams, while other enzymes inactivate tetracycline and aminoglycosides *via* acetylation, phosphorylation, or adenylation.

- **Active Drug Efflux**

Efflux pumps expel antimicrobial agents from bacterial cells, contributing to resistance. There are five main families of efflux pumps are ATP-Binding Cassette, Multidrug and Toxic Compound Extrusion, Small Multidrug Resistance, Major Facilitator Superfamily, and Resistance-Nodulation-Division family, which are particularly significant in Gram-negative bacteria. Efflux mechanisms can also confer intrinsic resistance in Gram-positive bacteria [39].

Genetic and Biochemical Mechanisms

Bacteria possess remarkable genetic plasticity that enables them to adapt to environmental threats, particularly antibiotics [45]. They employ two primary strategies for resistance.

- **Mutational Resistance**

Bacteria can develop mutations in genes associated with antibiotic action, allowing them to survive despite the presence of the drug. Once resistant mutants emerge, they can dominate the population as susceptible bacteria are eliminated. However, these mutations may be costly to the bacteria's overall fitness and are typically maintained only in environments where antibiotics are present. Resistance mechanisms include.

- Modifications of antibiotic targets (decreasing drug affinity)
- Reduced drug uptake
- Activation of efflux mechanisms to expel the drug
- Alterations in metabolic pathways through regulatory changes [46].

○ Horizontal Gene Transfer (HGT)

HGT is a key driver of bacterial evolution and a significant contributor to antibiotic resistance. Bacteria can acquire resistance genes from their environment, particularly from other organisms that produce antibiotics. The main mechanisms of HGT include.

- *Transformation:* Uptake of naked DNA, limited to a few bacterial species.
- *Transduction:* Gene transfer mediated by bacteriophages.
- *Conjugation:* Direct transfer of genetic material through cell contact, especially prevalent in the human gastrointestinal tract during antibiotic treatment [47].

Mobile genetic elements like plasmids and transposons play a crucial role in this genetic exchange. Integrons also facilitate the accumulation of resistance genes by incorporating mobile gene cassettes into bacterial chromosomes, driving further evolution and adaptability. Overall, bacteria's ability to utilize mutations and HGT significantly enhances their survival in the face of antibiotic pressure [48]. The AMR mechanism can be summarized in Fig.(**2**).

Role of Biofilms and Efflux Pumps

To interact with their surroundings and one another, complex microbial associations known as biofilms are anchored to biotic or abiotic surfaces and are embedded in the extracellular matrix that is created by the biofilms themselves. The ability of biofilms to withstand antimicrobial treatments better than planktonic cells is one of their primary characteristics [16]. It has been revealed that one of the mechanisms causing AMR in biofilm structures is efflux pumps. Many bacteria, including *Candida albicans, Escherichia coli,* and *Pseudomonas aeruginosa,* have been shown to provide evidence of the efflux pump's involvement in biofilm resistance [49].

The ability of bacteria in biofilms to withstand antimicrobial treatments better than planktonic cells is one of their primary characteristics. This characteristic poses a significant clinical challenge since it makes it difficult to treat illnesses brought on by bacteria that develop biofilms. The mature stage of biofilm formation has the highest level of resistance to antibiotics [50]. The AMR in biofilm structures is caused by several mechanisms.

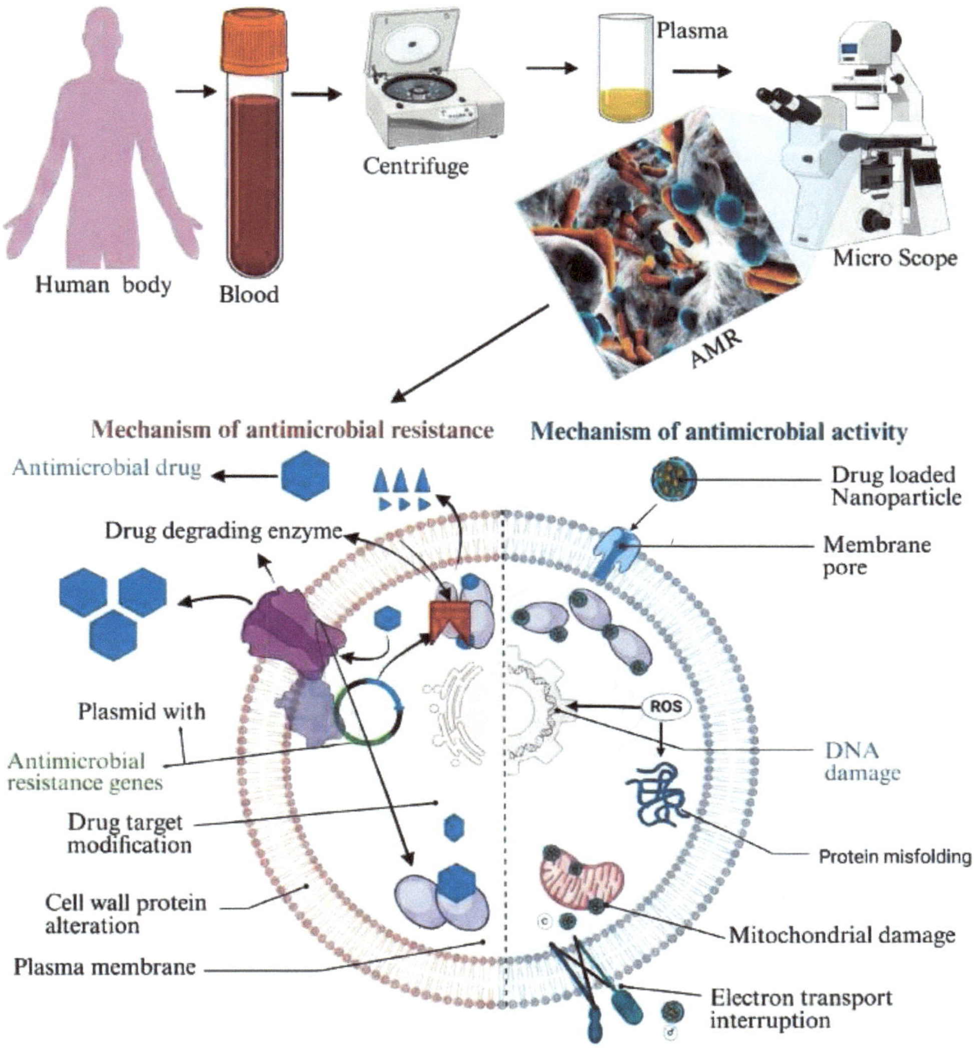

Fig. (2). Mechanism of AMR.

- Certain antibiotics can pass through the biofilm polysaccharide matrix, but there is insufficient antibiotic diffusion.
- Alterations in metabolism brought on by sluggish development and starvation reactions (oxygen, nutritional shortage, or environmental stress).
- Phenotypic alteration of the biofilm-forming cells.
- Quorum-sensing, however, their exact involvement is not clear.

- The efflux pumps' expression.
- Persisting cells are tiny portions of bacteria that are resistant to being killed by antibiotics. Mutants do not exist in the persistent cells [51].

One important mechanism of resistance in Gram-negative bacteria is drug efflux. Solutes are pumped out of the cell by these systems. Efflux pumps eliminate harmful compounds, such as metabolites, antibacterial agents, and quorum-sensing signal molecules, enabling microbes to control their internal environment. Efflux pumps can be made of one or multiple components; the latter type of pump is only present in Gram-negative bacteria [52].

Clinical Impact of AMR

AMR has several clinical consequences; some of the most important ones are listed here:

- The treatment of microbiological diseases, including bacterial, fungal, and viral infections, becomes more challenging due to antibiotic resistance.
- The emergence and transmission of novel resistance mechanisms threaten the range of therapies for many common diseases, such as upper respiratory tract infections, typhoid, flu, and urinary tract infections. Treatment failure, severe disability, or even death can result from these mechanisms.
- The effectiveness of cancer treatment, transplant surgery, and even basic dental procedures will be seriously threatened by AMR until new drugs are available [53].
- AMR infections require more extensive and expensive medical care, and they may require costly substitute drugs [54].

Drug Delivery Systems to Combat AMR: Overview of Drug Delivery Concepts

A pharmaceutical substance's transportation throughout the body to produce the intended therapeutic effect is referred to as drug delivery (DD). This includes formulations, technologies, and procedures. Drug delivery systems are technologically advanced devices intended to administer medicinal drugs to the body with precise control [55]. By focusing on certain bodily locations, regulating the release profile, and enhancing the bioavailability of the medications, these systems seek to maximize their effectiveness. Effective medication delivery methods are essential for enhancing treatment results and halting the emergence of resistance in the fight against AMR [14].

AMR and the Requirement for Innovative Drug Delivery Methods: When microorganisms, such as bacteria, fungi, and viruses, become resistant to the actions of drugs that were earlier successful against them, AMR develops. One of the main causes of AMR is the overuse and misuse of antimicrobial medicines [43]. Another is poor patient adherence. Drug delivery systems need to overcome several obstacles to solve AMR Table **2**, Fig.(**3**).

Table 2. Drug delivery used in AMR.

Drug Delivery Strategy	Description	Advantages in AMR	Challenges	Mechanism of Action	Result	Reference
NPs	Antimicrobial drugs are encapsulated in small particles. Include metallic NPs, polymeric NPs, and liposomes.	Better drug solubility and stability; enhanced targeting of infection sites; and controlled and sustained release.	Exorbitant development costs; Possible toxicity or immunological reaction.	Passive and active targeting of infection sites; enhanced cellular uptake.	Improved therapeutic efficacy and reduced resistance.	[57, 58]
Liposomes	Drug-carrying hydrophilic and hydrophobic biocompatible vesicles.	Preserving drugs against deterioration; Improving absorption and targeting.	Problems with storage and stability; Limited scalability.	Fusion with bacterial or host membranes to release the drug at the target site.	Enhanced delivery with minimized systemic exposure.	[59]
Polymeric NPs	Biodegradable polymer-based NPs with a steady drug release.	Controlled, continuous release that is both biocompatible and biodegradable.	Intricate production; Possibility of buildup inside the organism.	Slow degradation of the polymer allows timed drug release.	Prolonged antimicrobial activity at the site of infection.	[60]
Metallic NPs	Metallic NPs with inherent antibacterial qualities, such as those formed of gold or silver.	Direct antibacterial actions; the capacity to go beyond systems of microbial resistance.	Possible toxicity; Issues with the environment.	Disrupt bacterial membranes, produce reactive oxygen species (ROS).	Broad-spectrum killing, including drug-resistant bacteria.	[61, 62]
Microneedles/Transdermal Patches	Drugs are administered topically using tiny needles or patches to target specific locations or the bloodstream.	Low-invasive; Long-term; targeted medication administration; Diminished systemic adverse effects.	Skin rashes or discomfort, restricted to certain drugs.	Create microchannels in skin for direct drug diffusion.	Rapid systemic uptake with minimal pain or side effects.	[63]

(Table 2) cont.....

Drug Delivery Strategy	Description	Advantages in AMR	Challenges	Mechanism of Action	Result	Reference
Hydrogels	Substances that absorb water, swell, and may be infused with drugs to heal wounds or infections.	Keeps the wound-healing environment wet; Antimicrobials are released locally and slowly.	Contamination risk and restricted drug load capacity.	Localized, sustained release in a moist environment.	Accelerated wound healing and localized infection control.	[64, 65]
Phage Therapy	Using viruses called bacteriophages, which infect bacteria in place of antibiotics.	Extremely tailored to the target bacterium; Capable of coevolving with bacteria to avert resistance.	Developmental obstacles (manufacturing, phage selection); Possible defense reaction.	Phages bind and lyse specific bacterial cells.	Highly specific bacterial killing with minimal off-target effects.	[66]
Antibody-Drug Conjugates	Antibodies linked to antibiotics that target resistant bacteria alone.	Accurately targeting resistant germs; Decreased side effects.	Expensive and intricate manufacture; Possibility of immune-related adverse effects.	Antibodies bind to target bacteria, releasing the drug locally.	Targeted eradication of resistant pathogens with reduced collateral damage.	[67]
Solid Lipid Nanoparticles (SLNs)	Nanoparticles composed of solid lipids that encapsulate drugs.	High biocompatibility; Enhanced stability and controlled release.	Limited drug loading; Potential lipid oxidation.	Lipid matrix allows controlled release while avoiding burst release.	Improved bioavailability and sustained drug delivery.	[68]
Dendrimers	Branched, tree-like nanostructures with a central core used for drug conjugation.	High surface area for functionalization; Effective drug delivery.	High production cost; Toxicity at higher generations.	Surface functional groups enable targeted binding and drug release.	Enhanced penetration and activity against resistant bacteria.	[69]
Carbon Nanotubes (CNTs)	Cylindrical carbon-based nanostructures are used to deliver drugs or act as antimicrobial agents.	High drug-loading capacity; Strong penetration capability.	Cytotoxicity concerns; Biodegradability issues.	Piercing bacterial membranes and delivering drug payloads.	Effective against biofilms and persistent bacteria.	[70]
Quantum Dots (QDs)	Fluorescent semiconductor NPs with antibacterial surface modifications.	Diagnostic and therapeutic "theranostic" capabilities; Antibacterial action.	Toxicity due to heavy metals; Regulatory challenges.	Disruption of bacterial metabolism; ROS production	Dual use in detection and inhibition of pathogens.	[71]

(Table 2) cont.....

Drug Delivery Strategy	Description	Advantages in AMR	Challenges	Mechanism of Action	Result	Reference
Mesoporous Silica Nanoparticles (MSNs)	Nanoparticles with porous silica structures that encapsulate and protect drugs.	High surface area and loading; Controlled release profiles.	Potential biopersistence; Synthesis complexity.	Controlled drug diffusion from a porous structure.	Enhanced therapeutic concentration at infection sites.	[72]

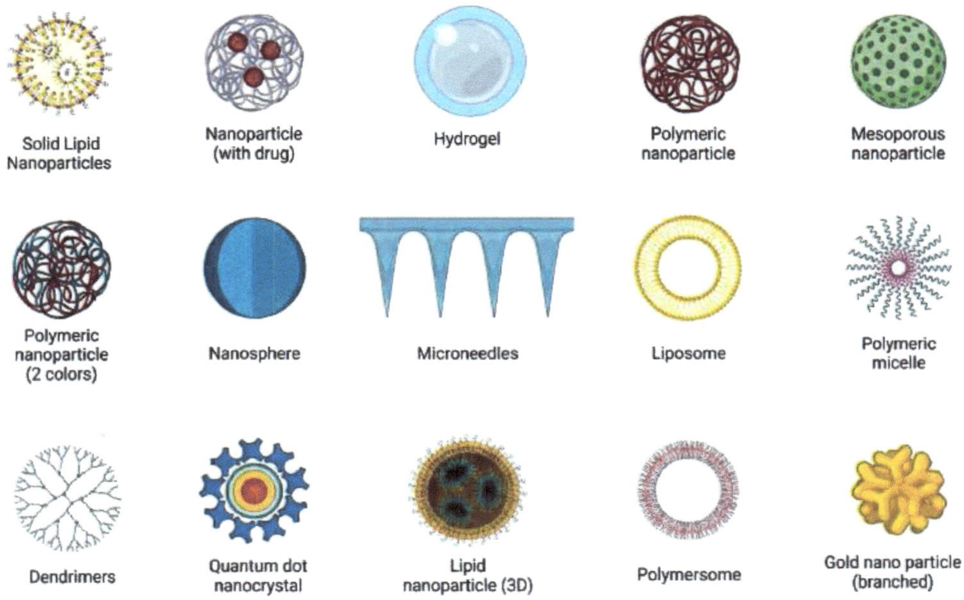

Fig. (3). Diagrammatic view of NDDS.

- Better targeting: Making certain that the right number of antimicrobials is present at the right infection location.
- Sustained release: It refers to delivering a regulated and continuous release of the medication to sustain therapeutic concentrations for prolonged durations.
- Reduction of side effects: Reducing toxicity and minimizing off-target effects to avoid killing off beneficial microorganisms.
- Enhanced permeability: It refers to the capacity to pass through physiological barriers that restrict medication penetration, such as biofilm layers or the blood-brain barrier (BBB).
- Reducing medications: Reducing the frequency and dosage of medications to prevent microbial adaptability and the development of resistance [56].

Importance of Targeted and Controlled Release

To combat AMR, targeted and controlled medication release is essential, as it maximizes the effectiveness of antimicrobial therapies while reducing the variables that lead to the development of resistance [56]. The following are the main justifications for the significance of these methods in the fight against AMR:

Improved Drug Efficacy at Infection Sites

- Antimicrobial drugs are concentrated at the site of infection instead of being dispersed throughout the body, thanks to targeted delivery. This enhances the efficacy of the therapy by producing greater local medication concentrations where the pathogens or germs are found [73].
- For example, antibiotics may be delivered directly to biofilms or certain bacterial indicators using liposomes or NPs that have been genetically modified to recognise them. This is especially useful for illnesses that are difficult to cure [74].

Reduced Side Effects and Toxicity

- By limiting the amount of exposure time of non-infected tissues to antimicrobial medicines, targeted medication delivery lowers toxicity and unintended side effects. Targeted systems assist in preserving general health and avert consequences like gastrointestinal disorders or organ damage by preserving healthy cells and the microbiota [75].
- With controlled release, systemic toxicity may be further decreased by allowing the medication to be given gradually over time, maintaining therapeutic drug levels without the need for frequent high doses [3].

Prevention of AMR Development

- Sub-therapeutic antibiotic doses or uneven dosages in traditional therapies may encourage the survival of resistant bacterial strains. With the use of controlled-release systems, infections are completely eradicated, and the likelihood of resistant bacteria surviving and proliferating is decreased. This is achieved by maintaining a consistent medication concentration within the therapeutic window [76].
- One of the main causes of resistance in bacteria is the selection pressure on the bacterium, which is minimised by targeted delivery systems by lowering the overall dosage of antibiotics utilised [25].

Overcoming Drug Resistance Mechanisms

- Certain bacteria use defence mechanisms against antibiotics, such as biofilm development or efflux pumps. To successfully overcome bacterial defences, targeted drug delivery systems may pierce these protective barriers and deliver larger quantities of the medicine where it is most required [77].
- To treat chronic and persistent infections that are resistant to traditional therapy, medications must be delivered directly to bacterial cells *via* the use of liposomes and NPs, which may penetrate biofilms [78].

Extended Drug Activity and Improved Patient Compliance

- By extending the duration of the drug's impact, controlled release technologies lower the frequency of doses. This helps avoid the development of resistance by ensuring that therapeutic medication levels are maintained for an extended period of time, in addition to improving patient compliance.
- Patients are more likely to comply with treatment regimens when given a once-daily or once-weekly dosage schedule *via* controlled-release devices, particularly in situations involving persistent infections [22].

Minimizing Overuse of Antibiotics

- Drug delivery systems help prevent the need for broad-spectrum antibiotics, which may hasten the development of resistance, by guaranteeing that antimicrobials are administered directly and in a regulated way to the site of infection. Targeted treatments help avoid overusing antibiotics and reduce the number of bacteria exposed to less-than-ideal medication concentrations [12].
- Example: A smaller dosage of a particular antibiotic may be enough in a well-targeted system, minimizing the likelihood of encouraging resistance in bacteria that are not the intended target.

Enhanced Penetration of Hard-to-Reach Areas

Treatment for infections in difficult-to-reach regions, such as the brain (because of the blood-brain barrier), the lungs, or deep tissue layers where bacteria may be more resistant, requires controlled and targeted delivery methods. In such places, these systems may be designed to increase the permeability of antimicrobial compounds. For instance, physiological barriers that often prevent antibiotics from penetrating the body may be crossed by NPs, allowing them to reach previously unreachable infection sites [79].

Combination Therapies

The use of combination therapy, in which several antibiotics or antimicrobial drugs are administered in a coordinated manner, is made easier by targeted and controlled release systems. By concurrently targeting numerous bacterial pathways, this strategy aids in the fight against illnesses that are resistant to multiple drugs. Combination treatments that use controlled release may guarantee that all medications remain effective over time and do not interfere with one another's therapeutic effects [80].

Advantages of NDDS in Combating AMR

Innovative methods known as NDDS were created to get beyond the drawbacks of traditional drug administration, especially in the battle against AMR. When treating illnesses caused by bacteria that are resistant to therapy, these methods provide substantial advantages [22]. The following are NDDS's main advantages in the fight against AMR.

Nanotechnology-Based Drug Delivery Systems

New approaches to disease prevention and treatment are made possible by the development of nano-drug delivery systems, or NDDSs. Inorganic NPs, liposomes, polymeric micelles, nanogels, and inorganic/organic (core/shell) NPs have all been utilized extensively as NDDS in preclinical and clinical research in recent years [37]. By extending the duration of action, enhancing targeting and efficacy, overcoming drug resistance, and lowering toxicity and immunogenicity, these systems can enhance the pharmacological and pharmaceutical properties of medications. NDDSs are being extensively used in preclinical and clinical stages these days [29, 81].

NPs and Nanocarriers

Nanomaterials are organic, inorganic, or hybrid particles, with some with a diameter of ≤100 nm, and others with a diameter of ≤ 500 nm18. Their shapes and structures are nearly infinite, ranging from rods to pyramids, fibrous networks, and spheres with solid or hollow interiors and smooth or rough surfaces [57]. Nanoscale materials differ from their bulk counterparts in several physicochemical properties, such as size, shape, and surface. The cell envelope has evolved into a physical barrier that keeps antimicrobials out. Bacterial surfaces are negatively charged due to the phosphate groups in lipopolysaccharide, which is present in the outer membrane of Gram-negative bacteria, and teichoic acids, which are found in the cell walls of Gram-positive bacteria. The activity of hydrophobic antimicrobials is compromised due to their limited ability to penetrate bacterial membranes in this highly polar environment [82].

Preferential electrostatic interactions with positively charged objects are made possible by the fact that bacterial cell surfaces are more negatively charged than those of mammalian cells [83]. Designing NPs to specifically damage bacterial membranes requires consideration of the charge density and hydrophobicity of the NP surface. Both extremely hydrophobic and highly cationic NPs can attach to the surface of mammalian cells, decreasing selectivity. Having a favorable amphiphilic balance allows cationic nanomaterials to have strong antibacterial properties with little cytotoxicity and hemolysis [84].

A range of nanomaterial-based strategies focuses on targeting the negatively charged surface of planktonic bacteria. The fabricated biodegradable cationic and amphiphilic polycarbonates self-assemble into cationic micellar NPs, killing MRSA. These polymeric NPs interact with bacteria through electrostatic interactions, disintegrating the membrane and causing cell lysis. 'Nanoknifes", materials with sharp-pointed edges, are particularly effective in compromising bacterial membrane integrity. In a study, single-walled carbon nanotubes and graphene oxide ruptured the cell surface of Ralstonia solanacearum, leading to cytoplasmic leakage and bacterial death. The ability of bacteria to develop resistance against therapeutics that damage the cell envelope is likely to be limited, making these strategies promising for long-term use with minimal risk of bacterial resistance [57].

Due to their inherent antibacterial activity and potential for use as drug delivery vehicles, NPs hold great promise as a means of combating AMR. Silver (AgNP) and gold (NPA) metal oxides, which are 10 nm in size, and polymer-based NPs, which are 200–400 nm in size, are examples of their range [61]. Whether aerosolized NPs are being delivered to the lungs or oral delivery is used for gastrointestinal infections, these nanocarriers can be customized to the route of administration and the accompanying pathophysiological barrier [85].

The surface charge, size, shape, or a combination of these elements determine how NPs carry out their antibacterial action. To rupture cellular membranes, cause leakage, and ultimately cause cell death, they can interact and interfere with the structure and integrity of proteins [86]. Antimicrobial-loaded NPs can disrupt mitochondrial activity, alter metabolic processes, and destroy pathogen DNA [84].

Metal NPs are widely used as antibacterial agents and drug delivery systems. They come in several forms, such as Ag-NPs, Au-NPs, Cu NPs, ZnO NPs, αFe_2O_3

NPs, and TiO_2 NPs. Chemical vapor deposition (CVD), pyrolysis, thermolysis, and sol-gel techniques can all be used to create metal NPs. They have the potential to provide additive or synergistic effects for strong bactericidal action, whether used alone or in combination with the right antibiotics. In conclusion, by offering a more effective and efficient delivery mechanism, NPs present a viable substitute for antibiotics in the fight against AMR [87, 88].

Lipid-Based Nanocarriers (Liposomes, Solid Lipid NPs)

Liposomes, first developed in the 1960s, are phospholipid vesicle systems that mimic human cell membranes, allowing for good biocompatibility and improved drug distribution. Composed primarily of phospholipids and cholesterol, liposomes can encapsulate both hydrophilic and lipophilic drugs, making them multifunctional carriers for anti-biofilm agents. Optimal liposome sizes for effective antimicrobial targeting range from 100 to 200 nm, facilitating enhanced cellular uptake through fusion with bacterial membranes, which creates transport channels instead of causing membrane rupture [59, 89].

The surface of liposomes can be modified with specific ligands for targeted delivery, and additional strategies can enhance their anti-biofilm activity by improving drug interactions with bacterial biofilms or inhibiting bacterial growth. However, achieving high drug loading, especially for hydrophobic compounds, while maintaining stability and an appropriate size distribution, remains a challenge [90]. Therefore, optimizing the composition and preparation methods of liposomes is essential for maximizing their therapeutic potential against biofilm. Lipids, excipients, and natural or synthetic polymers are used as carrier ingredients in the synthesis of organic NPs, sometimes referred to as polymeric or lipid-based NPs. Their superior features, including biocompatibility, biodegradability, and increased cargo transport with low systemic toxicity, make them superior to their inorganic counterparts. Lipid polymer hybrid nanocarriers, polyester, polyamides, and polymeric materials are other categories of polymer-based nanocarriers [91, 92].

Recent research on liposomal formulations has demonstrated their effectiveness in reducing bacterial biofilms. One study showed that combining Ps1G with tobramycin improved the antibiotic's activity against *Pseudomonas aeruginosa*, leading to a 20% reduction in biofilm biomass. Another formulation with lysozyme and gentamicin significantly decreased biofilm biomass and live bacterial counts in both *P. aeruginosa* and *Staphylococcus aureus*. Liposomes containing N-acetylcysteine and tobramycin were effective against *Escherichia coli*, *Acinetobacter baumannii*, and *Klebsiella pneumoniae*, enhancing biofilm inhibition. Azithromycin encapsulated in liposomes achieved a remarkable

93.22% reduction in biofilm at 1X MIC against a clinical isolate of *E. coli*. A combination of lysozyme, chlorhexidine, and lactoferrin inhibited biofilm formation in *Streptococcus mutans* and *Streptococcus sobrinus*. Finally, co-encapsulating serratiopeptidase with levofloxacin resulted in over 90% eradication of preformed biofilms in *S. aureus*-infected rats at sub-MIC concentrations. These findings underscore the potential of liposomal delivery systems in enhancing the efficacy of antimicrobials against biofilm-related infections [90].

PNPs

Polymeric NPs are nanoscale carriers, typically ranging from 1 to 1000 nm, composed of biocompatible and biodegradable polymers [93]. The main types include:

- NPs: Solid particles that encapsulate drugs within a polymer matrix.
- Nanocapsules: Vesicular systems that encapsulate drugs in a core surrounded by a polymeric membrane.
- Nanospheres: Continuous matrix systems that disperse drugs uniformly [94].

Common materials used in polymeric nanoparticles:

- PLGA (Poly (lactic-co-glycolic acid)): Known for its biodegradability and ability to control drug release.
- Chitosan: A natural polymer with antimicrobial properties that enhances drug solubility and stability.
- Alginate: Often used for its biocompatibility and ability to form gels [95].

Mechanisms of Action

PNPs enhance the effectiveness of antimicrobial agents through several mechanisms:

- Improved Solubility: PNPs can solubilize hydrophobic drugs, increasing their bioavailability.
- Targeted Delivery: Surface modification with targeting ligands directs NPs to specific sites, enhancing drug accumulation at infection sites.
- Sustained Release: PNPs facilitate the controlled release of drugs, maintaining therapeutic levels over extended periods and reducing dosing frequency.
- Combination Therapy: PNPs can co-deliver multiple agents to address various resistance mechanisms simultaneously [96].

Dendrimers and Their Applications

Dendrimers, characterized by their tree-like branched structures, offer unique properties for various applications in medicine and industry. Their precise control over structure, molecular weight, and surface functionalities allows for effective drug delivery and targeted therapeutic applications [97]. With a size range of 2 to 5 nm, dendrimers consist of a central core from which branched monomers extend, creating multiple functional groups for drug conjugation [98].

Dendrimers possess significant potential as antimicrobial agents due to their ability to enhance the effectiveness of conventional antibiotics and inhibit the growth of microbial pathogens. Their cationic nature enables strong electrostatic interactions with the negatively charged bacterial membranes, leading to membrane disruption and increased permeability [99]. High-generation cationic dendrimers, particularly polyamidoamine (PAMAM) types, demonstrate pronounced antibacterial activity, although they may exhibit cytotoxicity toward mammalian cells [100]. To mitigate toxicity while preserving antimicrobial effectiveness, researchers have explored various modifications. For example, nitric oxide-releasing dendrimers and the conjugation of PAMAM dendrimers with polyethylene glycol (PEG) have shown promise in reducing cytotoxicity. Additionally, the development of dendritic polyglycerol-chitosan constructs has yielded compounds effective against resistant strains like *Staphylococcus aureus* and *Pseudomonas aeruginosa* [101]. That dendrimer structure influences their ability to penetrate bacterial biofilms. The peripheral functional groups significantly affect the dendrimer's penetration and distribution within biofilms, with specific groups enhancing accumulation in acidic environments typical of biofilm settings [102].

Overall, dendrimers represent a versatile class of nanocarriers with the potential for developing new antimicrobial therapies, particularly through combination strategies that leverage their unique structural features and biocompatibility. Their ability to disrupt bacterial membranes, reduce the required dosages of conventional antibiotics, and target specific pathogens makes them a promising avenue in the fight against antimicrobial resistance [103].

Hydrogels

Multi-layered networks of polymer chains, known as hydrogels, can hold vast volumes of water or biological fluids [104, 105]. Given that they can be utilized to stop infections and inhibit bacterial growth, hydrogels are a viable material for reducing antimicrobial resistance [106]. Excellent antibacterial activities have been demonstrated by metal NPs mixed with hydrogels; metal oxide NPs have demonstrated low resistance and broad-spectrum effects. Metal oxides, however, have long-term toxicity and are difficult to discharge. Reducing antibiotic resistance and toxicity accumulation can be achieved by combining hydrogels with metal oxides. Zinc oxide nanoparticle (ZnO NPs) is a good option for wound dressings because of its low cytotoxicity and reported antibacterial activity. It is simple to combine copper oxide (CuO) NPs with polymers to create stable hydrogels with stable characteristics. The antibacterial activity of Poly (HEA-AAm)/WO_3 hydrogel containing WO_3 NPs has also been demonstrated against bacteria, including *Candida albicans*, *P. aeruginosa*, and *E. coli,*which cause bacterial keratitis. Additionally, the addition of magnesium oxide (MgO) NPs to the hydrogel of acrylic acid and polyvinyl alcohol (PAA/PVA) has demonstrated efficacious antibacterial properties [107]. This study created a hydrogel filled with antibacterial (mint) leaf juice MENVs derived from a plant leaf. A strong connection was observed between the injectable, biocompatible, self-healing hydrogel and bacterium cells. The results show reduced inflammation and faster healing [108].

Stimuli-Responsive Drug Delivery Systems

Exogenous Stimuli-Responsive Antibiotic Drug-Delivery Systems

The development of stimuli-responsive drug-delivery systems has focused on enhancing biomaterials, such as polymers and lipids, to respond to various stimuli—chemical (*e.g.*, pH, ionic strength), physical (*e.g.,* temperature, light), and biological (*e.g.,* proteolytic enzymes). A promising approach involves co-formulating metallic inorganic NPs like gold (Au), silver (Ag), and iron oxide (Fe_2O_3 and Fe_3O_4) with traditional delivery systems, including liposomes, polymersomes, and hydrogels. This integration leverages the advancements in synthesizing biocompatible, monodispersed inorganic NPs with diverse surface functionalities [109].

By utilizing the unique optical, magnetic, and physicochemical properties of these metallic NPs, researchers can achieve selective and controlled release of therapeutic agents in response to various stimuli such as light irradiation, magnetic fields, and pH changes. This strategy holds significant potential for enhancing the effectiveness of antibiotic delivery while minimizing side effects, marking a promising direction in the field of targeted drug delivery [110].

- ***Thermal Release***

Mechanisms in antibiotic drug-delivery systems leverage the unique optical and magnetic properties of inorganic NPs for the controlled release of therapeutics.

This is achieved through photothermal and magnetothermal methods, which enable the selective disruption of drug carriers via external stimuli like lasers or alternating magnetic fields [103].

Magnetic Release for Biofilm Eradication

Superparamagnetic iron oxide nanoparticles (SPIONs) offer a promising strategy for promoting antibiotic release in challenging environments like biofilms, where bacteria are protected by an extracellular polymeric matrix. Geilich *et al.* demonstrated the effectiveness of this approach using iron oxide polymersomes (IOPs), which were designed from methoxy poly (ethylene glycol)-b-poly (*d,l*-lactic acid) diblock copolymers. These IOPs co-encapsulated methicillin in the aqueous core and hydrophobic SPIONs in the membrane bilayer [111].

Biofilms of *Staphylococcus epidermidis* were grown on glass cover slips and treated with IOPs containing various concentrations of SPIONs and methicillin. When an external magnetic field was applied, the IOPs were effectively pulled through the biofilm, allowing for targeted delivery. This method resulted in a selective bactericidal effect in the areas influenced by the magnetic field, achieving complete biofilm eradication even at lower concentrations of methicillin than the minimum bactericidal concentration (MBC) of the free antibiotic. This research highlights the potential of magnetic release systems in overcoming antibiotic resistance within biofilms [103].

Endogenous Stimuli-Responsive Antibiotic Drug-Delivery Systems

Drug delivery systems that are redox-responsive, enzyme-responsive, pH-responsive, and ionic microenvironment-responsive are examples of the endogenous stimulation of biochemical and chemical origin. These DDSs initiate drug delivery by controlling the microenvironment of tissues, overexpression of certain enzymes, interactions between antibodies and antigens, and identification of host and guest moieties in particular states [112].

pH-Responsive Delivery Systems

PH-sensitive liposomes have emerged as promising alternatives to conventional liposomes for the targeted intracellular delivery of therapeutics, particularly in antimicrobial applications. Lutwyche *et al.* demonstrated the efficacy of gentamicin encapsulated in pH-sensitive liposomes against *Salmonella typhimurium* in macrophages, showing a 104-fold increase in antibacterial activity compared to free gentamicin. Similarly, Nasti *et al.* evaluated pH-sensitive liposomes containing nystatin for treating *Cryptococcus neoformans* infections, resulting in enhanced antifungal effects and reduced toxicity [113].

Despite the advantages of liposomes, such as high biocompatibility, significant drug-carrying capacity, and the ability to fuse with bacterial membranes, challenges remain due to their poor stability and tendency to fuse, leading to payload loss. While strategies like coating liposomes with PEG have been explored to enhance stability, these coatings often hinder the liposomes' ability to fuse with bacterial membranes [59]. To address this, Thamphiwatana and colleagues developed a novel approach using negatively charged doxycycline-loaded liposomes stabilized with cationic chitosan-coated gold (Au) NPs. This system leverages the protonation of chitosan at acidic pH for stabilization, which transitions to deprotonation at neutral pH, allowing the liposomes to fuse with bacterial membranes and release doxycycline effectively. Their findings indicated superior antibacterial efficacy against *Helicobacter pylori* compared to free doxycycline, showcasing the potential of pH-sensitive liposomal formulations for targeted antimicrobial therapy [103].

Enzyme-Responsive Systems

Highly selective and catalytically efficient enzyme-responsive materials have been widely used in the development of antibacterial compounds. Numerous enzymes have been employed in stimuli-responsive antibacterial theranostics, including lipase, phosphatase, hyaluronidase, β-lactamase, serine protease, urease, gelatinase, and nitroreductase. Enzymes accelerate reactions by reducing or oxidizing substrates and creating or breaking chemical bonds. Enzyme-responsive materials can identify bacterial infections, release antibiotics under control, improve the biocompatibility of antimicrobial peptides, and specifically destroy drug-resistant bacteria. Due to the widespread usage of β-lactam antibiotics in hospitals, a range of β-lactamase-activated antibacterial prodrugs has been developed to combat bacterial resistance to these medicines. To identify and tify and separate the bacteria rseparate the bacteria resistant to β-lactam antibiotics, certain β-lactamase-activated probes have also been created. Enzyme-responsive materials show enormous promise in realizing specific and selective antibacterial theranostics [114].

Light and Magnetic Field-Responsive Systems

Light-Responsive Systems

Light-responsive systems are materials or devices that react to light stimuli, often undergoing physical or chemical changes when exposed to specific wavelengths. These systems leverage photochemical reactions or changes in molecular conformation, allowing for applications in areas like photonics, sensing, and drug delivery. Common examples include photochromic compounds, which can change color or state when exposed to light, and polymeric materials that can undergo shape changes. The development of light-responsive systems has enabled advancements in fields such as smart materials and optoelectronics, where precise control over material behaviour is essential [115].

Magnetic Field-Responsive Systems

Magnetic field-responsive systems, on the other hand, are designed to respond to external magnetic fields, leading to changes in their properties or behaviours. These systems typically incorporate magnetic materials or NPs that can be manipulated by applying a magnetic field [116]. This responsiveness can manifest in various ways, including changes in alignment, movement, or even phase transitions. Applications range from targeted drug delivery using magnetic NPs to magnetic resonance imaging contrast agents [117]. The ability to control these systems remotely is a key feature [118, 116].

Integration with Antimicrobial Peptides

The potential use of antimicrobial peptides (AMPs) as a therapy approach against infections resistant to drugs is significant. Low molecular weight oligopeptides are known as AMPs. They possess wide-ranging antibacterial properties that combat harmful microbes. As the initial line of defense against invasive infections, AMPs are nonspecific and target components of microbes that aid in the immune response [119]. Because of their potency and diversity, AMPs are excellent options for alternative applications. For increased therapeutic activity, they can be utilized either alone or in conjunction with several different biomaterials. They are additionally useful for targeting drug-resistant bacteria in the manufacture of vaccines [120].

Synergistic Effects of NDDS and Antimicrobial Peptides

- **Combined Mechanisms for Increased Stability**

By preventing AMPs from degrading in biological settings, NDDS can lengthen their half-lives and boost their efficacy. For peptides that can be vulnerable to enzymatic breakdown, this is especially crucial [121].

- **Enhancement of Bioavailability**

AMPs can be more effectively delivered to infection sites with the help of NDDS, increasing their local concentration and lowering systemic exposure. Additionally, this focused strategy can reduce adverse consequences [29].

- **Managed Release**

For AMPs, NDDS can offer a regulated release mechanism that guarantees a long-lasting therapeutic benefit. This may assist in keeping the peptide at the infection site at effective concentrations without the need for regular dosages [122].

Biofilm-Targeted Delivery Systems

Technologies known as "biofilm-targeted delivery systems" are utilized to administer medications to treat microbial illnesses brought on by biofilms [16]. Biofilms are intricate formations that shield microorganisms from substances and procedures, making it challenging to eradicate and medicate those using antibiotics. By improving medication administration, dispersing biofilms, targeting dormant cells, and applying magnetic fields, biofilm-targeted delivery devices can aid in overcoming these obstacles [123].

Challenges of Biofilm-Associated Infections

Biofilm-associated infections present several challenges that complicate treatment and management. Here are some of the key difficulties:

- **Increased Resistance to Antimicrobial**
    - Reduced Penetration: The protective extracellular matrix of biofilms acts as a barrier, limiting the penetration of antimicrobials.
    - Altered Metabolism: Bacteria within biofilms often exhibit slower growth rates and metabolic changes, rendering them less susceptible to many antibiotics that target actively dividing cells.
    - Genetic Resistance: Biofilm bacteria can exchange genetic material, including genes that confer resistance, further complicating treatment efforts [124].

    - **Chronic Infections**
    - Persistence: Biofilms are often associated with chronic infections, as they can persist for long periods, leading to ongoing inflammation and tissue damage.
    - Recurrent Infections: Even if biofilm-associated bacteria are initially cleared, the resilient nature of biofilms can lead to reinfection or relapse [125].
    - **Immune Evasion**
    - Protection from Immune Response: The biofilm matrix can shield bacteria from the host's immune cells, making it difficult for the body to mount an effective defence.

- Inflammatory Response: Biofilms can elicit a chronic inflammatory response, which can lead to further tissue damage and complicate healing [126].

  - **Diagnosis Difficulties**

- Detection: Biofilm infections may be difficult to detect using standard diagnostic methods. Traditional cultures may not capture biofilm-forming bacteria, leading to misdiagnosis.
- Diverse Species: Biofilms can consist of multiple species, making it challenging to identify the causative organisms and select appropriate treatments [127].

  - **Biofilm Heterogeneity**

- Structural Variability: Biofilms can vary widely in structure, composition, and thickness, affecting their susceptibility to treatments.
- Spatial Variability: Different regions within a biofilm may have distinct microenvironments, impacting the effectiveness of antimicrobial agents [128].

  - **Limited Treatment Options**

- Conventional Antibiotics: Many antibiotics are ineffective against biofilm-associated bacteria, necessitating alternative therapeutic approaches.
- Lack of Approved Treatments: There are limited FDA-approved treatments specifically targeting biofilm infections, which can hinder clinical management [129].

  - **Impact on Medical Devices**

- Device-Related Infections: Biofilms frequently form on indwelling medical devices (*e.g.,* catheters, prosthetics), leading to device failure and increased risk of serious infections.
- Surgical Complications: Biofilm-associated infections can complicate surgical procedures, increasing morbidity and the need for additional interventions [130].

  - **Economic Burden**

- Healthcare Costs: The management of biofilm-associated infections often leads to increased healthcare costs due to longer hospital stays, additional treatments, and surgeries.
- Loss of Productivity: Chronic infections can result in a significant loss of productivity for affected individuals, impacting their quality of life [131].

Strategies to Combat Biofilms

- **Biofilms and Chronic Infections**

Multicellular clusters of bacteria that adhere to surfaces to create biofilms do so because they are resistant to dehydration, have mechanical strength, and can withstand antimicrobial agents. These biofilms, which are frequently associated with medical equipment, can result in long-term mucosal illnesses [132]. Antimicrobials are being delivered locally and physically removed as current treatment techniques. However, an alternative to antimicrobials is required to treat these diseases, as biofilm-related issues become more prevalent [128].

- **Biofilm Antimicrobial Tolerance**

Due to their transient, non-heritable physiological state known as antimicrobial tolerance, biofilms, a specific type of bacteria, are resistant to antimicrobials. Because of their distinct tolerance mechanisms, these biofilms can cause persistent infections that are challenging to treat. The inhibition of antimicrobial penetration, the buildup of enzymes that degrade antibiotics, eDNA presence, quorum sensing, up-regulating efflux pumps, altering growth rate, stress response, and the presence of persister cells are common reasons why antimicrobials fail in biofilms [133]. Additionally, concentration gradients found in biofilms provide both aerobic and anaerobic microenvironments that boost resistance to antimicrobial and antiseptic treatment. By upsetting these multicellular structures, antimicrobial efficacy and host defenses can both be increased [134].

- **Basic Strategies to Treat Biofilms**

The two ways to treat biofilms are dispersing biofilms to get rid of the ones that already exist and inhibiting biofilm formation to stop new ones from forming. Planktonic cells should not be allowed to adhere to surfaces or form early microcolonies to inhibit the formation of biofilms. To prevent microbial attachment, surface alterations or chemical pre-conditioning are other options. Controlling genes involved in biofilm formation is one way to hinder bacterial establishment or stop biofilm maturation [124].

- **NDDS Targeting Biofilm Matrix**

By attaching to particular ligands, NPs can be altered to specifically target elements of the biofilm matrix. Drug distribution can be enhanced by enzymatic methods, which degrade biofilm constituents. NPs with dual functions can both break the biofilm and deliver antimicrobial drugs. Synergistic combinations of antimicrobial drugs can be used to select against microorganisms associated with biofilms. Biofilms containing resistant strains can be targeted using tailored drug delivery methods [124, 135].

Case Studies

During this research, it was found that numerous case studies on antimicrobial resistance are being conducted; for instance, the World Health Organization and research agencies are involved in conducting a lot of case studies of WHO and NCT numbers across the world; some of them are as follows (Table **3**).

Table 3. Recent year clinical trials on ARM.

Sn	NCT Number	Title	Status	Intervention	Phase	Actual Enrolment	Population	Sponsor/Country	Result
1	NCT06305455	Resistance Profile of *Escherichia Coli* in infections of community origin: The importance of antimicrobial stewardship	Not yet recruiting	*Biological: Escherichia coli ESBL* To evaluate the change in the resistance profile of infections of community origin caused by *Escherichia coli* isolated from any culture material in patients admitted to the intensive care unit of a tertiary hospital.	-	200 18 Years and older (Adult, Older Adult)	200 18 Years and older (Adult, Older Adult)	José Raimundo Araujo de Azevedo	The study aims to describe the antimicrobial resistance profile of *Escherichia coli* isolated from community-acquired infections in patients admitted to the intensive care unit within 48 hours of hospital admission. It is sponsored by Hospital São Domingos Ltda.
2	NCT05734391	Surveillance of healthcare-associated infections & antimicrobial resistance	Enrolling by invitation	Diagnostic test: Routine infection control routine part of hospital IPC activities. Other names: Surveillance activity	Not Applicable	1500 (Child, Adult, Older Adult)	500 (Child, Adult, Older Adult)	University of Pennsylvania	This clinical trial is evaluating the antimicrobial peptide **PLG0206** for treating **periprosthetic joint infections (PJIs)**, which are commonly linked to **multidrug-resistant bacteria.**
3	NCT06632132	Antimicrobial resistance training for hemodialysis nurses	Completed	Other: Antimicrobial resistance training in hemodialysis units	Not Applicable	64 18 Years and older (Adult, Older Adult)	-	Jordan University of Science and Technology	An engineered antimicrobial peptide, for the treatment of periprosthetic joint infections (PJIs), has yielded promising interim results.

Applications

AMR is a danger to public health because it makes treating bacterial, viral, and fungal diseases more difficult. AMR has been tackled using a variety of creative strategies, with a special emphasis on NDDSs and other treatment breakthroughs [136].

- NDDS in Treating Specific Resistant Pathogens: NDDSs improve drug solubility, target particular areas, and overcome obstacles like biofilms to increase the effectiveness of antimicrobial therapies (Table **4**). By limiting side effects and lowering dose requirements, these methods may treat resistant bacteria more successfully [137].

Table 4. NDDS for certain resistant pathogens.

Pathogen	NDDS Used	Mechanism and Application
MRSA	NPs, Liposomes	Antibiotics are delivered directly to infection areas using NPs, such as lipid-based NPs, which improve the drug's capacity to break through biofilms and eradicate MRSA.
Pseudomonas aeruginosa (MDR strains)	Micelles, Hydrogels	To treat Pseudomonas biofilm infections in chronic wounds, antibiotics such as tobramycin may be effectively encapsulated and delivered using hydrogels and micellar drug carriers.
Mycobacterium tuberculosis	Polymeric NPs, Inhalable formulations	Anti-TB medications are administered via nanocarriers to the lungs, improving drug absorption and retention and overcoming resistance in lung infections.
Carbapenem-resistant Enterobacteriaceae (CRE)	Liposomes, Nanocarriers	Liposomal formulations provide higher penetration and effectiveness by improving the targeting of antibiotics such as polymyxins to CRE-caused illnesses.
VRE	NPs, Dendrimers	Vancomycin is being researched as a nanocarrier system, such as dendrimers, to ensure efficient delivery to VRE-infected areas.
Candida species (Fungal)	NPs, Liposomes, Hydrogels	NPs and liposomal amphotericin B formulations improve drug targeting and reduce systemic toxicity in treating resistant fungal infections.

CONCLUSION

This chapter provides a vast description of AMR and various NDDS used to overcome it. It includes an increasing problem in biofilm-associated disorders and AMR, which needs an innovative solution that utilizes nanotechnology and NDDS. NDDS reduces adverse effects and improves therapeutic efficacy by combining targeted and controlled release mechanisms. Details are provided on different qualities of biofilm, like their resistance to antibiotics, antimicrobials, and capacity for long-term infection. Combining antimicrobial peptides with NDDS creates a more effective therapeutic option that disrupts biofilm matrices and eliminates persistent infections. Improved drug delivery may be possible by analyzing nano-carriers such as polymers, liposomes, dendrimers, and many more novel formulations. To maximize the effectiveness, novel formulations of the drug must be used. To overcome the problem and enhance patient outcomes, ongoing research is essential.

REFERENCES

[1] Aslam B, Wang W, Arshad MI, *et al.* Antibiotic resistance: a rundown of a global crisis. Infect Drug Resist 2018; 11: 1645-58.
[http://dx.doi.org/10.2147/IDR.S173867] [PMID: 30349322]

[2] Yetisgin AA, Cetinel S, Zuvin M, Kosar A, Kutlu O. Therapeutic nanoparticles and their targeted delivery applications. Molecules 2020; 25: 1-31.
[http://dx.doi.org/10.3390/molecules25092193]

[3] Adepu S, Ramakrishna S. Controlled drug delivery systems: Current status and future directions. Molecules 2021; 26(19): 5905.
[http://dx.doi.org/10.3390/molecules26195905] [PMID: 34641447]

[4] Bello OA, Ayanda OI, Aworunse OS, Olukanmi BI. Pharmacogn Rev 2018; 1(2): 57-72.

[5] Iskandar K, Murugaiyan J, Hammoudi Halat D, *et al.* Antibiotic Discovery and Resistance: The Chase and the Race. Antibiotics (Basel) 2022; 11(2): 182.
[http://dx.doi.org/10.3390/antibiotics11020182] [PMID: 35203785]

[6] Devi NS, Mythili R, Cherian T, *et al.* Overview of antimicrobial resistance and mechanisms: The relative status of the past and current. Microbe 2024; 3: 100083.
[http://dx.doi.org/10.1016/j.microb.2024.100083]

[7] Morel CM, Edwards SE, Harbarth S. Preserving the 'commons': addressing the sustainable use of antibiotics through an economic lens. Clin Microbiol Infect 2017; 23(10): 718-22.
[http://dx.doi.org/10.1016/j.cmi.2017.08.002] [PMID: 28811243]

[8] Barathe P, Kaur K, Reddy S, Shriram V, Kumar V. Antibiotic pollution and associated antimicrobial resistance in the environment. Journal of Hazardous Materials Letters 2024; 5: 100105.
[http://dx.doi.org/10.1016/j.hazl.2024.100105]

[9] Ahmed SK, Hussein S, Qurbani K, *et al.* Antimicrobial resistance: Impacts, challenges, and future prospects. Journal of Medicine, Surgery, and Public Health 2024; 2: 100081.
[http://dx.doi.org/10.1016/j.glmedi.2024.100081]

[10] Prestinaci F, Pezzotti P, Pantosti A. Antimicrobial resistance: a global multifaceted phenomenon. Pathog Glob Health 2015; 109(7): 309-18.
[http://dx.doi.org/10.1179/2047773215Y.0000000030] [PMID: 26343252]

[11] Goel N, Fatima SW, Kumar S, Sinha R, Khare SK. Antimicrobial resistance in biofilms: Exploring marine actinobacteria as a potential source of antibiotics and biofilm inhibitors. Biotechnol Rep (Amst) 2021; 30: e00613.
[http://dx.doi.org/10.1016/j.btre.2021.e00613] [PMID: 33996521]

[12] Muteeb G, Rehman MT, Shahwan M, Aatif M. Origin of antibiotics and antibiotic resistance, and their impacts on drug development: A narrative review. Pharmaceuticals (Basel) 2023; 16(11): 1615.
[http://dx.doi.org/10.3390/ph16111615] [PMID: 38004480]

[13] Khan J, Tarar SM, Gul I, Nawaz U, Arshad M. Challenges of antibiotic resistance biofilms and potential combating strategies: a review. 3 Biotech 2021; 11(4): 1-15.

[14] Terreni M, Taccani M, Pregnolato M. New antibiotics for multidrug-resistant bacterial strains: Latest research developments and future perspectives. Molecules 2021; 26(9): 2671.
[http://dx.doi.org/10.3390/molecules26092671] [PMID: 34063264]

[15] Mabilat C, Gros MF, Nicolau D, *et al.* Diagnostic and medical needs for therapeutic drug monitoring of antibiotics. Eur J Clin Microbiol Infect Dis 2020; 39(5): 791-7.
[http://dx.doi.org/10.1007/s10096-019-03769-8] [PMID: 31828686]

[16] Sharma S, Mohler J, Mahajan SD, Schwartz SA, Bruggemann L, Aalinkeel R. Microbial biofilm: A review on formation, infection, antibiotic resistance, control measures, and innovative treatment. Microorganisms 2023; 11(6): 1614.
[http://dx.doi.org/10.3390/microorganisms11061614]

[17] Egorov AM, Ulyashova MM, Rubtsova MY. Bacterial Enzymes and Antibiotic Resistance 2018; 10(39): 33-48.

[18] Cyphert EL, Wallat JD, Pokorski JK, Recum HA, Von . Erythromycin Modification That Improves Its Acidic Stability while Optimizing It for Local Drug Delivery. 2017.
[http://dx.doi.org/10.3390/antibiotics6020011]

[19] Huemer M, Shambat SM, Brugger SD. Antibiotic resistance and persistence — Implications for human health and treatment perspectives 2020; 1-24.

[20] Salam A, Al-amin Y, Salam MT, Pawar JS. Antimicrobial Resistance : A Growing Serious Threat for Global. 2023; 1-20.

[21] Annunziato G. Strategies to Overcome Antimicrobial Resistance (AMR) Making Use of Non-Essential Target Inhibitors: A Review. Int J Mol Sci 2019; 20(23): 5844.
[http://dx.doi.org/10.3390/ijms20235844] [PMID: 31766441]

[22] Ezike TC, Okpala US, Onoja UL, *et al.* Advances in drug delivery systems, challenges and future directions. Heliyon 2023; 9(6): e17488.
[http://dx.doi.org/10.1016/j.heliyon.2023.e17488] [PMID: 37416680]

[23] Tekade RK, Maheshwari R, Soni N, Tekade M, Chougule MB. Nanotechnology for the Development of Nanomedicine. Nanotechnology-Based Approaches for Targeting and Delivery of Drugs and Genes 1(3): 61. 2017 Jan.
[http://dx.doi.org/10.1016/B978-0-12-809717-5.00001-4]

[24] Wang L, Hu C. The antimicrobial activity of nanoparticles : present situation and prospects for the future. 2017; 1227-49.
[http://dx.doi.org/10.2147/IJN.S121956]

[25] de Oliveira DV, Van Der Sand ST. Phenotypic tests for the detection of β-lactamase-producing enterobacteriaceae isolated from different environments. Curr Microbiol 2016; 73(1): 132-8.
[http://dx.doi.org/10.1007/s00284-016-1036-6] [PMID: 27071981]

[26] Mirghani R, Saba T, Khaliq H, Mitchell J, Do L, Chambi L. Biofilms : Formation , drug resistance and alternatives to conventional approaches 2022; 8(june): 239-77.

[27] Gupta A, Jain P, Nagori K, Adnan M. Ajazuddin. Treatment strategies for psoriasis using flavonoids from traditional Chinese medicine. Pharmacological Research -. Zhongguo Xiandai Zhongyao 2024; 12: 100463.

[28] Worthington RJ, Melander C. NIH Public Access 2014; 31(3): 177-84.

[29] Zong T xin, Silveira AP, Vasconcelos A, Sampaio MC, Muehlmann LA, Zhang J, *et al.* Recent Advances in Antimicrobial Nano-Drug Delivery Systems. 2022.

[30] Hussain S, Joo J, Kang J, Kim B, Braun GB, She Z gang, *et al.* HHS Public Access 2018; 2(2): 95-

103.

[31] Rajgopal B, Gupta SK, Deshmukh R, Gupta A, Patel A, Sakure K, *et al.* Emerging trends in hydrogels for the treatment of vaginal candidiasis: A comprehensive review. Recent Advances in Anti-Infective Drug Discovery 20.
[http://dx.doi.org/10.2174/0127724344348928250220063431]

[32] Eleraky NE, Allam A, Hassan SB, Omar MM. Nanomedicine Fight against Antibacterial Resistance : An Overview of the Recent Pharmaceutical Innovations 1-51.

[33] Manuscript A. NIH Public Access 2015; 157(1): 121-41.

[34] Gaurav A, Bakht P, Saini M, Pandey S, Pathania R. Role of bacterial efflux pumps in antibiotic resistance, virulence, and strategies to discover novel efflux pump inhibitors. 2023; 1-13.
[http://dx.doi.org/10.1099/mic.0.001333]

[35] Kumar V, Yasmeen N, Pandey A, Chaudhary AA, Alawam AS, Rudayni HA, *et al.* Antibiotic adjuvants : synergistic tool to combat multi-drug resistant pathogens. 2023; 1-14. (December)
[http://dx.doi.org/10.3389/fcimb.2023.1293633]

[36] Ventola CL. Antibiotic Resistance Crisis Part 1 : Causes and Threats 2015; 40(4): 277-83.

[37] Kumar D, Gupta SK, Verma A. Ajazuddin. Transferosome as Nanocarrier for Drug Penetration Enhancement Across Skin: A Comparison with Liposome and Ethosome. Curr Nanomed 2024; 15.

[38] Wen H, Jung H, Li X. Drug Delivery Approaches in Addressing Clinical Pharmacology-Related Issues: Opportunities and Challenges. AAPS J 2015; 17(6): 1327-40.
[http://dx.doi.org/10.1208/s12248-015-9814-9] [PMID: 26276218]

[39] Reygaert WC. An overview of the antimicrobial resistance mechanisms of bacteria. 2018; 482-501. 4(June).
[http://dx.doi.org/10.3934/microbiol.2018.3.482]

[40] Allen HK, Levine UY, Looft T, Bandrick M, Casey TA. Treatment, promotion, commotion: antibiotic alternatives in food-producing animals. Trends Microbiol 2013; 21(3): 114-9.
[http://dx.doi.org/10.1016/j.tim.2012.11.001] [PMID: 23473629]

[41] Manyi-Loh C, Mamphweli S, Meyer E, Okoh A. Antibiotic use in agriculture and its consequential resistance in environmental sources: Potential public health implications. Vol. 23. Molecules 2018; 23(4): 795.
[http://dx.doi.org/10.3390/molecules23040795] [PMID: 29601469]

[42] Verraes C, Van Boxstael S, Van Meervenne E, *et al.* Antimicrobial resistance in the food chain: a review. Int J Environ Res Public Health 2013; 10(7): 2643-69.
[http://dx.doi.org/10.3390/ijerph10072643] [PMID: 23812024]

[43] Uddin TM, Chakraborty AJ, Khusro A, *et al.* Antibiotic resistance in microbes: History, mechanisms, therapeutic strategies and future prospects. J Infect Public Health 2021; 14(12): 1750-66.
[http://dx.doi.org/10.1016/j.jiph.2021.10.020] [PMID: 34756812]

[44] Lade H, Kim JS. Bacterial targets of antibiotics in methicillin-resistant *Staphylococcus aureus.* Antibiotics (Basel) 2021; 10(4): 398.
[http://dx.doi.org/10.3390/antibiotics10040398] [PMID: 33917043]

[45] Jian Z, Zeng L, Xu T, *et al.* Antibiotic resistance genes in bacteria: Occurrence, spread, and control. J Basic Microbiol 2021; 61(12): 1049-70.
[http://dx.doi.org/10.1002/jobm.202100201] [PMID: 34651331]

[46] Coculescu B ioan. Antimicrobial resistance induced by genetic changes 2009; 2(2): 114-23.

[47] Michaelis C, Grohmann E. Horizontal Gene Transfer of Antibiotic Resistance Genes in Biofilms. 2023.
[http://dx.doi.org/10.3390/antibiotics12020328]

[48] Partridge SR, Kwong SM, Firth N, Jensen SO. crossm Mobile Genetic Elements Associated with Antimicrobial Resistance 2018; 31(4): 1-16.

[49] Soto SM. Role of efflux pumps in the antibiotic resistance of bacteria embedded in a biofilm. 2013; 223-9.
[http://dx.doi.org/10.4161/viru.23724]

[50] Zhao A, Sun J, Liu Y. Understanding bacterial bio fi lms : From de fi nition to treatment strategies 2023; 1-23. (April)

[51] Srinivasan R, Santhakumari S. Bacterial biofilm inhibition : A focused review on recent therapeutic strategies for combating the biofilm mediated infections. 2021; 1-19. 12(May).
[http://dx.doi.org/10.3389/fmicb.2021.676458]

[52] Manuscript A. NIH Public Access. 2010; 69: pp. 1555-623.

[53] Gidwani B, Gupta SK, Sahu J. A Panoptic Review on Improvement in Chemothera-peutic Properties of Cytotoxic Drugs through Calixarene. International Journal of Pharmaceutical Sciences and Nanotechnology(IJPSN) 2023; 16(3): 6546-55. [IJPSN].
[http://dx.doi.org/10.37285/ijpsn.2023.16.3.8]

[54] Lin TZ, Jayasvasti I, Tiraphat S, Pengpid S, Jayasvasti M, Borriharn P. The Predictors Influencing the Rational Use of Antibiotics Among Public Sector : A Community-Based Survey in Thailand. 2022; 27-36. (March).
[http://dx.doi.org/10.2147/DHPS.S339808]

[55] Tewabe A, Abate A, Tamrie M, Seyfu A, Abdela Siraj E. Targeted drug delivery — from magic bullet to nanomedicine: Principles, challenges, and future perspectives. J Multidiscip Healthc 2021; 14: 1711-24.
[http://dx.doi.org/10.2147/JMDH.S313968] [PMID: 34267523]

[56] Majumder MAA, Rahman S, Cohall D, *et al.* Antimicrobial stewardship: Fighting antimicrobial resistance and protecting global public health. Infect Drug Resist 2020; 13: 4713-38.
[http://dx.doi.org/10.2147/IDR.S290835] [PMID: 33402841]

[57] Makabenta JM V, Nabawy A, Li C hsuan, Schmidt-malan S, Patel R, Rottelo VM. bacterial infections 2022; 19(1): 23-36.

[58] Tiwari P, Prajapati SK, Dixit V, Raza MA, Ajazuddin , Gupta SK, *et al.* Recent advancements in nanoparticle drug delivery systems to cure neurological disorders *via* the nasal route. Neurología Argentina 2025 Jun.

[59] Nsairat H, Khater D, Sayed U, Odeh F, Al Bawab A, Alshaer W. Liposomes: structure, composition, types, and clinical applications. Heliyon 2022; 8(5): e09394.
[http://dx.doi.org/10.1016/j.heliyon.2022.e09394] [PMID: 35600452]

[60] Gagliardi A, Giuliano E, Venkateswararao E, Fresta M. Biodegradable polymeric nanoparticles for drug delivery to solid tumors 2021; 12(February): 1-24.

[61] Wahab S, Salman A, Khan Z, Khan S, Krishnaraj C. Metallic Nanoparticles A Promising Arsenal against Antimicrobial Resistance — Unraveling Mechanisms and Enhancing Medication Efficacy 2023.

[62] Banchhor R, Patel A, Sharma MK, *et al.* Advances in Green Synthesis of Zinc Oxide Nanoparticles: A Promising Nanotechnology Approach for Diabetes Mellitus Management. Drug Deliv Lett 2025; 15: 15.
[http://dx.doi.org/10.2174/0122103031350147250310032617]

[63] Jung JH, Jin SG, Jin G. Microneedle for transdermal drug delivery: current trends and fabrication. J Pharm Investig 2021; 51(5): 503-17.
[http://dx.doi.org/10.1007/s40005-021-00512-4] [PMID: 33686358]

[64] Yang D, Chen H, Wei H, Liu A, Wei DX, Chen J. Hydrogel wound dressings containing bioactive

compounds originated from traditional Chinese herbs: A review. Smart Materials in Medicine 2024; 5(1): 153-65.
[http://dx.doi.org/10.1016/j.smaim.2023.10.004]

[65] Zaffar S, Saha S, Agrawal T, *et al.* Improved Diabetic Wound Healing *via* Flower Extracellular Vesicles and Carbon-Dot-Infused Alginate-Polyethylenimine Antibacterial Hydrogel. ACS Biomater Sci Eng 2025; 11(7): 4219-30.
[http://dx.doi.org/10.1021/acsbiomaterials.5c00443] [PMID: 40384057]

[66] Lin DM, Koskella B, Lin HC, Lin DM, Lin HC, Gastroenterology S. Phage therapy : An alternative to antibiotics in the age of multi-drug resistance 2017; 8(3): 162-73.

[67] Darbandi A, Abdi M, Dashtbin S, Yaghoubi S, Sholeh M, Kouhsari E. Antibody – Antibiotic Conjugates : A Comprehensive Review on Their Therapeutic Potentials Against Bacterial Infections 2024; 1-11.

[68] Arabestani MR, Bigham A, Kamarehei F, *et al.* Solid lipid nanoparticles and their application in the treatment of bacterial infectious diseases. Biomed Pharmacother 2024; 174: 116433.
[http://dx.doi.org/10.1016/j.biopha.2024.116433] [PMID: 38508079]

[69] Gholap AD, Bhowmik DD, Deshmukh AY, Hatvate NT. Quintessential impact of dendrimer bioconjugates in targeted drug delivery. In 2023. 257-302.
[http://dx.doi.org/10.1016/bs.coac.2023.02.009]

[70] Das S, Roy S, Dinda SC, *et al.* Carbon nanotubes in brain targeted drug delivery: A comprehensive review. Results in Chemistry 2025; 15: 102206.
[http://dx.doi.org/10.1016/j.rechem.2025.102206]

[71] Daby TPM, Modi U, Yadav AK, Bhatia D, Solanki R. Bioimaging and therapeutic applications of multifunctional carbon quantum dots: Recent progress and challenges. Next Nanotechnology 2025; 8: 100158.
[http://dx.doi.org/10.1016/j.nxnano.2025.100158]

[72] Fatima R, Katiyar P, Kushwaha K. Recent advances in mesoporous silica nanoparticle: synthesis, drug loading, release mechanisms, and diverse applications. Frontiers in Nanotechnology 2025; 7 2025 Mar 18
[http://dx.doi.org/10.3389/fnano.2025.1564188]

[73] Belete TM. Novel targets to develop new antibacterial agents and novel alternatives to antibacterial agents. Hum Microbiome J 2019; 11: 100052.
[http://dx.doi.org/10.1016/j.humic.2019.01.001]

[74] Takallu S, Aiyelabegan HT, Zomorodi AR, *et al.* Nanotechnology improves the detection of bacteria: Recent advances and future perspectives. Heliyon 2024; 10(11): e32020.
[http://dx.doi.org/10.1016/j.heliyon.2024.e32020] [PMID: 38868076]

[75] Murugaiyan J, Kumar PA, Rao GS, *et al.* Progress in Alternative Strategies to Combat Antimicrobial Resistance: Focus on Antibiotics. Antibiotics (Basel) 2022; 11(2): 200.
[http://dx.doi.org/10.3390/antibiotics11020200] [PMID: 35203804]

[76] Helmy YA, Taha-Abdelaziz K, Hawwas HAEH, *et al.* Antimicrobial Resistance and Recent Alternatives to Antibiotics for the Control of Bacterial Pathogens with an Emphasis on Foodborne Pathogens. Antibiotics (Basel) 2023; 12(2): 274.
[http://dx.doi.org/10.3390/antibiotics12020274] [PMID: 36830185]

[77] Zhang F, Cheng W. The Mechanism of Bacterial Resistance and Potential Bacteriostatic Strategies. Antibiotics (Basel) 2022; 11(9): 1215.
[http://dx.doi.org/10.3390/antibiotics11091215] [PMID: 36139994]

[78] Panthi VK, Fairfull-Smith KE, Islam N. Liposomal drug delivery strategies to eradicate bacterial biofilms: Challenges, recent advances, and future perspectives. Int J Pharm 2024; 655: 124046.
[http://dx.doi.org/10.1016/j.ijpharm.2024.124046] [PMID: 38554739]

[79] Upadhyay RK. Drug delivery systems, CNS protection, and the blood brain barrier. Biomed Res Int 2014.

[80] Nishant Shinde, Akhilesh S. Chauhan, Sanjay K. Gupta, Surendra H. Bodakhe, Devi Prasad Pandey, Antifertility studies of curcumin and andrographolide combination in female rats, Asian Pacific Journal of Reproduction, Volume 4, Issue 3, 2015, Pages 188-194, ISSN 2305-0500. [http://dx.doi.org/10.1016/j.apjr.2015.06.012]

[81] Wang T, Zhang D, Sun D, Gu J. Current status of *in vivo* bioanalysis of nano drug delivery systems. J Pharm Anal 2020; 10(3): 221-32. [http://dx.doi.org/10.1016/j.jpha.2020.05.002] [PMID: 32612868]

[82] Silhavy TJ, Kahne D, Walker S. The Bacterial Cell Envelope. Cold Spring Harb Perspect Biol 2010; 2(5): a000414. [http://dx.doi.org/10.1101/cshperspect.a000414]

[83] Fischbach MA. Combination therapies for combating antimicrobial resistance. Curr Opin Microbiol 2011; 14(5): 519-23. [http://dx.doi.org/10.1016/j.mib.2011.08.003] [PMID: 21900036]

[84] Thambirajoo M, Maarof M, Lokanathan Y, *et al.* Potential of Nanoparticles Integrated with Antibacterial Properties in Preventing Biofilm and Antibiotic Resistance. Antibiotics (Basel) 2021; 10(11): 1338. [http://dx.doi.org/10.3390/antibiotics10111338] [PMID: 34827276]

[85] Roy I, Vij N. Nanodelivery in airway diseases: Challenges and therapeutic applications. Nanomedicine 2010; 6(2): 237-44. [http://dx.doi.org/10.1016/j.nano.2009.07.001] [PMID: 19616124]

[86] Bruna T, Maldonado-Bravo F, Jara P, Caro N. Silver nanoparticles and their antibacterial applications. Int J Mol Sci 2021; 22(13): 7202. [http://dx.doi.org/10.3390/ijms22137202] [PMID: 34281254]

[87] Sánchez-López E, Gomes D, Esteruelas G, *et al.* Metal-based nanoparticles as antimicrobial agents: An overview. Nanomaterials (Basel) 2020; 10(2): 292. [http://dx.doi.org/10.3390/nano10020292] [PMID: 32050443]

[88] Modi SK, Gaur S, Sengupta M, Singh MS. Mechanistic insights into nanoparticle surface-bacterial membrane interactions in overcoming antibiotic resistance. Front Microbiol 2023; 14(April): 1135579. [http://dx.doi.org/10.3389/fmicb.2023.1135579] [PMID: 37152753]

[89] Liu P, Chen G, Zhang J. A Review of Liposomes as a Drug Delivery System: Current Status of Approved Products, Regulatory Environments, and Future Perspectives. Molecules 2022; 27(4): 1372. [http://dx.doi.org/10.3390/molecules27041372] [PMID: 35209162]

[90] Makhlouf Z, Ali AA, Al-Sayah MH. Liposomes-Based Drug Delivery Systems of Anti-Biofilm Agents to Combat Bacterial Biofilm Formation. Antibiotics (Basel) 2023; 12(5): 875. [http://dx.doi.org/10.3390/antibiotics12050875] [PMID: 37237778]

[91] Ferreira M, Ogren M, Dias JNR, *et al.* Liposomes as antibiotic delivery systems: A promising nanotechnological strategy against antimicrobial resistance. Molecules 2021; 26(7): 2047. [http://dx.doi.org/10.3390/molecules26072047] [PMID: 33918529]

[92] Gupta SK, Vyawahare NS, Kagathara VG, Patil MN, Pujari RR. Assessment of antihypertensive activity of novel synthetic hybrid compound on 2K1C induced hypertensive rats. Pharmacologyonline 2009; 2.

[93] Yadav HKS, Almokdad AA, Shaluf SIM, Debe MS. Polymer-Based Nanomaterials for Drug-Delivery Carriers. Nanocarriers for Drug Delivery: Nanoscience and Nanotechnology in Drug Delivery 531-6. 2019 Jan 1. [http://dx.doi.org/10.1016/B978-0-12-814033-8.00017-5]

[94] Rajesh S Jr. JWL. Nanoparticle-based targeted drug delivery. Exp Mol Pathol 2000; 86(3): 215-23.

[95] Hayee R, Iqtedar M, Albekairi NA, *et al.* Levofloxacin loaded chitosan and poly-lactic-co-glycolic acid nano-particles against resistant bacteria: Synthesis, characterization and antibacterial activity. J Infect Public Health 2024; 17(5): 906-17.
[http://dx.doi.org/10.1016/j.jiph.2024.03.023] [PMID: 38569270]

[96] Aleksandra Zieli nska 1 2, Filipa Carreiró 1, Ana M, *et al.* Polymeric Nanoparticles: Production, Characterization, Toxicology and Ecotoxicology. Molecules 2020; 25(3731).

[97] Pandita D, Madaan K, Kumar S, Poonia N, Lather V. Dendrimers in drug delivery and targeting: Drug-dendrimer interactions and toxicity issues. J Pharm Bioallied Sci 2014; 6(3): 139-50.
[http://dx.doi.org/10.4103/0975-7406.130965] [PMID: 25035633]

[98] Pérez-Ferreiro M, M Abelairas A, Criado A, Gómez IJ, Mosquera J. Dendrimers: Exploring their wide structural variety and applications. Polymers (Basel) 2023; 15(22): 4369.
[http://dx.doi.org/10.3390/polym15224369] [PMID: 38006093]

[99] Paul S, Verma S, Chen YC. Peptide dendrimer-based antibacterial agents: Synthesis and applications. ACS Infect Dis 2024; 10(4): 1034-55.
[http://dx.doi.org/10.1021/acsinfecdis.3c00624] [PMID: 38428037]

[100] Fox LJ, Richardson RM, Briscoe WH. PAMAM dendrimer - cell membrane interactions. Adv Colloid Interface Sci 2018; 257: 1-18.
[http://dx.doi.org/10.1016/j.cis.2018.06.005] [PMID: 30008347]

[101] Falanga A, Del Genio V, Galdiero S. Peptides and dendrimers: How to combat viral and bacterial infections. Pharmaceutics 2021; 13(1): 101.
[http://dx.doi.org/10.3390/pharmaceutics13010101] [PMID: 33466852]

[102] Ezeh CK, Dibua MEU. Anti-biofilm, drug delivery and cytotoxicity properties of dendrimers. ADMET DMPK 2024; 12(2): 239-67.
[http://dx.doi.org/10.5599/admet.1917] [PMID: 38720923]

[103] Canaparo R, Foglietta F, Giuntini F, Della Pepa C, Dosio F, Serpe L. Recent Developments in Antibacterial Therapy : and Therapeutic Nanoparticles. Molecules 2019; 24: 1-15.
[http://dx.doi.org/10.3390/molecules24101991] [PMID: 31137622]

[104] Ali A, Saroj S, Saha S, Gupta SK, Rakshit T, Pal S. Glucose-responsive chitosan nanoparticle/poly(vinyl alcohol) hydrogels for sustained insulin release *in vivo*. ACS Appl Mater Interfaces 2023; 15(27): 32240-50.
[http://dx.doi.org/10.1021/acsami.3c05031] [PMID: 37368956]

[105] Akash Gupta, Sanjay Kumar Gupta, Interplay of novel formulation- based treatment strategies for psoriasis: Advancing therapeutic outcomes, Next Research 2025 2(3): 100731.
[http://dx.doi.org/10.1016/j.nexres.2025.100731]

[106] Wahid F, Zhong C, Wang HS, Hu XH, Chu LQ. Recent advances in antimicrobial hydrogels containing metal ions and metals/metal oxide nanoparticles. Polymers (Basel) 2017; 9(12): 636.
[http://dx.doi.org/10.3390/polym9120636] [PMID: 30965938]

[107] Tang Y, Xu H, Wang X, *et al.* Advances in preparation and application of antibacterial hydrogels. J Nanobiotechnology 2023; 21(1): 300.
[http://dx.doi.org/10.1186/s12951-023-02025-8] [PMID: 37633883]

[108] Saroj S, Saha S, Ali A, Gupta SK, Bharadwaj A, Agrawal T, *et al.* Plant extracellular nanovesicle-loaded hydrogel for topical antibacterial wound healing *in vivo*. 2024; 8-12.

[109] Wells CM, Harris M, Choi L, Murali VP, Guerra FD, Jennings JA. Stimuli-responsive drug release from smart polymers. J Funct Biomater 2019; 10(3): 34.
[http://dx.doi.org/10.3390/jfb10030034] [PMID: 31370252]

[110] Armenia I, Cuestas Ayllón C, Torres Herrero B, *et al.* Photonic and magnetic materials for on-demand

local drug delivery. Adv Drug Deliv Rev 2022; 191: 114584.
[http://dx.doi.org/10.1016/j.addr.2022.114584] [PMID: 36273514]

[111] Álvarez E, Estévez M, Gallo-Cordova A, *et al.* Superparamagnetic iron oxide nanoparticles decorated mesoporous silica nanosystem for combined antibiofilm therapy. Pharmaceutics 2022; 14(1): 163.
[http://dx.doi.org/10.3390/pharmaceutics14010163] [PMID: 35057058]

[112] Raza A, Rasheed T, Nabeel F, Hayat U, Bilal M, Iqbal HMN. Endogenous and exogenous stimuli-responsive drug delivery systems for programmed site-specific release. Molecules 2019; 24(6): 1117.
[http://dx.doi.org/10.3390/molecules24061117] [PMID: 30901827]

[113] Alrbyawi H, Poudel I, Annaji M, *et al.* pH-Sensitive Liposomes for Enhanced Cellular Uptake and Cytotoxicity of Daunorubicin in Melanoma (B16-BL6) Cell Lines. Pharmaceutics 2022; 14(6): 1128.
[http://dx.doi.org/10.3390/pharmaceutics14061128] [PMID: 35745701]

[114] Wang X, Shan M, Zhang S, Chen X, Liu W, Chen J. Stimuli-responsive antibacterial materials : Molecular structures, design principles, and biomedical applications 2022; 2104843: 1-25.

[115] Clerc M, Sandlass S, Rifaie-graham O, Peterson JA, Bruns N. Visible light-responsive materials : the (photo) chemistry and applications of donor – acceptor Stenhouse adducts in polymer science 2023; 1-77.

[116] Gupta SK, Verma A. Magnetic hydrogel and its biomedical applications. In: Ganguly S, Margels S, Das P, Eds. Magnetic polymer composites and their emerging applications. 1st ed., Boca Raton: CRC Press 2024.
[http://dx.doi.org/10.1201/9781003454236-8]

[117] Verma A, Gupta SK. History and techniques of bioimaging. In: Rajabzadeh AR, Srinivasan S, Das P, Ganguly S, Eds. Magnetic quantum dots for bioimaging. 1st ed. New York: CRC Press 2023; p. 22.
[http://dx.doi.org/10.1201/9781003319870-5]

[118] Longo R, Gorrasi G. Electromagnetically Stimuli-Responsive Nanoparticles-Based Systems for Biomedical Applications : Recent Advances and Future Perspectives 2021.

[119] Mba IE, Nweze EI. Antimicrobial Peptides Therapy: An Emerging Alternative for Treating Drug-Resistant Bacteria. An Emerging Alternative for Treating Drug-Resistant Bacteria 2022; 95(4): 445-63.
[PMID: 36568838]

[120] Gera S, Kankuri E, Kogermann K. Antimicrobial peptides – Unleashing their therapeutic potential using nanotechnology. Pharmacol Ther 2022; 232: 107990.
[http://dx.doi.org/10.1016/j.pharmthera.2021.107990] [PMID: 34592202]

[121] Zhang QY, Yan ZB, Meng YM, *et al.* Antimicrobial peptides: mechanism of action, activity and clinical potential. Mil Med Res 2021; 8(1): 48.
[http://dx.doi.org/10.1186/s40779-021-00343-2] [PMID: 34496967]

[122] Xuan H, Truong T, Hiep T. Since January 2020 Elsevier has created a COVID-19 resource centre with free information in English and Mandarin on the novel coronavirus COVID- 19. The COVID-19 resource centre is hosted on Elsevier Connect, the company ' s public news and information. Life Sci 2020; (January): 118407.

[123] Sousa A, Phung AN, Škalko-Basnet N, Obuobi S. Smart delivery systems for microbial biofilm therapy: Dissecting design, drug release and toxicological features. J Control Release 2023; 354: 394-416.
[http://dx.doi.org/10.1016/j.jconrel.2023.01.003] [PMID: 36638844]

[124] Roy R, Tiwari M, Donelli G, Tiwari V. Strategies for combating bacterial bio films : A focus on anti-bio film agents and their mechanisms of action. 2018; 9(1): 522-4.

[125] Vestby LK, Grønseth T, Simm R, Nesse LL. Bacterial biofilm and its role in the pathogenesis of disease. Antibiotics (Basel) 2020; 9(2): 59.
[http://dx.doi.org/10.3390/antibiotics9020059] [PMID: 32028684]

[126] Donlan RM, Costerton JW. Biofilms: survival mechanisms of clinically relevant microorganisms. Clin Microbiol Rev 2002; 15(2): 167-93.
[http://dx.doi.org/10.1128/CMR.15.2.167-193.2002] [PMID: 11932229]

[127] Shenoy VP, Harika K, Narasimhaswamy N, Chawla K. Detection of biofilm production and its impact on antibiotic resistance profile of bacterial isolates from chronic wound infections. J Glob Infect Dis 2020; 12(3): 129-34.
[http://dx.doi.org/10.4103/jgid.jgid_150_19] [PMID: 33343163]

[128] Woodworth BA, Cohen NA, Palmer JN. Biofilms. Rhinology and Facial Plastic Surgery 2009; pp. 241-6.

[129] Alaoui Mdarhri H, Benmessaoud R, Yacoubi H, *et al.* Alternatives therapeutic approaches to conventional antibiotics: Advantages, limitations and potential application in medicine. Antibiotics (Basel) 2022; 11(12): 1826.
[http://dx.doi.org/10.3390/antibiotics11121826] [PMID: 36551487]

[130] Mishra A, Aggarwal A, Khan F. Medical Device-Associated Infections Caused by Biofilm-Forming Microbial Pathogens and Controlling Strategies. Antibiotics (Basel) 2024; 13(7): 623.
[http://dx.doi.org/10.3390/antibiotics13070623] [PMID: 39061305]

[131] Assefa M, Amare A. Biofilm-Associated Multi-Drug Resistance in Hospital-Acquired Infections: A Review. Infect Drug Resist 2022; 15(August): 5061-8.
[http://dx.doi.org/10.2147/IDR.S379502] [PMID: 36068834]

[132] Arunasri K, Mohan SV. Biofilms: Microbial Life on the Electrode Surface. Biomass, Biofuels, Biochemicals: Microbial Electrochemical Technology Sustainable Platform for Fuels, Chemicals and Remediation 295-313. 2019 Jan 1.

[133] Uruén C, Chopo-Escuin G, Tommassen J, Mainar-Jaime RC, Arenas J. Biofilms as promoters of bacterial antibiotic resistance and tolerance. Antibiotics (Basel) 2020; 10(1): 3.
[http://dx.doi.org/10.3390/antibiotics10010003] [PMID: 33374551]

[134] Shree P, Singh CK, Sodhi KK, Surya JN, Singh DK. Biofilms: Understanding the structure and contribution towards bacterial resistance in antibiotics. Medicine in Microecology 2023; 16: 100084.
[http://dx.doi.org/10.1016/j.medmic.2023.100084]

[135] Wille J, Coenye T. Biofilm dispersion: The key to biofilm eradication or opening Pandora's box? Biofilm 2020; 2: 100027.
[http://dx.doi.org/10.1016/j.bioflm.2020.100027] [PMID: 33447812]

[136] Ayukekbong JA, Ntemgwa M, Atabe AN. The threat of antimicrobial resistance in developing countries: causes and control strategies. Antimicrob Resist Infect Control 2017; 6(1): 47.
[http://dx.doi.org/10.1186/s13756-017-0208-x] [PMID: 28515903]

[137] Huang L, Huang XH, Yang X, *et al.* Novel nano-drug delivery system for natural products and their application. Pharmacol Res 2024; 201: 107100.
[http://dx.doi.org/10.1016/j.phrs.2024.107100] [PMID: 38341055]

SUBJECT INDEX

A

B

Mukesh Kumar Singh, Gurdeep Singh, Amrendra Pratap Yadav & Papiya Bigoniya (Eds.)

C

D

E

F

G

H

I

K

L

M

N

O

P

Q

R

S

T

U

V

W

Z

www.ingramcontent.com/pod-product-compliance
Lightning Source LLC
LaVergne TN
LVHW070950210926
848482LV00002B/161